Nutritional Concerns of Women

Nutritional Concerns of Women

Edited by

Ira Wolinsky, Ph.D.

Department of Human Development
University of Houston
Houston, Texas

Dorothy Klimis-Tavantzis, Ph.D.

Department of Food Science
and Human Nutrition
University of Maine
Orono, Maine

CRC Press
Boca Raton   New York   London   Tokyo

Library of Congress Cataloging-in-Publication Data

Nutritional concerns of women / edited by Ira Wolinsky, Dorothy Klimis
-Tavantzis.
      p. cm. -- (Modern nutrition)
      Includes bibliographical references and index.
      ISBN 0-8493-8502-4 (alk. paper)
      1. Nutritionally induced diseases--Sex factors. 2. Women
    – Nutrition. 3. Women--Diseases. 4. Women--Health and hygiene.
I. Wolinsky, Ira. II. Klimis-Tavantzis, Dorothy J. III. Series:
Modern nutrition (Boca Raton, Fla.)
RC622.N8932 1996
616'.0082--dc20   95-42174
                                                                CIP

© 1996 by CRC Press, Inc.
No claim to original U.S. Government works
International Standard Book Number 0-8493-8502-4
Library of Congress Card Number 95-42174
Printed in the United States of America 1 2 3 4 5 6 7 8 9 0
Printed on acid-free paper

Dedicated to our students.

SERIES PREFACE FOR MODERN NUTRITION

The CRC Series in Modern Nutrition is dedicated to providing the widest possible coverage to topics in nutrition. Nutrition is an interdisciplinary, inter-professional field par excellence. It is noted by its broad range and diversity. We trust that the titles and authorship in this series will reflect that range and diversity.

Published for a scholarly audience, the volumes of the CRC Series in Modern Nutrition are designed to explain, review, and explore present knowledge and recent trends, developments, and advances in nutrition. As such, they will also appeal to the educated layman. The format for the series will vary with the needs of the author and the topic, including, but not limited to, edited volumes, monographs, handbooks, and texts.

My colleague, Dorothy J. Klimis-Tavantzis, and I are most pleased to have had the opportunity of working together to bring you the very timely volume, *Nutritional Concerns of Women*.

Ira Wolinsky, Ph.D.
Series Editor

PREFACE

We are pleased to bring you this volume as a part of the *CRC Series in Modern Nutrition*. We hope it will be useful to the educational, scientific, and lay communities in evaluating the existing body of knowledge on nutritional issues for women.

We mean this volume to be a scholarly effort, well grounded in physiology and nutrition. We trust that the information presented will facilitate the recommendation of appropriate food choices by women. We have assembled an excellent roster of chapter authors, each an expert in his/her field, and we, the editors, are pleased to appear alongside them. We have tried to be as comprehensive as possible in the selection of topics. For the pregnancy and lactation chapter, only the highlights are given, since each of these subjects could easily be the subject of an entire volume. If any of the readers feel that an important topic(s) has been left out, please let us know your thoughts for possible inclusion in future editions or in other volumes in this series. We have attempted to minimize overlapping among the chapters but deemed that some of it was important for its reinforcement value and for different interpretation by the author(s).

During the past few years, the nutrition of women has gained in interest and controversy as witnessed by accelerated research and inclusion of female subjects into nutritionally related women's health initiatives. Hopefully this book will facilitate nutrition recommendations for women and their caregivers and help American and Canadian women integrate nutrition and women's health issues into principles to follow in everyday life.

Ira Wolinsky, Ph.D.
Houston, Texas

Dorothy J. Klimis-Tavantzis, Ph.D.
Orono, Maine

THE EDITORS

Ira Wolinsky, Ph.D. is a Professor of Nutrition at the University of Houston. He received his B.S. degree in Chemistry from the City College of New York in 1960 and his M.S. (1965) and Ph.D. (1968) degrees in Biochemistry from Kansas University. He has served in research and teaching positions at the Hebrew University, (Medical School and Faculty of Agriculture), the University of Missouri, and Pennsylvania State University, as well as conducting basic research in NASA life sciences facilities.

Dr. Wolinsky is a member of the American Institute of Nutrition and the American Society for Clinical Nutrition, among other scientific organizations.

Dr. Wolinsky has contributed numerous nutrition research papers. His current major research interests include the nutrition of bone and calcium and sports nutrition. He has been the recipient of research grants from both public and private sources.

Dr. Wolinsky has co-authored a book on the history of the science of nutrition, *Nutrition and Nutritional Diseases. The Evolution of Concepts,* and edited the CRC Press volume *Nutrition in Exercise and Sport.* He is also editor of the *CRC Series in Modern Nutrition* and the *CRC Series in Nutrition in Exercise and Sport* and co-editor of the *CRC Series in Methods in Nutrition Research.*

Dorothy J. Klimis-Tavantzis, Ph.D., is Associate Professor of Clinical Nutrition at the Food Science and Human Nutrition Department at the University of Maine, Orono. Dr. Klimis-Tavantzis received her undergraduate training in Biology (Honors) at Beaver College, Glenside, Pennsylvania. She obtained her M.S. in Human Physiology and Ph.D. in Nutrition at The Pennsylvania State University.

Dr. Klimis-Tavantzis is a member of Sigma Delta Epsilon, American Institute Nutrition, Society for Clinical Nutrition, Graduate Women in Science, The American Dietetic Association, The Society of Nutrition Education, The Atherosclerosis Council of the American Heart Association, Maine Affiliate. Her current major research interests relate to basic investigations on the possible role of manganese in chronic diseases such as atherosclerosis, and to applied investigations utilizing nutritional interventions to reduce cardiovascular disease risk in children and adolescents. She has received research funding from the American Heart Association and the U.S. Department of Agriculture and was a Fulbright Fellow in the National Centre for Nutrition, Athens, Greece, 1995–1996. Dr. Klimis-Tavantzis is editor of the CRC book *Manganese in Health and Nutrition.*

CONTRIBUTORS

Irene Alton, M.S., R.D.
Coordinator of Nutrition Services
Health Start Inc.
St. Paul, Minnesota

John J. B. Anderson, Ph.D.
Department of Nutrition
University of North Carolina
School of Public Health
Chapel Hill, North Carolina

Eldon W. Askew, Ph.D.
Division of Foods and Nutrition
University of Utah
Salt Lake City, Utah

Carolyn K. Clifford, Ph.D.
National Cancer Institute
National Institutes of Health
Bethesda, Maryland

Nancy Boucot Cummings, M.D.
National Institute of Diabetes and
* Digestive and Kidney Diseases*
National Institutes of Health
Bethesda, Maryland

Janet M. Friedmann, M.S., R.D.,
** CNSD**
Department of Nutrition
The Pennsylvania State University
University Park, Pennsylvania

Lisa Gaetke, Ph.D., R.D.,
Department of Internal Medicine
University of Kentucky
College of Medicine
Lexington, Kentucky

Betsy Haughton, Ed. D., R.D.
Department of Nutrition
University of Tennessee
Knoxville, Tennessee

Kelly Hill, M.D.
Department of Psychiatry
University of Kentucky
College of Medicine
Lexington, Kentucky

Catherine G. Ratzin Jackson,
Ph.D., F.A.C.S.M.
School of Kinesiology
* and Physical Education*
University of Northern Colorado
Greeley, Colorado

Gordon L. Jensen, M.D., Ph.D.
Department of Gastroenterology
* and Nutrition*
Geisinger Medical Center
Danville, Pennsylvania

Nancy King, Ph.D., R. D.
Nutrition Care Division
Brooks Army Medical Center
Fort Sam Houston, Texas

Dorothy Klimis-Tavantzis, Ph.D.
Human Nutrition and Foods
University of Maine
Orono, Maine

Priscille G. Massé, Ph.D.
School of Nutrition
* and Family Studies*
University of Moncton
Moncton, New Brunswick, Canada

Craig J. McClain, M.D.
Department of Internal Medicine
University of Kentucky
College of Medicine
Lexington, Kentucky

Barbara C. Pence, Ph.D.
Department of Pathology
Texas Tech University
Health Science Center
Lubbock, Texas

Susan P. Robbins, D.S.W.
Graduate School of Social Work
University of Houston
Houston, Texas

Jaime S. Ruud, M.S., R.D.
Nutrition Consultant
Lincoln, Nebraska

Antoinette Saddler, M.D.
Department of Internal Medicine
University of Kentucky
College of Medicine
Lexington, Kentucky

Kelley S. Scanlon, Ph.D., R.D.
Division of Nutrition
Centers for Disease Control and
* Prevention*
Atlanta, Georgia

Helen Smiciklas-Wright, Ph.D.
Department of Nutrition
The Pennsylvania State University
University Park, Pennsylvania

Irene M. Soucy, M.S., R.D., CNSD
Department of Nutrition
The Pennsylvania State University
University Park, Pennsylvania

Judith S. Stern, Sc.D.
Departments of Nutrition and
* Internal Medicine*
University of California - Davis
Davis, California

Mary Story, Ph.D., R.D.
Public Health Nutrition
School of Public Health
University of Minnesota
Minneapolis, Minnesota

Paul R. Thomas, Ed.D.
Center for Food and Nutrition Policy
Georgetown University
Washington, D.C.

Ira Wolinsky, Ph.D.
Department of Human Development
University of Houston
Houston, Texas

Ray Yip, M.D., M.P.H.
Division of Nutrition
Centers for Disease Control
* and Prevention*
Atlanta, Georgia

Paula C. Zemel, Ph.D., R. D.
Department of Nutrition
University of Tennessee
Knoxville, Tennessee

TABLE OF CONTENTS

Chapter 1

WOMEN'S HEALTH AND NUTRITION RESEARCH: U.S. GOVERNMENTAL CONCERNS

Nancy Boucot Cummings

CONTENTS

I. INTRODUCTION

With an increasing focus on women's rights starting in the 1970s in the U.S.[1] came a concern about women's health. The practice of medicine had been primarily a male-dominated one, so that many of the major concerns for women's health and nutrition appeared to have been neglected. Women were not included in major clinical trials. Research tended to be conducted on male animals because of stated concerns that the variations in the menstrual cycle would make interpretation of experimental results difficult.

1

In the 1980s a number of efforts to evaluate the place of women and their health in research, treatment, and prevention of disease were spearheaded by the government. The Assistant Secretary for Health of the Department of Health and Human Services appointed a Task Force on Women's Health Issues. When the report of this task force was issued, responsibilities for implementation were delegated to the government agencies in accord with their mandates. The National Institutes of Health (NIH) developed an Advisory Committee on Women's Health Issues. The Government Accounting Office conducted a study of the inclusion of women in clinical trials. With NIH support, the Institute of Medicine of the National Academy of Science convened a Planning Panel for Including Women in Clinical Trials. The U.S. Public Health Service developed an Action Plan for Women's Health. The NIH developed and the Congress called for establishment of an Office of Research on Women's Health. The Director of the NIH announced the Women's Health Initiative, a clinical trial of major proportions, which would address significant women's health issues involving morbidity and mortality in post-menopausal women: cardiovascular disease, breast and colon cancer, and osteoporosis, along with risk factors affecting these diseases such as obesity, poor nutrition, and tobacco use.

Women's health research has become a major commitment of the NIH, the Public Health Service, and, more broadly, the U.S. Congress. The panoply of initiatives addressing women's health concerns is both welcome and exciting. There is complexity in the interaction between the people and the government, especially when there are broad concerns about such a significant issue as the interface between medicine, nutrition, and women's health research.

After the report of the Task Force on Women's Health Issues[2] was published in 1985, the NIH organized an Advisory Committee on Women's Health Issues. This committee assessed NIH's involvement in women's health research and made recommendations for implementation and/or expansion of this research. Within 2 months of the committee's inception, a recommendation was made that women be included in clinical trials. The NIH and most of its institutes, centers, and divisions support a great deal of research devoted to diseases which affect only women, women primarily, and both sexes. Women were not included in significant clinical studies for a prolonged period of time for two reasons: (1) concerns about the hazards of experimentation for women during the reproductive years and (2) difficulties in interpretation of variations in results because of hormonal effects. In fact, most laboratory research on mammals was conducted on male rats.

II. INCIDENCE AND PREVALENCE
OF DISEASES IN WOMEN

A brief survey of data about incidence and prevalence from the U.S. National Center for Health Statistics provides an objective picture of the diseases and risk factors women encounter. These data address the five leading causes of death and some risk factors. The data come from 29 tables of morbidity and mortality derived from several different National Center for Health Statistics sources.

Of the five leading causes of death for males and females, both white and black, rates of death from heart disease lead all other causes for all groups, with malignant neoplasms a close second. Lesser death rates are observed for cerebrovascular disease, accidents, chronic obstructive pulmonary disease, pneumonia, and diabetes mellitus, for which rates differ between the groups.

For black women, ages 25 to 85+ years, heart disease, cerebrovascular disease, and malignant neoplasms are the leading causes of death. Other prominent causes among the top five for specified age groups include accidents and liver disease. In a comparison of death rates for ischemic heart disease and acute myocardial infarction in all females, white females, and black females, deaths for black females are low throughout all age groupings. Deaths from heart failure for all females and white females are almost the same.

Breast cancer rates for all women, white women, and black women are comparable throughout age groups. The age-adjusted death rates/100,000 population for those countries for which data are available show a linear correlation with dietary intake of fat in grams/day. As Japanese women aged 50 to 59 years have increased their fat intake from 1955 to 1975, their breast cancer death rate has increased.[3]

Women have three major risk factors: obesity, cigarette smoking, and alcohol. While 25 to 45% of all women aged 20 to 74 are overweight, black women are significantly more overweight in every age group. About 60% of black women from ages 45 to 54 are overweight. Over 25% of women over 18 years of age smoke cigarettes. Five percent more black than white women in the 25- to 44-year group are smokers.

The National Center for Health Statistics Health Interview Survey reported that 45% of women said they abstained from alcohol, 35% were light drinkers, 15% were moderate drinkers, and 4% were heavier drinkers. Due to reticence to admit drinking habits, percentages for light/moderate/heavy drinking are apt to be artificially low.

III. HEALTH MAINTENANCE: WHO'S "ESSENTIAL ELEMENTS"

In addition to considering disease, it is vitally important to view health maintenance as a potential means for decreasing the occurrence and morbidity of disease. Americans often focus on treatment of illness rather than on disease prevention. In the U.S. as well as worldwide, women tend to be responsible not only for their own health care, but also for that of their family. Hence, emphasis is on primary health care, of which nutrition and nutrition education should be major components. In the late 1970s, the following eight essential elements for primary health care were delineated by the World Health Organization:[4]

1. Education concerning primary health problems and methods of preventing and controlling them
2. Promotion of food supply and proper nutrition
3. Adequate supply of safe water and basic sanitation
4. Maternal and child health care, including family planning
5. Immunization against major infectious diseases
6. Prevention and control of locally endemic diseases
7. Appropriate treatment of common diseases and injuries
8. Provision of essential drugs

IV. THE U.S. PUBLIC HEALTH SERVICE

A. TASK FORCE ON WOMEN'S HEALTH ISSUES (1983 TO 1985)

In 1983, the Assistant Secretary for Health gave a charge to the Task Force on Women's Health Issues that it was to assess problems of women's health in the context of contemporary American women's lives. After identification of women's health issues of contemporary societal significance, these issues were integrated with Public Health Service priorities. Recommendations of the task force[2] were organized as follows:

1. Promotion of a safe, healthful, physical, and social environment
2. Provision of services for prevention and treatment of disease
3. Research and evaluation
4. Recruitment and training of health care personnel
5. Public education and dissemination of research information
6. Design of guidelines for legislative and regulatory measures

Fifteen subcategories were designated under these six recommendations. The three major recommendations[2] for conduct of research and evaluation (recommendation 3) were

1. Expansion of biomedical and behavioral research with emphasis on conditions and diseases unique to, or more prevalent in, women in all age groups
2. Expansion of research and development for more effective, acceptable, and safe contraceptive methods for both men and women
3. Expansion of studies of causes, prevention, improved diagnosis, and treatment of debilitating diseases such as breast and other reproductive system cancers; sexually transmitted diseases; arthritic diseases including systemic lupus erythematosus, osteoporosis, and certain mental disorders

The following other research categories were included under the recommendations for research and evaluation: baseline data, diagnostic methods, nutritional requirements, care settings, psychosocial factors, pharmacokinetics, chronic conditions, safety and efficacy of estrogen and other therapies for treatment of menopausal and postmenopausal symptoms and osteoporosis, mental illnesses, risk factors, socioeconomic issues affecting women and especially older women, and the effects of gender differences on longevity. Emphasis throughout the report was on the impact of societal changes on women's lives and the effect of human behavior as shaped by cultural and social values upon health and disease.

Following publication of the task force report and its summary, a National Conference on Women's Health (June 1986)[5] was sponsored by the Public Health Service Coordinating Committee on Women's Health Issues and the Food and Drug Administration. The main topics of this conference were (1) women's health (a course of action, nutrition, issues in mental health, alcoholism and substance abuse, pregnancy and childbirth); (2) older women's health (contemporary and emerging health issues); (3) taking charge (how to make a difference, cancer, menstrual cycle, osteoporosis); and (4) women and their health care providers (a matter of communication).

B. NIH ADVISORY COMMITTEE ON WOMEN'S HEALTH ISSUES

The U.S. Public Health Service Task Force's mandate included establishment of groups within each agency to implement the recommendations according to their appropriate responsibilities. The Advisory Committee on Women's Health Issues, established in 1985, has produced two reports on the NIH support of research related to women's health and disease, identified the limited inclusion of women in clinical trials, and recommended policies to correct this shortage. These policies were published in the NIH Guide to Grants and Contracts in 1986, 1987, and 1989.[6]

C. GOVERNMENT ACCOUNTING OFFICE STUDY

Many congressional hearings focused on various aspects of women's health. Congress also has formed a Women's Health Caucus. Three members of Congress requested a study by the Government Accounting Office to address the concerns about failure to include women in most of the major clinical trials. There were special concerns about long-term trials focused on cardiovascular diseases such as the Multiple Risk Factor Intervention Trial (MRFIT)[7] and the Harvard Physicians Trials.[8] The Government Accounting Office report was presented at a hearing in June 1990. At that time, NIH reemphasized its policy of commitment to and emphasis on research pertinent to women and their illnesses. This policy requires research grant applicants to justify exclusion or underrepresentation of women in clinical trials.

D. OFFICE OF RESEARCH ON WOMEN'S HEALTH

Creation of the Office of Research on Women's Health was announced by the acting director of NIH in September 1990 at an NIH hearing. The Director of the National Institute of General Medical Sciences, who had chaired the Task Force on Women's Health, was appointed acting director of this new office, and immediately organized a public hearing about women's health (June 1991). Public testimony from 62 organizations interested both in women's health and in the need for research on women's health was accepted. Written testimony was received from an additional 30 organizations.

A workshop entitled "Opportunities for Research on Women's Health: What We Know and What Needs to Be Done" was held in September 1991. The first director of the Office of Research on Women's Health was appointed. The workshop set a scientific agenda for women's health across the life span: birth to young adulthood, young adulthood to perimenopausal years, perimenopausal to mature years, and mature years. The agenda also included cross-cutting areas of science: reproductive biology, early developmental biology, cardiovascular diseases, malignant neoplasms, immune and infectious diseases, and aging. The workshop addressed the current status of research on women's health and gaps in research, identified biomedical research opportunities, and recommended approaches and options for research on women's health.

With NIH support, an Institute of Medicine Planning Panel for "Including Women in Clinical Trials[9]" was convened in March 1991. The goal of this panel was to determine whether a study to develop policies allowing orderly progress toward inclusion of women in clinical research was needed, timely, feasible, and suited to the capabilities of the Institute of Medicine. The panel included experts in relevant areas of science and clinical trials methodology, as well as persons knowledgeable about ethics, law, Institutional Review Boards, the Food and Drug Administration, and concerns of women and minorities. The report of this 2-day meeting distills the major issues of women's health research. Inadequate representation of women in clinical research had been highlighted by the Government Accounting Office, some segments of the research community, the media, and women's advocacy groups, among others. Major studies were cited which failed to include women: the Physicians Health Study,[6] Multiple Risk Factor Intervention Trials,[7] the Baltimore Longitudinal Study,[10] the trials of AIDS therapy, as well as other drug trials.[11]

Six reasons for exclusion of women from the study populations of some trials, or for the failure to include gender analyses in publications, were identified. These were

1. Cyclical hormonal changes occurring in women
2. Inclusion of women with men making the study population less homogeneous

3. Significant increase in cost of trials if the study population were enlarged enough to allow testing gender hypotheses or subgroup analyses
4. Increase in cost and accrual burdens of the trial if representative numbers of women were included in the trial for conditions in which the incidence is lower in women than in men
5. Ethical reasons to avoid exposing existing, or potential, fetuses to harm
6. Legal and financial consequences if the fetus or child were harmed as a result of the mother's participation in a clinical trial

The panel voiced a major concern about the need to use funds efficiently by targeting priority areas for data analysis by gender, testing gender-specific hypotheses, and identifying research areas critical for women's health.

The relative neglect of concerns pertinent to the health of women in clinical research included:

1. A pervasive sense in the research community that women's issues are of secondary importance, and that the need for fetal protection overrides other values such as women's autonomous decision making
2. The overwhelming proportion of men in biomedical science whose perspectives may be different from those of women
3. The longer lifespan of women and their lesser or later representation in some major diseases, leading to the perception that women are healthier and less in need of study
4. Attitudinal stances which must be altered if gender equity in research is to be achieved

Three questions raised were

1. When are gender-specific hypotheses relevant?
2. When is women's reproductive health likely to be affected?
3. What subgroup analyses pertinent to gender are needed?

The panel study concluded that three fundamental questions persist:

1. Are there problems in the use of women in clinical trials and in the design of trials that are retarding the contribution of biomedical science to the health of women?
2. If problems are identified, are they amenable to solution?
3. Are there agencies, institutions, or groups whose policies and activities have an effect on the ways in which relevant research is conducted, and to whom a study would address its recommendations?

The panel identified other questions related to barriers to inclusion of women in research and proposed two general investigations: examination of the language commonly used to discuss women as research subjects, and examination of the political factors which influence science policy. This study viewed its audience as broad, and the groups which should provide answers to the questions as numerous.

The Director of NIH gave women's health research a high priority. In her testimony before the U.S. House of Representatives' Committee on Energy and Commerce, Subcommittee on Health and Environment, a month after her (1991) confirmation hearing, the director emphasized her "deep personal commitment to research on women's health...and that [she was] encouraged that the critical issues related to research on women's health [were] receiving the spirited consideration of Congress." She announced[12] a "far-reaching Women's Health Study which would take a comprehensive approach to the three major sources of morbidity and mortality in women of all socioeconomic strata: cancer, cardiovascular diseases, and disorders such as osteoporosis, which leads to fractures, and severe musculoskeletal frailty in aging women."

E. U.S. PUBLIC HEALTH SERVICE ACTION PLAN FOR WOMEN'S HEALTH

The U.S. Public Health Service Action Plan for Women's Health (September 1991) provided a sweeping plan for improvement of women's health through prevention, research, treatment, services, education, information, and policy. The plan established substantive goals which reflected the U.S. Public Health Service commitment to maintain and to forward the health and quality of life of American women and to implement these goals within the limited resources available. All U.S. Public Health Service agencies and program offices, in line with their respective missions, have established goals and action steps addressing the breadth of women's health issues across age, biology, and sociocultural issues. The Office of Women's Health, Office of Assistant Secretary for Health, bears the responsibility for monitoring implementation of the action plan using annual progress reports which identify accomplishments, barriers, modifications, and other related U.S. Public Health Service initiatives, as well as utilizing a computerized system to track the status of specific goals and actions by intervention categories, priority health issues, and target populations. Each of the 12 agencies and offices is responsible for 1 to 5 of the 38 goals.

The Healthy People 2000 — National Health Promotion and Disease Prevention Objectives[13] campaign has the goal of developing a national strategy to improve significantly the health of the nation over the coming decade by addressing the prevention of major chronic illnesses, injuries, and infectious diseases. Among objectives and targets are: physical activity and obesity; tobacco and heart disease; lung cancer; cigarette smoking; breast cancer and mammography; maternal, child health, and prenatal care.

F. FOOD AND DRUG ADMINISTRATION

Women are recipients of about 70% of prescriptions and frequently hold health responsibilities for children and spouses, so that women's understanding and health information are important for the majority of people. Under the "Healthy People 2000"[13] initiative of the Department of Health and Human Services, the Food and Drug Administration has the lead responsibility for increasing communications between primary care providers and elderly patients. The implementation of this plan is multifaceted and includes work with private groups such as the National Council on Patient Information and Education, presentations to both professional and consumer organizations, and publication of relevant articles. This initiative focuses on a team approach and recognizes the unique position of pharmacists, in the health care provider relationship.

Under the Omnibus Budget Reconciliation Act of 1990,[14] a Drug Use Review Program was mandated that requires states to provide counseling for all Medicaid patients, and a drug use review program to assure that prescriptions are appropriate, medically necessary, and unlikely to produce adverse effects.

A Campaign on Women and Medicines, whose purpose was to ensure safer and more effective use of medicines through improved communication between women and health care providers (e.g., doctors, pharmacists, nurses), was initiated by the Food and Drug Administration. Women use more medicines than do men and serve as "medicine managers" for other family members. The interaction of foods, alcohol, and medicines, timing of medications, side effects, and adverse actions of medications are important informational aspects of this campaign. While this campaign focuses on all women's concerns, it is directed especially toward concerns of pregnant and lactating women, menopausal women, and special populations such as minorities and the elderly. The National Council on Patient Information and Education, which cooperates with the Food and Drug Administration in its educational mission, has published information[15] about women and medicines, counseling women about medicines and diseases and conditions common to women.

V. OFFICE OF RESEARCH ON WOMEN'S HEALTH

The Office of Research on Women's Health is responsible for assuring that research conducted and supported by NIH adequately addresses issues regarding women's health and that there is appropriate participation of women in clinical research, especially in clinical trials. The three main ORWH goals are:

1. To strengthen and enhance NIH efforts to improve prevention, diagnosis, and treatment of illness in women
2. To assure that research conducted and supported by the NIH addresses issues regarding women's health appropriately
3. To assure that there is appropriate participation of women in clinical studies

The Office of Research on Women's Health also has the charge to set the NIH research agenda for women's health and provide the relevant NIH tracking system, monitor recruitment, retention, promotion, and follow-up of women in science and of women in biomedical research, involve the scientific community, and include medical, legal, and ethical issues.

The codification of the requirement to include women in clinical trials has been announced in the NIH Guide to Grants and Contracts. It specifies that:[16]

1. Adequate numbers of women proportional to their prevalence in the condition under study shall be included in clinical studies.
2. Failure to include an adequate number of women without compelling justification will be considered to affect the investigator's ability to answer the scientific question being posed.
3. Any justification for excluding women in such studies will be evaluated by the peer review group and factored into the relative level of merit given the proposal.
4. No application or proposal for any application excluding women will be approved for funding unless compelling justification has been provided.

Activities of Office of the Research on Women's Health in the past year have included supplemental funding and plans for future workshops. In 1991 and 1992, the Office of Research on Women's Health provided administrative supplements to ongoing clinical studies which enhanced the number of women or provided for inclusion of women in these studies. Twenty supplemental grants totaling over $800,000 were awarded and over half of the principal investigators on these grants in 1991 were women.

The Office of Research on Women's Health has two cooperative projects in process: one with the Institute of Medicine to address the medical, legal, and ethical barriers to inclusion of women in clinical studies, and one with the National Academy of Science to support a task force considering recruitment and promotion of women in science and engineering.

A. WOMEN'S HEALTH INITIATIVE

The Women's Health Initiative addresses the three leading causes of death and disability among American women over 45 years of age: cardiovascular diseases, cancer, and osteoporosis. The three study components are epidemiological surveillance, a clinical trial, and a community prevention trial. The Women's Health Initiative addresses three of the leading health problems for women: cardiovascular disease, breast and colon cancer, and osteoporosis, with its sequelae of bone fractures. The Clinical Trial's Coordinating Center in Seattle was selected for the Women's Health Initative. Sixteen Vanguard Centers were chosen and another 30 centers followed within a year. The NIH Women's Health Initiative provides an integrated, multidisciplinary approach to the prevention of some of the most common causes of disability, mortality, and death in postmenopausal women. Clinical trials, observational studies, and community trials will be used. These will address the evaluation of benefit and risk in prevention as well as adverse effects. There is a paucity of research on conditions and treatments unique to, or of greater concern for, women. There have been no preventive clinical trials assessing the effect of dietary change on prevention of breast and colon cancer, or of coronary heart disease, using these diseases as end points. Clinical trials of hormone replacement therapy, using coronary heart disease, stroke, and osteoporosis as end points are also, lacking. There is a paucity of longitudinal data on predictors and markers of disease development in women, yet a considerable gap exists between the established value of healthy behavior and adoption of these behaviors, especially among minorities and the medically underserved.

A Women's Health Initiative Oversight Committee is monitoring the progress of the entire program. Three important considerations for the Women's Health Initiative are that proposed studies: (1) build on other studies, and (2) do not supplant; or (3) compete with them. Measurements, especially clinical outcomes, will be comparable to those in similar studies, and opportunities exist for ancillary studies that could use the unique opportunity provided by this large cohort of women.

The Clinical Trials, in three integrated trials, are evaluating hormone replacement therapy, calcium and vitamin D, and dietary modification of fat and fiber. The Community Trials will implement known interventions in over 30,000 residents. Postmenopausal women, aged 50 to 79, will be invited to participate in either the clinical trial or the observational study. The clinical trial is a large randomized control trial of women which involves 45 clinics, one coordinating center, two to three central laboratories, and a drug distribution center.

It is anticipated that the benefit of the Women's Health Initiative will exceed the risks. The clinical outcomes expected on hormone replacement therapy are a decrease in coronary heart disease and in fractures, which will be greater than the possible increase in breast and endometrial cancers. Dietary modification will decrease breast and colorectal cancer, diabetes, and coronary heart disease. The potential of calcium and vitamin D to decrease fractures and colorectal cancer is anticipated to be greater than that to increase the incidence of renal calculi. Total mortality, quality of life, and side effects will be evaluated.

B. COMMUNITY RANDOMIZED TRIAL

The purpose of the Community Randomized Trial is to evaluate strategies to achieve healthful behaviors, including improved diet, nutritional supplementation, smoking prevention and cessation, increased physical activity, and early disease detection for women of all races, ethnic groups, and socioeconomic strata. Selection for the Community Randomized Trial will be from geopolitical regions of 30,000 or more adult residents of both sexes and where the intervention must be able to reach an inclusive sample of the population. At least 20% of the Community Randomized Trial participants will be minority or "underserved" persons. The observational studies will provide estimates of risk factors and disease prevalence and incidence for comparison with the clinical trial cohort, as well as for women of those age cohorts in general. The Community Randomized Trial evaluation strategies include cross-sectional samples, an estimated 500 women/sample/community, comparison of the first and last samples, and use of a middle sample for intervention corrections. The approach to the communities will involve community participation; established, modified, or new community channels; and potential channels including health care providers, work sites and organizations, public education, food services, and media.

There is an acute awareness of the need to address the issue of minority representation, since health maintenance and disease prevention are particularly important in these groups which have a statistically higher morbidity and mortality. It is recognized that some of this morbidity and mortality may be related to the fact that in 1993 over 40.9 million nonelderly Americans had no health coverage[17] and a similar number had inadequate coverage. Further, psychosocial and behavioral aspects will be assessed, since they are potential predictors both of compliance and of future disease and disability.

VI. SUMMARY

There is excitement and vibrancy in the area of women's health. Not only is it an idea whose time has come, perhaps tardily, but it is a concept of vital importance to more than half of the American population who are women, and to the rest of the population who need and are dependent upon women. Of major significance is the recognition of the importance of prevention and of health maintenance — both modalities for which the importance of good nutrition is key.

Under the leadership of the U.S. Public Health Service and with the recommendations included in its action plan, all of its agencies and offices are moving to encourage interventions that include prevention, research, treatment and services, education, information, and policy.

The accomplishments in women's health and in relevant research that we will see in the next decades will be dramatic. The anticipated cooperative efforts across health care disciplines and among the many organizations concerned with women's health give promise of great advances.

REFERENCES

1. Cummings, M. C., Jr. and Wise, D., *Democracy Under Pressure,* 7th Ed., Fort Worth, TX, 1993, 142.
2. Women's Health, Report of the Public Health Service Task Force on Women's Health Issues, Vol. I, 100:73–106, Washington, D.C.: U.S. Government Printing Office, 461–1950:37708, Washington, D.C., 1985.
3. National Cancer Institute, personal communication.
4. Mahler, H., Blueprint for Health for All, *WHO Chron.,* 31, 491, 1980.
5. Women's Health, J. U.S. Public Health Service, Supplement to July-August Issue, 1986. PHS 86-50193 (U.S. Public Health Service 324–990), DHHS, Washington, D.C.
6. NIH Guide to Grants and Contracts, 1986, 1987, 1988.
7. Multiple Risk Factor Intervention Trial: risk factor changes and mortality results, *J.A.M.A.* 248, 1465, 1982.
8. Steering Committee of the Physicians Health Study Research Group, Final report on the aspirin component of the ongoing Physicians Health Study, *N. Engl. J. Med.,* 321, 129, 1989.
9. Institute of Medicine, Planning Panel for Including Women in Clinical Trials, March, 1991, Washington, D.C.
10. Hallfrisch, J., Muller, D., Drinkwater, D., Tobin, J., and Andres, R., Continuing diet trends in men: the Baltimore Longitudinal Study of Aging (1961–1987), *J. Gerontol.,* 45, M186, 1990.
11. Clinical Trials conducted by the National Institute of Heart, Lung and Blood Diseases; National Institute on Aging; National Institute of Allergy and Infectious Diseases, National Institutes of Health (over several decades with numerous articles published).
12. USHR Committee on Energy and Commerce, Subcommittee on Health and Environment, Dr. Bernadine Healy's testimony.
13. Healthy People 2000, National Health Promotion and Disease Prevention Objectives, U.S. Department of Health and Human Services, DHHS Publication No. (PHS) 91–50213, U.S. Government Printing Office, Washington, D.C.
14. Omnibus Reconciliation Act of 1990, P.L. 101–508, Paragraph 4401 (g).
15. Talk about Prescriptions Month, p. 4, October 1991.
16. NIH Guide to Grants and Contracts, 20, 1, 1991.
17. Snider, S. and Fronstin, P., Sources of Health Insurance and Characteristics of the Uninsured: Analysis of March 1994 Current Population Survey, EBRI Special Report SR-28, Issue Brief Number 158, February 1995.

Chapter 2

MAJOR DIET-RELATED RISK FACTORS IN AMERICAN WOMEN

Carolyn K. Clifford

CONTENTS

I. INTRODUCTION

Women and men share the same basic nutritional concerns, but women have considerable additional needs related to menarche, reproduction, lactation, and menopause that justify an emphasis on the nutritional concerns of women in any discussion of nutrition and health issues. Prior to the 20th century, health statistics related to women were not recorded in any regular or standardized manner, and the data were of questionable quality. Discussions of women's health centered almost exclusively on childbearing capabilities and complications. Generally less educated than men, women had little knowledge of or interest in themselves as individuals with specific health and nutritional needs. The social mores of the day influenced the members of the medical community, who believed that women's health complaints originated from "nervous conditions" rather than physical or pathological causes.[1] Many

0-8493-8502-4/96/$0.00+$.50
© 1996 by CRC Press, Inc.

of these early attitudes have not been easily abandoned. Some women have demanded both recognition of the need for and action toward equal status for women in health considerations and biomedical research for many years. Only recently, however, have scientists, clinicians, and women in the general population discussed concerns such as breast cancer, eating disorders, and menopause freely and openly and acknowledged these concerns as both personal and public health issues.[1]

II. NUTRITIONAL CONSIDERATIONS IN HEALTH AND DISEASE

A normal diet should "...supply all essential nutrients in adequate amounts; supply a physiologic quantity of bulk and fluids, be easily digestible and confer a feeling of satiety; it should be readily available from the standpoint of both supply and cost; it should live up to the gustatory expectations of the prospective consumer and conform to the gastronomic customs of the group."[2] Within this framework, an infinite variety of dietary patterns are possible that will result in adequate nutrition for the majority of healthy individuals. Individuals, however, differ in their genetic makeup and in physiologic aspects, including endocrine activity, metabolic efficiency, and specific nutritional requirements. Even in normal circumstances, women's nutritional needs differ from those of men, requiring special focus on calcium and iron. Menarche, childbearing, lactation, and menopause produce specific metabolic and physiologic differences that separate women from men. Pregnancy and lactation are accompanied by physiologic, biochemical, and physical changes that result in required increases in daily intake of most nutrients.[3] Menorrhagia and pregnancy are the most prevalent causes of iron-deficiency anemia among young women. Aging in women also is accompanied by changes that may compromise nutritional status. Decline in circulating estrogen after menopause, for example, can affect calcium balance and is associated with an accelerated decrease in bone mass that can result in osteoporosis.[4]

For both women and men, the three leading causes of death in the U.S. are heart disease, cancer, and stroke; women, however, may be more susceptible to certain risk factors associated with these diseases or may be affected differently than men, partly because of differences in hormonal status.[5] Consider obesity, a condition that has been found to affect more women than men in almost all reported studies. Evidence suggests that obesity is an independent factor for the development of atherosclerotic cardiovascular disease, hypertension, diabetes, gallbladder disease, and some cancers.[4] Breast cancer, estimated to be the second leading cause of cancer death in women in the U.S. in 1994,[6] following lung cancer, has been the focus of numerous studies relating this cancer to body weight. Epidemiologic studies have demonstrated a significant direct association between body weight and breast cancer for postmenopausal women in contrast to a significant inverse association for premenopausal women.[7,8] Chronic diseases such as heart disease, cancer, and osteoporosis increase with age. Osteoporosis, for example, afflicts 24 million Americans, primarily women, including one third to one half of all postmenopausal women and 90% of women over 75 years of age.[9] Women now constitute approximately 52% of the general U.S. population and 59% of the population ages 65 and greater. Among individuals ages 85 and above — a group expected to double in the coming decade — women make up nearly 75% of the population.[9] Demographic studies project that there will be increasing numbers of elderly women during the first part of the 21st century. More women than men, therefore, will face the health problems that accompany advanced age.

III. RECOMMENDED DIETARY ALLOWANCES AND DIETARY RECOMMENDATIONS/GUIDELINES

The importance of proper dietary intake in health maintenance and chronic disease risk reduction cannot be emphasized too strongly and has been recognized by numerous organizations that actively endorse good nutrition as an integral part of health. The first recommended dietary allowances (RDAs) for intake of energy and nutrients, developed by the Food and Nutrition Board of the National Research Council, were established in 1943 and have been revised periodically since then to include new research results, with the most recent edition published in 1989.[10] The current RDAs, which have been established for protein, 11 vitamins, and 7 minerals, represent an estimated, rather than absolute, standard for essential nutrients judged to be adequate to meet the known nutritional needs of almost all healthy individuals of both genders and different ages. RDAs are usually higher for men than women, except for women who are pregnant or lactating; for these women, the recommended allowances are usually higher than for men. Since many dietary components are involved in diet and optimal health relationships, translating the RDAs into a universally applicable, eating pattern is a challenge.

Defining food choices and eating patterns that best fulfill nutrient requirements has been a goal of many federal agencies and private health organizations that have developed dietary recommendations and guidelines during the past decade. The Dietary Guidelines for Americans[11] recommend that to stay healthy one should eat a variety of foods; maintain healthy weight; choose a diet low in total fat, saturated fat, and cholesterol; choose a diet with plenty of vegetables, fruits, and grain products; use sugars only in moderation; use salt and sodium only in moderation; and if alcoholic beverages are consumed, do so in moderation.

In 1990, a national strategy for improving the health of the U.S. population, called "Healthy People 2000: National Health Promotion and Disease Prevention Objectives",[12] was established. The goals of this strategy for Americans are to increase the span of healthy life, to reduce health disparities among population groups, and to achieve access to prevention services. One section specific to nutrition includes 21 objectives related to health status, risk reduction, and services and protection. Many of these objectives relate to women and target reductions in coronary heart disease, cancer, overweight, total fat and saturated intake, salt and sodium intake, and iron deficiency. Other objectives target increases in the consumption of complex carbohydrate and fiber-containing foods, calcium intake, and use of food labels to make nutritious food choices that are low fat/low calorie and consistent with the Dietary Guidelines for Americans.

IV. DIET-DISEASE RELATIONSHIPS

Extensive scientific evidence demonstrates associations between foods or eating patterns and health maintenance or chronic diseases. Epidemiologic data from international correlation, migrant, and time-trend studies suggest a positive relationship between total fat consumption or consumption of animal fat and increased risk of several cancers, as well as a positive relationship between saturated fat and coronary heart disease.[3,4,13,14] One of the most consistent epidemiologic findings indicates that populations consuming diets high in plant foods have lower risk of some types of cancer and coronary heart disease.[3,4,15-17] These diets are usually low in total fat, saturated fat, and cholesterol, and high in dietary fiber and antioxidants, including vitamin C and the precursors of vitamin A, such as β-carotene and other carotenoids.

Inadequate calcium intake is a contributing nutritional risk factor in the development of osteoporosis in later life. Epidemiologic and clinical studies have characterized osteoporosis as an asymptomatic reduction in bone mass.[3,4] Osteoporosis occurs most frequently in postmenopausal white women; as bone mass decreases, the risk of fractures increases. Calcium balance usually reflects the degree to which bone formation is coupled with resorption and depends on the amount of calcium in the diet and the efficacy of calcium absorption by the intestine. Scientific evidence also suggests a role of dietary calcium in blood pressure regulation.

V. DIETARY INTAKE OF WOMEN

Dietary guidance, community nutrition intervention programs, and nutrition policy aimed at improving the diets of women depend on the knowledge of what women eat. The National Health and Nutrition Examination Surveys (NHANES) provide a national reference source for periodic information on the dietary, nutritional, and health status of the U.S. population. Recent results from the third National Health and Nutrition Examination Survey (NHANES III), Phase I[18,19] — conducted between 1988 and 1991 — indicate that females (all ages) of all race-ethnic groups consumed 34% of their total energy intake from total fat and 12% from saturated fat. These data suggest that the intake of both total fat and saturated fat exceeds the current dietary guidelines. Mean dietary fiber intake was 12.75 g in females of all ages, which is much lower than the 20 to 30 g daily recommended by the National Cancer Institute (NCI).[3]

The mean calcium intake among females of all ages was 744 mg, which is below the RDAs of 1200 mg for females ages 11 to 24 and pregnant and lactating women, and 800 mg for women ages 25 and over. Mean iron intake was 12.37 mg for females of all ages, compared with the RDAs of 15 mg for women under age 50 years and for lactating women; 10 mg for women ages 51 and older; and 30 mg for pregnant women.

Vitamin A intake for females of all ages was 884 retinol equivalents (RE), which is above the RDA of 800 RE for all women except lactating women, whose RDA is 1200 to 1300 RE. Mean vitamin C intake was 95 mg for females of all ages, well above the RDA of 60 mg for all women, except pregnant and lactating women. Further data analyses are currently under way to compare the food sources of energy and nutrients consumed by different population groups in NHANES III to results from earlier national surveys.

VI. SOCIETY'S IMPACT ON NUTRITION

Extensive changes in eating patterns, food choices, and methods of food preparation have occurred in the U.S. over the last 50 years, including marked increases in eating away from home. An increase in women working outside the home has contributed to a decrease in the time spent on food preparation in the home. This, coupled with trends that include an increasing number of people dining alone and the prevalence of less formal life-styles, has resulted in increasing demand for and reliance on "fast" and convenience foods, beginning at young ages.[20]

Along with their desire for convenience, consumers are developing an increasing awareness of and interest in the relationship between diet and health.[3,4] Nutrition is currently a marketable commodity, as reflected by the proliferation of health and fitness clubs, the presence of fresh fruit and salad bars in both fast-food and full-service restaurants, and the increase in food products that project a "healthy", "fresh", "natural", and "lite" image. The food industry has taken aggressive steps to meet consumer demands for health and fitness foods — "fat-free" has become a nutritional preoccupation for many consumers. Restaurants are highlighting selections, such as the use of egg substitutes, that meet the American Heart Association's recommendations for cholesterol and saturated fats. The ready-to-eat cereal market is a vehicle for promoting fiber, raisins and other fruits, calcium, "no-salt, no-sugar, no-preservatives", and reduced fat. The soft-drink industry is promoting "healthy" by adding fruit juice, adding vitamins and minerals, removing caffeine and sugar, and introducing sport-drink products to its list of formulations.[20]

As an adjunct to the fitness movement, the use of vitamin supplementation by the American public, particularly women, has increased dramatically, with a 25% increase in 1993 compared with 1985. This was led by a strong increase in the sales of antioxidants, specifically vitamins C and E. Data indicate that vitamin sales were skewed toward women (46% had used vitamin supplements in the last month vs. 38% for men). Overall, individuals ages 45 years and greater, college-educated, and living in the western U.S. purchase vitamin supplements more than other groups.[21]

The print and electronic media have prominently promoted and advertised the concept of diet and health. There is a never-ending flow of information — from the results of preventive clinical research trials and the best food sources of antioxidants to news releases and press conference coverage concerning the type and amount of fat found in various popular ethnic foods and movie theater popcorn. However, along with the concept of "good health", the media has also projected the "right size and shape" to American women. Often this image is one of an overly thin woman that contradicts the need for regular and well-balanced dietary intake based upon a variety of foods. The desirability of this physical appearance becomes paramount and often fuels the development of inappropriate self-image and eating disorders, potentially jeopardizing some women's health and nutritional status.[5]

VII. WOMEN'S HEALTH AS A RESEARCH FOCUS

The randomized controlled clinical trial design has been viewed as the "gold standard" in clinical research, but has only been used to a limited extent in testing nutrition and chronic disease hypotheses. Most large-scale clinical trials evaluating the effects of drugs or devices have not traditionally included women. Often women have been excluded from participation in large-scale clinical trials because of lower event rates, later age of disease onset, and cyclic hormonal changes that introduce additional study variables. For example, the incidence of coronary heart disease is lower in premenopausal women than in postmenopausal women or men. Thus, an intervention study of coronary heart disease in premenopausal women would require a larger sample size and longer study duration to achieve sufficient statistical power than if a similar study were conducted in men. Further, potential pregnancy and the possible teratogenic effects of drugs or devices on an unborn child in certain studies may increase risks to an unacceptably high level.

Most biomedical knowledge about the causes, expression, and treatment of diseases such as heart disease, cancer, and stroke is derived from studies of men and subsequently applied to women, with the supposition that there are no differences between men and women. To the contrary, there are differences — in body mass, composition, and blood volume; in responses to drugs; and in possible variable pharmokinetic effects as a result of the menstrual cycle, menopause, and/or use of oral contraceptives. As the statistics on mortality and morbidity specific to women were integrated into biomedical knowledge and interpreted, it became apparent that the health problems of women were becoming more severe and that the knowledge necessary to reverse this trend was not currently available.[9]

Concerns like these have prompted the demands made by advocacy groups, members of Congress, health professionals, and the public that stipulate health issues related to women must be recognized and become a focus of future research. In response, the Office of Research on Women's Health (ORWH) was established at the NIH (NIH) in September 1990.[5] This action was part of a vigorous and continuing effort to strengthen and enhance research related to diseases, disorders, and conditions that affect women and to ensure that women are appropriately represented in biomedical and biobehavioral research studies. The ORWH research agenda for the coming decade calls for women's health issues to be viewed across scientific disciplines and medical specialties, as well as for the investigation of possible gender and racial differences in the conditions that affect both men and women, but that have been previously studied primarily in men.

The NIH Revitalization Act of 1993 adds new dimension to policies for inclusion of women and minorities in clinical research funded by the NIH. This law requires the NIH to ensure that women and members of minority groups are included in each clinical research project. The NIH must also ensure that clinical trials are designed and carried out in a manner that provides valid analysis of whether the variables studied affect women or members of minority groups differently than other subjects. Exclusion is permitted only if substantial scientific data exist that demonstrate no significant differences in effects of variables among women, men, and minority groups.[22] The new provisions additionally specify that the term "minority group" includes subpopulations of minority groups and that the NIH, in consultation with the director of the ORWH and the Office of Research on Minority Health, must conduct outreach programs for the recruitment of women and minorities meeting study requirements.

Socioeconomic status and urban vs. rural residence are additional relevant factors to be considered in biomedical research on women's health. The socioeconomically disadvantaged woman, for example, may present a very different health profile from her economically secure counterpart.[23] The recruitment and retention of minorities, women, appropriate subpopulations, and the underserved are imperative to ensure the application of research findings to all Americans. Two examples of ongoing clinical trials that focus on preventing disease and improving the health and quality of life for women are described below.

Begun in fall 1993, the Women's Health Initiative (WHI)[24] is a 10-year randomized controlled trial in postmenopausal women that will examine the effects of a low-fat eating pattern, calcium and vitamin D supplementation, and hormone replacement therapy on cardiovascular disease, cancer, and osteoporosis. The dietary modification aims to decrease total calories from fat to 20%, decrease total calories from saturated fat to less than 7%, and increase complex carbohydrates and fiber-containing foods to five or more servings of vegetables/fruits and six or more servings of grain products daily. This clinical trial will enroll approximately 63,000 postmenopausal women 50 to 79 years of age at 40 clinical centers throughout the U.S. In addition to the randomized clinical trial component, the WHI includes a prospective observational study in an additional 100,000 women to determine the etiologic factors and predictors of chronic disease. A third trial component will involve community-based intervention studies that seek effective ways to promote behaviors aimed at preventing cancer, cardiovascular disease, and osteoporosis.

The Harvard Women's Health Study (WHS) is a double-blind, placebo-controlled, randomized trial designed to evaluate the risks and benefits of low-dose aspirin and β-carotene and vitamin E supplements in the primary prevention of cardiovascular disease and cancer in healthy postmenopausal women in the U.S.[25,26] Begun in 1992, the WHS will enroll approximately 40,000 female health professionals with no previous history of the two diseases.

VIII. FINAL COMMENTS

The interrelationships among nutrition, health promotion, and disease prevention are evident throughout an individual's life cycle. It has, however, become apparent that women do have specific nutritional needs and concerns that are different from those of men. The chapters that follow demonstrate that nutritional status is an integral part of a woman's overall health status at every age and contributes to many aspects of her life. Overall, the authors' contributions emphasize the role of nutrition in women's health and disease. The roles of diet and nutrition in the major life events such as menarche, contraception issues, pregnancy, lactation, menopause, and aging, as well as chronic diseases including cardiovascular disease, cancer, and osteoporosis, are discussed. Nutrition is also explored as a component of self-image, body weight, eating disorders, and physical fitness. Though an optimal diet has yet to be defined, more concerted strategies are needed to assist women in modifying their eating habits to achieve dietary patterns that are consistent with the dietary guidelines for improving health and have the potential for reducing the morbidity and mortality of several diet-related chronic diseases. The public health implications are not limited to women alone, but will likely improve the health of their families and the nation.

REFERENCES

1. LaRosa, J. H. and Pinn, V. W., Gender bias in biomedical research, *J. Am. Med. Women's J.*, 48, 145, 1993.
2. Burton, B. T., *Human Nutrition*, Blakiston Publication, New York, 1976, 153.
3. U.S. Department of Health and Human Services, The Surgeon General's Report on Nutrition and Health, NIH Publ. No. 88-50210, Public Health Service, U.S. Government Printing Office, Washington, D.C., 1988, 539.
4. National Academy of Sciences, National Research Council, Commission on Life Sciences, Food and Nutrition Board, *Diet and Health. Implications for Reducing Chronic Disease Risk*, National Academy Press, Washington, D.C., 1989, 615
5. Pinn, V. W., Women's health issues: a U.S. perspective, *Can. J. OB/GYN Women's Health Care*, 6, 671, 1994.

6. Boring, C. C., Squires, T. S., Tong, T., and Montgomery, S., Cancer statistics, 1994, *CA Cancer J. Clin.*, 44, 7, 1994.

7. Howe, G. R., Hirohata, T., Hislop, T. G., Iscovich, J. M., Yuan, J.-M., Katsouyanni, K., Lubin, F., Marubini, E., Modan, B., Rohan, T., Toniolo, P., and Shunzhang, Y., Dietary factors and risk of breast cancer: combined analysis of 12 case-control studies, *J. Natl. Cancer Inst.*, 82, 561, 1990.

8. Albanes, D., Caloric intake, body weight, and cancer: a review, *Nutr. Cancer*, 9, 199, 1987.

9. Report of the National Institutes of Health: Opportunities for Research on Women's Health, NIH Publ. No. 92-3457A. U.S. Department of Health and Human Services, Washington, D.C., 1992, 1.

10. National Research Council, *Recommended Dietary Allowances*, 10th ed., National Academy Press, Washington, D.C., 1989, 1.

11. U.S. Department of Agriculture and U.S. Department of Health and Human Services, *Dietary Guidelines for Americans*. Washington, D.C., 1990, 1.

12. U.S. Department of Health and Human Services, Public Health Service, *Healthy People 2000 — National Health Promotion and Disease Prevention Objectives*, U.S. Public Health Service, DHHS Publ. No. (PHS) 91-50212, 1991, 111.

13. Hursting, S. D., Thornquist, M., and Henderson, M. M., Types of dietary fat and the incidence of cancer at five sites, *Prev. Med.*, 19, 242, 1990.

14. Willett, W. C., Diet and health: what should we eat?, *Science*, 264, 532, 1994.

15. Weisburger, J. H., Nutritional approach to cancer prevention with emphasis on vitamins, antioxidants, and carotenoids, *Am. J. Clin. Nutr.*, 53, 226s, 1991.

16. Ziegler, R. G., Subar, A. F., Craft, N. E., Ursin, G., Patterson, B. H., and Graubard, B. I., Does β-carotene explain why reduced cancer risk is associated with vegetable and fruit intake?, *Cancer Res.*, 52, 2060s, 1992.

17. Block, G., Vitamin C and cancer prevention: the epidemiologic evidence, *Am. J. Clin. Nutr.*, 53, 270s, 1991.

18. McDowell, M. A., Briefel, R. R., Alaimo, K., Bischof, A. M., Caughman, C. R., Carroll, M. D., Loria, C. M., and Johnson, C. L., Energy and macronutrient intakes of persons ages 2 months and over in the U.S.: Third National Health and Nutrition Examination Survey, Phase 1, 1988–91, *Adv. Data*, 255, 1, 1994.

19. Alaimo, K., McDowell, M. A., Briefel, R. R., Bischof, A. M., Caughman, C. R., Loria, C. M., and Johnson, C. L., Dietary intake of vitamins, minerals, and fiber of persons ages 2 months and over in the U.S.: Third National Health and Nutrition Examination Survey, Phase 1, 1988–91, *Adv. Data*, 258, 1, 1994.

20. Smith, R. E., Food demands of the emerging consumer: the role of modern food technology in meeting that challenge, *Am. J. Clin. Nutr.* 58(Suppl.), 307s, 1993.

21. Council for Responsible Nutrition, *1993 Overview of the Nutritional Supplement Market*, Washington, D.C., 1994, 1.

22. NIH guidelines on the inclusion of women and minorities as subjects in clinical research, *Fed. Reg.*, 59, 14509, 1994.

23. Kumanyika, S. K., Women and health research: rewriting the rules, *Perspect. Appl. Nutr.*, 2, 10, 1994.

24. Office of Research on Women's Health, *Women's Health Initiative: Overview Statement*, National Institutes of Health, Bethesda, MD, 1994, 1.

25. Buring, J. E. and Hennekens, C. H., The Women's Health Study: summary of the study design, *J. Myocardial Ischemia*, 4, 27, 1992.

26. Buring, J. E. and Hennekens, C. H., The Women's Health Study: rationale and background, *J. Myocardial Ischemia*, 4, 30, 1992.

Chapter 3

Women's Self-Conception of Nutrition: Societal Influences on Eating Behavior

Susan P. Robbins

CONTENTS

I. INTRODUCTION

The pursuit of physical beauty and the idealization of the human body is endemic to Western culture and has been traced to the ancient Greek conception of humans as being godlike. The definition of beauty and the ideal body shape, however, varies across cultures and has changed over time.[1,2] Since beauty is judged by one's physical appearance, societal norms governing appearance are a critical factor in how others judge us and, consequently, how we judge ourselves.

In contemporary American society, the physical ideal is embodied by youth, fitness, and thinness. This ideal is created, supported, and perpetuated to a large extent by the media and the modern advertising industry which continually stress the importance of being or becoming attractive. Other major industries such as fashion, cosmetics, cosmetic surgery, diet, and fitness also play a central role in sustaining this cultural ideal. They, in turn, are supported by the ongoing quest for youth and beauty.[2,3]

II. APPEARANCE NORMS AND
THE STIGMA OF OVERWEIGHT

From an early age, children are socialized to social and cultural expectations regarding appropriate masculine and feminine behavior.[4-6] However, the expectations for men and women are different regarding socially acceptable appearance. Body shape and weight, in particular, are more central aspects of attractiveness for women than men. Schur[3] has pointed out that while descriptive terms such as "portly", "stocky", and "heavy-set" are commonly used to refer to fat men, comparable terms do not exist for fat women. According to Goffman,[7] larger male figures used in advertising reflect a more positive definition of male weight that is symbolic of the "social weight" (power, prestige) that society accords men. As the pressure to attain the ideal has intensified in the past two decades, both men and women are becoming increasingly dissatisfied with their appearance.[1,7,9] Women, however, are under particular pressure to be thin.

Numerous authors have pointed out that appearance norms have a greater impact on women than on men.[1-3,10-12] According to Schur,[3] girls are taught from the beginning of childhood that their looks are a commodity and appearance is a key factor in their future success or failure. Concern about attaining the ideal becomes a pervasive focus in women's lives, and appearance norms play a central role in women's self-conceptions.[2,3,8] In our culture, beauty is synonymous with thinness.

Perhaps most damaging to women's physical and mental health is the fact that the cultural ideal is not based on any realistic sense of the normal varieties of the female body.[2,10,13] Goffman[7] has noted that women are constantly exposed to unrealistic role models. Although the ideal female figure has undergone periodic transformations since the 1920s, the ideal has been largely unattainable for most women. From the voluptuous, slim-waisted *Playboy* model in the early 1950s, to the slender, boyish Twiggy in the 1960s, to the aerobically muscular Susan Powter in the 1990s, the cultural ideal has shown a trend toward increasing thinness over the past 20 to 30 years.[12,14,15] Ironically, Rodin and Larson[1] have pointed out that during this time period, body weight for the average woman under 30 years old has actually increased.

The ideal female body shape (and the obsession to attain it) has been closely linked to significant social, political, and economic changes of the 20th century.[2,10,13,16] According to Wolf,[10] women's preoccupation with dieting and thinness began around 1920 when women gained the right to vote. With increasing occupational and educational opportunities for women since the 1960s, the ideal emphasized a more athletic, muscular, and androgynous shape, consistent with a professional business look.[2,13] Tavris[13] notes that the number of books and articles on dieting increases astronomically during egalitarian times, as do eating disorders among women and girls. Although the standard for the 1990s promoted by the media is a more voluptuous, "ultra-feminine" look, Seid[2] cautions that this does not mean that we are about to accept a bigger body ideal; female role models continue to be extremely slender. She contends that we have erroneously come to believe that this distorted ideal is the norm.

Increasingly, over the last several decades, the standard of acceptable public appearance has been based on the widely accepted notion of a "desirable" or "ideal" weight. The concept of "ideal weight" was developed by insurance companies in the 1920s and, by the 1950s, health experts began to warn the public that excess fat (defined as 15 to 20% above one's ideal weight) was associated with serious disease and a shorter life expectancy. With the advent of the new insurance tables, average-weight people were now redefined as overweight or, in some cases, as obese.[2] More recently, appearance norms have become even more rigid as contemporary concerns about nutrition and "wellness" have interchangeably linked health, diet, thinness, and fitness.[2,13] Despite our growing concern with weight, investigators are now raising serious questions about the validity of links between overweight, illness, and mortality for all but the seriously obese.[17,18] However, according to Millman,[19] health concerns have never been the primary factor in the social rejection of overweight people. Fatness is seen not only as a physical condition, but it implies a character flaw as well. She notes that women, in particular, suffer more from the social and psychological stigma of obesity than from the weight itself.

The stigma of overweight has been well documented in numerous studies. Negative attitudes toward fat and obese people have been found in young children, adolescents, and adults alike.[20-26] DeJong[27] has suggested that the extent to which we hold people responsible for their appearance may be related to the degree of stigma that is attached to their obesity. Clinard and Meier[28] have noted that implicit in these negative attitudes is a moral implication that overweight people are simply unwilling to control their behavior. This belief is now buttressed by a health and fitness industry which stresses personal responsibility in achieving the ideal body size and shape.

Schur[3] has stressed that societal emphasis on female appearance places extreme pressure on *all* women not to violate even the most restrictive appearance norms. In fact, Wolf (p. 200) has suggested that dieting has become "the essence of contemporary femininity."[10] Unfortunately, rigid social stereotypes of female beauty are often incorporated into a woman's self-concept and this can have serious consequences for nutrition and physical and mental health.

III. PERSONAL IDENTITY, SELF-CONCEPT, AND BODY IMAGE

As part of the normal maturational process, adolescents in contemporary society begin to solidify their *personal identity* as they move from adolescence to young adulthood. Four interrelated aspects of personal identity have been identified in the literature: *biological* (involving, for example, body shape and weight), *intellectual* (such as cognitive and academic abilities), *psychological* (encompassing self-concept, self-esteem, and body image), and *social* (including interpersonal relationships and sociocultural norms). When these aspects are brought together, personal identity is formed.[29] According to Brackney,[29] many of the developmental conflicts that females encounter during identity formation are related to social definitions of behavioral expectations and future adulthood roles for women. She contends that, unlike boys (p. 155), the majority of adolescent girls experience "conflicts within and among the biological, psychological, intellectual, and social aspects of identity."[29] Negative stereotypes about women and appearance norms that are unattainable for most females often have an adverse effect on adolescent identity formation. As personal identity becomes solidified in adulthood, the way in which people come to define themselves and the feelings associated with those definitions are central to their feelings of self-worth.

Social theorist Cooley's[30] concept of the *looking glass self* demonstrates the way in which interaction with others shapes all self-conception. The process of self-conception involves three phases: first, we imagine how we appear to others; second, we imagine their judgments of that appearance; finally, the self-feelings that we develop (such as pride or shame) incorporate these perceptions.[30] In sum, we see ourselves, in part, as others see us. Appearance norms that are shaped by cultural ideals play a crucial influence both in how others see us and how we see ourselves.

Self-concept is the stable image of oneself that is formed in the quest for personal identity.[29] Included in self-concept are feelings of self-esteem, self-worth, and one's body image. *Body image* specifically refers to the feelings, perceptions, thoughts, and reactions that a person has about his or her body size, shape, weight, and appearance; it is the way a person subjectively experiences his or her body.[1,31,32] Body image is a critical factor in how a person feels about him- or herself and often has a significant impact on feelings of self-esteem and self-worth. Negative body image can lead to a variety of social, health, and psychological problems including shyness, eating and nutrition problems, and depression.[13,31,33]

The social importance of appearance and, particularly, attractiveness has been found to be related to a person's sense of self-worth and self-acceptance.[35,36] However, research has demonstrated that body image and attractiveness are more important dimensions of self-concept for women than for men.[37] Given our cultural ideals that equate female beauty with thinness, development of a positive body image is particularly difficult for women who are overweight.

In a review of the literature, Rodin and Larson[1] traced the developmental determinants of body image for men and women throughout the life span. They found that adolescents are particularly sensitive to appearance norms and that girls show more concern with their appearance than do boys.[38] In addition, girls generally see themselves as less attractive, and this negative perception has been found to be related to lower body esteem and self-esteem.[38,39]

Compounding problems of perception, normal adolescent weight gain associated with physical maturation brings boys "closer to their ideal", while taking girls "further away" from theirs (p. 152).[1] Physiological differences between men and women further exacerbate this situation. Cross-culturally, from birth, females not only begin life with a higher percentage of body fat than males, but they also experience more fat storage and weight gain as a part of their natural development.[10] This is especially true during puberty when growth in boys usually adds weight in the form of lean tissue, while girls, in contrast, gain a significant increase in fat tissue.[1,40-42] This increase in fat tissue is important for sexual maturation and fertility.[10] Tavris[13] notes that most white teenage girls regard normal adolescent weight gain as a sign of fatness.

Adolescents are extremely aware of and sensitive to sociocultural norms regarding appearance and they incorporate these into their definition of the "ideal" physique.[25] However, a recent study found cultural differences between black and white female adolescents in their description of the "ideal" American girl.[43] In contrast to white teenagers, whose ideal reflected the slim Barbie doll physique and focused primarily on physical features, the ideal for black adolescents was not related to physical characteristics. Instead, a "nice personality", a "personal sense of style", and "getting along well with others" were among the items that topped their list. When pressed to describe physical traits, they listed a "small waist", "fuller hips", and "large thighs". Parker[43] notes that these are physical characteristics valued by black men. Seventy percent of the black teens in this study reported being satisfied with their weight, whereas the overwhelming majority (90%) of white teens was dissatisfied. For the white adolescents, weight was a critical factor in self-concept.[43]

Not surprisingly, research has shown that girls who are dissatisfied with their weight typically want to be thinner; boys, on the other hand, want to be heavier.[25,44] Studies have shown that many adolescent girls are increasingly unhappy with their bodies, with a majority believing that they are too fat.[2,10,34] A study of over 2000 adolescent girls in Michigan found dieting and dissatisfaction with body image to be a common response to physical changes during puberty.[45] Concern with weight and dieting is now spreading to younger age groups, as evidenced by a 1986 study. In this study, 50 to 80% of girls age 9 through 11 reported that they were too fat.[23,24] As a result of our national obsession with weight, dieting and eating disorders are becoming increasingly prevalent among adolescent girls.[1,2,23]

Concerns about weight and negative body attitudes are prevalent not only in adolescent girls, but in adult women as well. As a normal part of adult female development, the physiological changes associated with pregnancy and menopause also encourage weight gain and fat storage.[1] Many women, however, have come to view pregnancy as a "distortion" of the body due to their fear and dread of weight gain.[2] Further, as women age, they also experience a larger increase in body fat and greater declines in their basal metabolic rate.[46-49] Although weight gain with age is cross-culturally typical for both men and women,[10] metabolic differences do not taper off until old age.[50]

These normal life cycle changes serve to reinforce women's apprehension about their appearance. Many women come to believe that weight is the central issue in their lives;[2] for some, their entire identity is placed on their weight.[51] Having little sense of who they are, they often report feeling empty, confused, and dissatisfied, and many regard their weight as the primary obstacle to happiness and self-realization.[2,51] Concern with weight has been noted to be a chronic stressor in women[53] that often leads to a collapse of self-esteem and a diminished sense of effectiveness.[53,54] This is consistent with studies that have shown a significant relationship among low self-esteem, body dissatisfaction, and dieting.[55-57]

Studies by Rubin,[58] Lakoff and Scherr,[59] and Wooley and Wooley[53] have revealed a surprising prevalence of distorted body image. The degree to which women perceive themselves to be overweight has been found to bear little relationship to their actual weight. For example, in Wooley and Wooley's national survey of 33,000 women for *Glamour Magazine,* 75% of their respondents felt that they were too fat, although only 25% were medically overweight.[53] More surprising is that 45% of the women who were *underweight* also believed that they were too fat. Seid[2] contends that the widespread distortion of body image among women and the resulting low self-esteem, if not self-loathing, is similar to that found in anorexics and bulimics. Although body distortion is now spreading among men as well, it is primarily women who diet and exhibit eating disorders.[2,60-62]

IV. THE EFFECT OF NEGATIVE SELF–CONCEPTION ON NUTRITION AND EATING BEHAVIOR

Although the majority of women do not starve themselves to anorexic extremes, negative self-concept and distorted body image do lead women to engage in frequent dieting.[2,53,58] Fad diets are commonplace and women are much more likely than men to join group dieting programs.[61,62] Diets, however, are often counterproductive to proper nutrition. Wolf[10] suggests, in fact, that the term "diet" is a trivializing word for self-inflicted semistarvation. Chronic dieting and undernutrition have been found to create both biological and emotional distress.[2,52,63,64]

In a University of Minnesota study on semistarvation, physiologist Keys[65] documented the psychological, behavioral, and physical effects of an extended low calorie diet on a healthy group of young men. In addition to predictable weight loss, the undernourishment produced ravenous appetites, food obsessions and cravings, depression, social withdrawal, decreased sexual interest, and lethargy in most of the subjects. Some even exhibited patterns of binge eating followed by vomiting and feelings of guilt, typical of bulimia. In a review of the literature on starvation studies and the literature on dieting problems, Bruch[66] found similarities in the physical and psychological effects caused by dietary restriction. Perhaps most significantly, she found uniform changes of behavior and personality, similar to those found in Keys' subjects, that do not disappear until weight gain is resumed.[66]

Chronic undernutrition leaves people chronically hungry and Wolf[10] maintains that hunger teaches women to erode their self-esteem through their hatred of their bodies. Some researchers believe that chronic hunger may cause neuroendocrine abnormalities that contribute to compulsive dieting.[2,62] There is an increasing recognition that dieting itself may, in fact, be a primary cause of both eating disorders and obesity.[2,52]

V. CONCLUSIONS

The social and cultural forces that equate female beauty with thinness have led to an increasing prevalence in negative and distorted body image, dieting, and eating disorders among women. Body dissatisfaction leads women to restrictive eating and chronic dieting in an attempt to be fashionably thin. The hunger caused by dieting, however, has been found to further perpetuate subsequent weight gain, obsessions with food, and biological and emotional stress.

Consequently, nutritionists and dietitians should be cautious about advising women who are chronic dieters to further restrict their caloric intake.[57] It has also been suggested that an assessment of the accuracy of body weight perception is an important component of evaluation.[31,57] In addition, education is necessary for women to understand the difference between an unrealistic "ideal" weight and a healthy maintainable weight.[57] Finally, on a cultural level, we must redefine appearance norms so that they more accurately reflect the reality of women's bodies.

ACKNOWLEDGMENT

The author would like to thank Carolyn Brooks for her assistance in the preparation of this book chapter.

REFERENCES

1. Rodin, J. and Larson, L., Social factors and the ideal body shape, in *Eating, Body Weight and Performance in Athletes: Disorders of Modern Society*, Brownell, K. D., Rodin, J., and Wilmere, J. H., Eds., Lea & Febiger, Philadelphia, 1992, chap. 10.
2. Seid, R. P., *Never Too Thin: Why Women Are at War with Their Bodies*, Prentice-Hall, New York, 1989.
3. Schur, E. M., *Labeling Women Deviant: Gender, Stigma and Social Control*, Random House, New York, 1984, 66.
4. Stone, G. P., Appearance and the self, in *Human Behavior and Social Processes*, Rose, G. P., Ed., Houghton Mifflin, Boston, 1962, 88.

5. Stone, G. P., Appearance and the self: a slightly revised version, in *Life as Theatre: A Dramaturgical Source Book*, Brissett, D. and Edgley, C., Eds., Aldine deGruyter, New York, 1990, 141.

6. Dorenkamp, A. G., McClymer, J. F., Moynihan, M. M., and Vadum, A. C., Eds., *Images of Women in American Popular Culture*, Harcourt Brace Jovanovich, New York, 1985, chap. 3.

7. Goffman, E., *Gender Advertisements*, Harper Colophon Books, New York, 1979.

8. Neimark, J., The beefcaking of America, *Psychol. Today*, 27, 32, 1994.

9. Pertschuk, M., Trisdorfer, A., and Allison, P. D., Men's bodies: the survey, *Psychol. Today*, 27, 35, 1994.

10. Wolf, N., *The Beauty Myth: How Images of Beauty Are Used Against Women*, Anchor Books, New York, 1992.

11. Silverstein, B., Perdue, L., Peterson, B., Vogel, L., and Fantini, D. A., Possible causes of the thin standard of bodily attractiveness for women, *Int. J. Eating Disorders*, 5, 135, 1986.

12. Silverstein, B., Peterson, B., and Perdue, L., Some correlates of the thin standard of bodily attractiveness in women, *Int. J. Eating Disorders*, 5, 145, 1986.

13. Tavris, C., *The Mismeasure of Woman*, Simon & Schuster, New York, 1992, chap. 1.

14. Garner, D., Garfinkle, P., Schwartz, D., and Thompson, M., Cultural expectations of thinness in women, *Psychol. Rep.*, 47, 483, 1980.

15. Silverstein, B., Carpman, S., Perlick, D., and Perdue, L., Nontraditional sex role aspirations, gender identity conflict and disordered eating among college women, *Sex Roles*, 23, 687, 1990.

16. Orbach, S., *Fat is a Feminist Issue*, Berkeley Books, New York, 1985.

17. Bennett, W. and Gurin, J., *The Dieter's Dilemma: Eating Less and Weighing More*, Basic Books, New York, 1982.

18. Stewart, A. L. and Brook, R. H., Effects of being overweight, *Am. J. Public Health*, 73, 171, 1983.

19. Millman, M., *Such a Pretty Face: Being Fat in America*, Norton, New York, 1980.

20. Richardson, S. A., Goodman, N., Hastorf, A. H., and Dornbush, S. M., Cultural uniformity in reaction to physical disabilities, *Am. Sociol. Rev.*, 26, 241, 1961.

21. Kalisch, B. J., The stigma of obesity, *Am. J. Nursing*, 72, 1124, 1972.

22. Mayer, J., Dwyer, J., and Feldman, J. J., The social psychology of dieting, *J. Health Soc. Behav.*, 11, 269, 1970.

23. Mellin, L. M. and Petitti, D. B., Chaotic family system associated with adolescent obesity, *Int. J. Obesity*, 11, A437, 1987.

24. Mellin, L. M., Irwin, C. E., Jr., and Scully, S., Prevalence of disordered eating in girls: A survey of middle–class children, *J. Am. Diet. Assoc.*, 92, 851, 1992.

25. Cohen L., Adler, N., and Irwin, C., Body figure preferences in male and female adolescents, *J. Abnorm. Psychol.*, 3, 276, 1987.

26. Maddox, G. L., Back, K. W., and Liederman, V., Overweight as social deviance and disability, *J. Health Soc. Behav.*, 9, 287, 1968.

27. DeJong, W., The stigma of obesity: the consequences of naive assumptions concerning the causes of physical deviance, *J. Health Soc. Behav.*, 21, 75, 1980.

28. Clinard, M. B. and Meier, R. F., *Sociology of Deviant Behavior*, Harcourt Brace Jovanovich, New York, 1992, 436.

29. Brackney, B., The psychology of female adolescence: identity and conflict, in *The American Woman: Her Past, Her Present, Her Future*, Richmond-Abbott, M., Ed., Holt, Rinehart & Winston, New York, 1979, chap. 6.

30. Cooley, C. H., *Social Organization*, Schocken Books, New York, 1962.

31. Body image and weight control, *Diet. Curr.*, 20, 1, 1993.

32. Fisher, S., *Development and Structure of the Body Image*, Vol. 1, Lawrence, Hillsdale, NJ, 1986.

33. Donovan, M. E. and Sanford, L. T., The elements of self-esteem, in *Every Woman's Emotional Well-Being*, Tavris, C., Ed., Prentice-Hall, New York, 1986, 33.

34. Orenstein, P., *Schoolgirls: Young Women, Self–Esteem, and the Confidence Gap*, Doubleday, New York, 1994.

35. Adams, G. R., Physical attractiveness research, *Hum. Dev.*, 20, 217, 1977.

36. Story, I., Factors associated with more positive body self- concepts in pre-school children, *J. Soc. Psychol.*, 108, 49, 1979.

37. Lerner, R. M. and Karabenick, S. A., Physical attractiveness, body attitudes, and self-concept in late adolescents, *J. Youth Adolesc.*, 3, 307, 1974.

38. Simmons, R. G. and Rosenberg, F., Sex, sex roles and self image, *J. Youth Adolesc.*, 4, 229, 1975.

39. Marino, D. D. and King, J. C., Nutritional concerns during adolescence, *Pediatr. Clin. North Am.*, 27, 125, 1980.

40. Beller, A. S., *Fat and Thin: A Natural History of Obesity*, Farrar, Straus and Giroux, New York, 1977.

41. Tanner, J. M., Sequence and tempo in the somatic changes in puberty, in *Control of the Onset of Puberty*, Grumbach, M. M., Grave, G. D., and Mayer, F. E., Eds., John Wiley & Sons, New York, 1974, 100.

42. Faust, M. S., Alternative constructions of adolescent growth, in *Girls at Puberty*, Brooks-Gunn, J. and Petersen, A. C., Eds., Plenum Press, New York, 1983, 105.

43. Nichter M. and Parker, P., cited in Body image: white weight, *Psychol. Today*, September/October 27, 9, 1994.

44. Tobin-Richards, M. H., Boxer, A. M., and Petersen, A. C., The psychological significance of pubertal change: sex differences in perceptions of self during early adolescence, in *Girls at Puberty*, Brooks-Gunn, J. and Petersen, A. C., Eds., Plenum Press, New York, 1983, 127.

45. Drewnowski, A. and Yee, D. K., Adolescent dieting: fear of fatness and the role of puberty, presented at the annual meeting of the American Psychological Association, Atlanta, 1988, 1.

46. Young, C. M., Blondin, J., Tensuan, R., and Freyer, J. H., Body composition studies of "older" women, thirty-seven years of age, *Ann. N.Y. Acad. Sci.*, 110, 589, 1963.

47. Young, C. M., Martin, M. E. K., Chihan, M., and McCarthy, M., Body composition of young women: some preliminary findings, *J. Am. Diet. Assoc.*, 38, 332, 1961.

48. Forbes, G. and Reina, J. C., Adult lean body mass declines with age: some longitudinal observations, *Metabolism*, 19, 653, 1970.

49. Wessel, J. A., Ufer, A., Van Huss, W. D., and Cederquist, D., Age trends of various components of body composition and functional characteristics for women aged 20–69 years, *Ann. N.Y. Acad. Sci.*, 110, 608, 1963.

50. Brownmiller, S., *Femininity*, Fawcett Columbine, New York, 1985, 21.

51. Chernin, K., *The Hungry Self: Women, Eating and Identity*, Harper & Row, New York, 1985.

52. Attie, I. and Brooks-Gunn, J., Weight concerns as chronic stressors in women, in *Gender and Stress*, Barnett, R. C., Biener, L., and Baruch, G. K., Eds., Free Press, New York, 1987, 237.

53. Wooley, O. W. and Wooley, S. W., Feeling fat in a thin society: 33,000 women tell how they really feel about their bodies, *Glamour*, 198, 251, February 1994.

54. Fallon, P., Katzman, M. A., and Wooley, S. C., Eds., *Feminist Perspectives on Eating Disorders*, Guilford, New York, 1993.

55. Tuschl, R., Platte, P., Laessle, R., Stichler, W., and Pirke, K., Energy expenditure and everyday eating behavior in healthy young women, *Am. J. Clin. Nutr.*, 52, 81, 1990.

56. Tuschl, R., Laessle, R., Platte, P., and Pirke, K., Differences in food-choice frequencies in restrained and unrestrained eaters, *Appetite*, 14, 9, 1990.

57. Mortenson, G. M., Hoerr, S. L., and Garner, D. M., Predictors of body satisfaction in college women, *J. Am. Diet. Assoc.*, 93, 1037, 1993.

58. Rubin, L., cited in Chernin, K., *The Obsession: Reflections on the Tyranny of Slenderness*, Harper & Row, New York, 1981, 35.

59. Lakoff, R. and Scherr, R., *Face Value: The Politics of Beauty*, Routledge & Kegan Paul, London, 1984.
60. Haynes, G., Study shows men as unhappy as women about weight gain, *Lansing State J.*, January 18, 4B, 1988.
61. Schwartz, H., *Never Satisfied: A Cultural History of Diets, Fantasies, and Fat*, Free Press, New York, 1986.
62. Brumberg, J. J., *Fasting Girls: The Emergence of Anorexia Nervosa as a Modern Disease*, Harvard University Press, Cambridge, MA, 1988.
63. Striegel-Moore, R. H., Silberstein, L. R., and Rodin, J., Toward an understanding of risk factors for bulimia, *Am. Psychol.*, 41, 246, 1986.
64. Ross, C. E., Overweight and depression, *J. Health Soc. Behav.*, 35, 63, 1994.
65. Keys, A., Brozek, J., Henschel, A., Michelson, O., and Taylor, H. L., *The Biology of Human Starvation*, University of Minnesota Press, Minneapolis, 1950.
66. Bruch, H., *Eating Disorders*, Basic Books, New York, 1973, chap. 1 and 2.

Chapter 4

DIET AND OSTEOPOROSIS

John J. B. Anderson

CONTENTS

0-8493-8502-4/96/$0.00+$.50
© 1996 by CRC Press, Inc.

I. INTRODUCTION

The relationships among several nutrients and bone mass, as measured by modern instruments, have been evolving over recent decades so that scientists can make reasonable estimates of the amounts of nutrients needed to meet the requirements for developing and maintaining bone tissues. The optimal amounts of many nutrients needed by bone tissues during the life cycle, however, have not yet been established. This chapter will focus on research findings bearing on the nutrient-bone relationships of women beyond menopause, including the elderly period of life, i. e., 60 years of age and older. Fracture end points, such as of the hip, are commonly used to serve as surrogate measures of osteoporosis.

Because bone tissue and the cells that make it and degrade it are so inextricably linked to nutrition, some background information on bone physiology and biochemistry is necessary. First, a few basic definitions of terms pertinent to bone are given and then descriptions of bone development and turnover are provided. Then, bone changes throughout the life cycle are reviewed, and finally nutrient and other risk factors for osteoporosis are highlighted. Although hereditary contributions to bone are considered to be greater during the developmental years, they continue to remain important into late life.[1]

II. DEFINITIONS

This section gives several defintions of terms related to bone and bone changes across the life cycle.

bone—a mineralized tissue containing an organic matrix (osteoid) which mineralizes and forms hydroxyapatite crystals
   bone as a tissue—mature bone tissue exists as cancellous (trabecular) tissue and cortical (compact) tissue in the *same* bone
   bone as an organ—individual bones such as the femur and a single vertebra in the spinal column make up the skeleton

bone modeling—the building of bone from a genetic program; osteoblasts which form bone dominate over osteoclasts which degrade bone

bone remodeling—the restructuring of bone after the cessation of growth and throughout adulthood; the normal sequence is first activation of the osteoclasts which degrade bone and then osteoblasts attempt to form new bone and in so doing replace the bone lost during degradation; in older individuals the amount of bone formed is *not* enough to replace the amount lost, which results in a net decrement of bone mass

bone turnover—the degrading and building of bone tissue; the rates of these two processes vary at different stages of the life cycle, being higher during the early growth phases and in the early postmenopausal years and low during late life

fracture—the actual fracture of a bone by external forces

    minimal trauma (fragility) fracture—fracture which occurs as a result of minor trauma, such as falling, coughing, or other activities of daily living

    traumatic fracture—fracture which results from a large force (strain) such as being thrown by a horse, being in an auto accident, or other high-impact collisions

osteopenia—low bone mass; similar in meaning to osteoporosis, but not specific

osteoporosis—low bone mass at 2.5 standard deviations below the mean values for young healthy adults,[3] plus poor bone quality at the microscopic level

    primary osteoporosis of type I and II—classes of osteoporosis related to low gonadal hormones (type I) and late life (type II)

    secondary osteoporosis—associated with drug therapy or another disease

    idiopathic osteoporosis—osteoporosis of unknown etiology

peak bone mass (PBM)—the greatest amount of bone at any time of life, typically accrued by 30 years of age or thereafter

III. EPIDEMIOLOGY OF OSTEOPOROSIS

The bone sites which most commonly fracture include the wrists (Colles' fractures of the radius and ulna), the lumbar spine (vertebrae), the ribs, and the hips (proximal femur), but practically any skeletal site can fracture as a result of low bone mass and poor bone quality at the microarchitectural level. For convenience, osteoporotic fractures have recently been classified according to the stage of the life cycle to which an individual belongs.[2] In addition, another class called idiopathic osteoporosis, or low bone mass and quality of unknown origin, exists, but the clinical nature of this class is beyond this review. The major types of osteoporosis are characterized in Table 1.

The major fracture which affects women so greatly in terms of morbidity and mortality is that of the hip. Fractures of the vertebrae may be symptomatic,

TABLE 1
Major Types of Osteoporosis

	Type I	Type II
Period	Postmenopausal	Senescent or senile
Gender	Female[a]	Female and male
Bone tissue	Cancellous	Cortical and cancellous
Fractures	Vertebrae and wrist (proximal forearm)	Vertebrae, hips, and other sites
Etiology	Loss of estrogens (menopause[b])	Multiple factors, including aging

[a] Males with low gonadal hormones also suffer occasionally from this type.

[b] Natural or surgical menopause and amenorrhea from any cause contribute to low circulating estrogen concentrations in blood.

Modified from Riggs, B.L. and Melton, L. J., III, *N. Engl. J. Med.*, 314, 1676, 1986.)

i.e., produce pain and other effects, but typically they are not. Therefore, it is difficult to identify vertebral fractures from radiologic or other evidence. Most of this review will emphasize the devastating effects of hip fractures and an attempt will be made to provide support for the importance of primary prevention through healthy early-life behaviors. Information on the potential worldwide problem of the projected incidence rates of hip fractures in the next few generations has been published.[3,4]

The increasing incidence of hip fracture will make an already major public health problem more severe within the next 30 years. The lifetime risk for women to suffer a hip fracture is as high as 15%. Approximately 2.5 million hip fracture cases will occur annually by the year 2025 in the world compared to an annual rate of 800,000 today. The risk of a woman suffering a hip fracture is approximately twice that of a man. The longer the life expectancy, the more fractures will occur. The risk of hip fracture by a postmenopausal woman is doubled every 7 years as she grows older. The occurrence of a hip fracture in an individual also implies a substantial increase in mortality as well as morbidity.

The hospital-related costs for a hip fracture amount to $15,000 to 20,000 or more per patient per week, but rehabilitation and other related costs after the first 7 d postsurgical repair would be additional. Hospital discharges in the U.S.A. for fractures for patients 85 years and older rank second, only behind cardiovascular diseases. Therefore, projected costs for hip fractures will increase enormously over the next several decades as the elderly represent almost 25% of the total American population by 2030.

IV. BONE STRUCTURES AND MEASUREMENTS OF BONE MASS

Bone is a dynamic tissue, but with a slow turnover, and it is composed of two types of bone tissue, cancellous (trabecular) and cortical (compact). Individual bones are formed by a process called bone modeling, and each bone contains differing proportions of cancellous and cortical bone. For example, vertebral bones of the spinal column contain much higher amounts of cancellous bone tissue than other bones. Long bones, such as the femur, contain much more cancellous tissue at the ends, i. e., hips and knees, than in the shaft region. Cancellous bone typically is more metabolically active than cortical bone tissue, and therefore it turns over faster than cortical tissue. This fact takes on greater importance after menopause when the higher rates of resorption of bone tissue, especially of the vertebrae, the hips, and wrists, result in the loss of bone mass and set the stage for the development of osteoporosis.

The development of bones early in life is referred to as modeling. After skeletal growth (height) is completed by approximately 16 to 18 years in girls and 20 to 22 years in boys, modeling is also over and remodeling becomes the sole process through which bones change (see below). Modeling of the long bones of the limbs results from new cell formation at epiphyses and the subsequent formation of cartilage which is then replaced by bone (mineralized) tissue. Modeling is dominated by the formation of bone, even though some resorption of bone tissue within an individual bone must also occur to increase the length of bones and to give them the shape they need for the supporting and movement functions of the body. Thus, the normal sequence of bone activity during growth and development is first formation and then resorption.

Bone remodeling is the process through which bone is lost at any age, but primarily after skeletal growth (height) has been completed. In this process, bone resorption by osteoclasts precedes bone formation by osteoblasts, but the net effect is a loss of bone mass because osteoblasts in the elderly cannot form as much bone during each remodeling cycle as is removed by osteoclasts. The rates of bone loss vary during the last decades of life, according to the status of each woman. Table 2 provides estimates of relative gains of bone mass (mineral content) early in life and losses later in life by females.

The measurement of bone mineral content (BMC) and the estimation of bone mineral density (BMD) are commonly made today with a machine known as a dual-energy X-radiographic absorptiometer (DEXA). X-rays of two different energies are used to correct for soft tissues surrounding bone at different sites of the skeleton. With DEXA instruments, total-body bone mass (TBBM), hip mass, forearm mass, and vertebral mass measurements can be made. (Mass means BMC.) Other machines, such as single-photon absorptiometry (SPA), have previously been used to measure forearm and calcaneus bone mass. Because this instrument requires the use of a radioactive source with a relatively short life, the long-lasting X-ray machines have become dominant in clinical and research use and SPA instruments are seldom employed today.

TABLE 2
Bone Mass Accrual Early in Life and
Loss Later in Life: Females in
Developed Nations

Age (years)	Relative Gain (%)	Relative Loss (%)
0–8	45	—
8–16	45	—
17–30	10	—
30–50[a]	—	0–5
50–60	—	10–20[b]
60–80	—	20–30[c]
Totals	100%	30–55%

[a] Menopause is assumed to begin at approximately age 50, but some small amount of bone loss may occur in the decades prior to menopause.
[b] Bone loss related to type I osteoporosis.
[c] Bone loss related to type II osteoporosis.

V. NUTRIENT NEEDS AND BONE LOSS AFTER MENOPAUSE

Women require numerous nutrients to maintain their bone tissue, even after the beginning of the menopausal transition.

A. LOSS OF BONE MASS: EARLY POSTMENOPAUSE

The loss of bone mass during the early postmenopausal period is inevitable, as it results from a cessation of ovarian production of estrogens. This period of life is when type I osteoporosis occurs as a result of the loss of ovarian estrogens. Furthermore, this bone loss typically occurs during early postmenopause—a period lasting only 5 years or so—*despite* an adequate intake of calcium. Recent reports have shown selective skeletal benefits of calcium supplements beyond the first 5 years following menopause;[5] the nearly universal exception is that the vertebrae of early postmenopausal women do not respond to additional amounts of calcium as supplements. Several studies have clearly demonstrated that the effect of calcium alone on bone mass is not nearly as potent as that of estrogen during the first 5 years after menopause.

In general, women who achieved higher peak bone mass prior to menopause track at a higher level during the early postmenopausal period. The benefit to women who track at a higher level of bone mass through the first postmenopausal decade is that they reach the risk ranges for fractures, i.e., 2.5 standard deviations below the mean values for healthy young adults (20 to 29 years), at a considerably later time in life than those who enter menopause with low bone mass. Entry into the fracture risk range could be delayed by as much as a decade!

B. LOSS OF BONE MASS: SENESCENCE

Several investigators have shown the positive effect of calcium on bone mass in elderly female subjects who are at least a decade beyond menopause. The beneficial effect of calcium to women has been shown to be a significantly greater bone mass and density, and presumably a lower fracture rate, compared to low-calcium-consuming women. Still other investigators have supported the contention that an adequate long-term or lifetime calcium consumption from dairy products leads to greater bone mass in older women. Lactoovovegetarian Seventh-Day Adventist (SDA) women have not been shown, however, to have greater bone mass values than similarly aged omnivorous women.[6,7]

A 5-year prospective study of elderly Caucasian women between the ages of 76 and 81, on average, demonstrated that radial bone mass was lost over this half-decade period at a rate of almost 1% per year, much higher than anticipated, despite an adequate calcium intake of approximately 900 mg/d over the 5-year time frame.[8] It is noteworthy that the low-calcium consumers (650 mg/d or less) tracked below the high-calcium consumers (greater than 950 mg/d) in bone mass over the 5-year study. These results imply that the tracking phenomenon continues into late life for most women and that calcium intake remains an important contributor to bone mass, but they also suggest that the relatively calcium-independent occurrence of bone loss at this elderly age must be greatly affected by other determinants, such as ambulatory capacity, cognitive state, drug usage, and other physical, social, and psychological factors.

The bone mass of postmenopausal Boston women consuming very low amounts of calcium daily (400 to 500 mg) was shown to benefit from a 500-mg supplement each day over a 2-year period, as recently reported.[5] The usual diets of these women had been clearly deficient in calcium and, thus, their modest gain in bone mass of approximately 1% per year during their mid-60s indicates that women with poor calcium intakes can improve their bone mass and reduce their likelihood of fractures from this simple measure. Women with adequate calcium in their diets, on the other hand, are less likely to benefit from calcium supplementation. The reason for this diminishing return is that higher amounts of calcium in the diet already are at, or exceed, the threshold or saturation level for calcium absorption, and that very little additional calcium will be absorbed with additional consumption of calcium.[9] The increased quantities of calcium absorbed, however, are dependent on reasonably bioavailable food sources and supplements of calcium, as well as several physiological variables.[10]

In summary, many reports, especially over the past few years, provide strong evidence that intakes of dietary calcium at the adult RDA of 800 mg/d, or even somewhat higher amounts, exert a positive influence on bone mass in elderly women. It is presumed that adequate amounts of bone mass in elderly women help them maintain the microscopic architecture of cancellous bone tissue and help them resist fragility fractures, especially those of the hips. An additional important factor associated with the retention of bone mass, not previously discussed, and which may serve as a surrogate for physical activity integrated over a lifetime, is lean body mass. The maintenance of lean body mass goes hand-in-hand with the the retention of skeletal mass in the elderly.

VI. CALCIUM METABOLISM
AFTER MENOPAUSE

Calcium homeostasis is the maintenance of the blood calcium concentration at a set level through the actions of calcium-regulating hormones, especially parathyroid hormone (PTH) and the vitamin D hormone, 1,25-dihydroxyvitamin D. PTH is secreted by the parathyroid glands whenever the blood calcium ion concentration becomes lowered. This increase in circulating PTH results in several actions, including the removal of calcium ions (and phosphate ions) from the skeleton and the production of 1,25-dihydroxyvitamin D by the kidney. The result is a net loss of mineral (calcium) from the skeleton. If the diet does not provide enough calcium, too little calcium (quantity) will be absorbed even with the enhancement of calcium absorption through the intestinal action of 1,25-dihydroxyvitamin D. In postmenopausal women, the efficiency of calcium absorption is depressed because of the lack of ovarian estrogens (see below).

The generalization about the postmenopausal status of women, then, is that decay and inefficiency of the homeostatic mechanisms follow within a decade or so the loss of ovarian function, and without estrogen (or estrogen/gestagen) replacement therapy, postmenopausal women will soon have depressed calcium absorption, increased PTH-induced bone resorption, and a net rate of loss of bone mass throughout the skeleton. The trabecular tissue of vertebrae, the hips, the distal forearm (wrists), and other sites of the skeleton undergo relatively greater resorption than cortical tissue, and this decreases the strength of bone tissue at these specific skeletal sites, where fragility fractures are most likely to occur.

Elderly individuals have several changes in calcium metabolism which contribute to less efficient utilization of calcium, negative calcium balance, and continued loss of bone mass. These changes include a decline in intestinal calcium absorption, a tendency for PTH concentrations to increase with age, enhanced urinary losses of calcium, and reductions in bone formation. Each of these alterations alone, or combinations of them, can hasten the rate of bone loss, largely independent of other factors such as specific nutrients.

Gastrointestinal function declines in most elderly subjects, and in postmenopausal women this decline is thought to begin shortly after menopause. Part of the decrement in calcium absorption results from a reduction in gastric acid secretion,[11] i.e., hypochlorhydria, and part from the less efficient transport of calcium ions across the epithelial mucosa.[12-14] The latter decline may result from a poor vitamin D adaptation to low calcium intake[15] or from a partial intestinal cell inhibition to the action of the hormonal form of vitamin D in the elderly.[16]

PTH concentrations tend to be elevated in older subjects.[17-22] Most, but not all, investigators are in agreement on this point. In a study of 494 women, the PTH concentration increased significantly at age 65, at the same age when 1,25-dihydroxyvitamin D decreased significantly. In late postmenopausal women, PTH seems to be more effective than in premenopausal females in stimulating calcium transfer from bone to blood (extracellular fluid or ECF), whether the calcium ions are derived from bone resorption or from increased movement of ions from the bone fluid compartment across bone lining cells to the ECF. In part, the enhanced PTH effect is considered to result from the relative absence of circulating estrogens in elderly women and a decline in absorption associated not only with the loss of estrogens, but also with age.[22] A persistent elevation of circulating PTH means that bone is continuously lost during the period of elevation.

Renal reabsorption of calcium ions also declines in elderly individuals. In women, this decrement in reabsorptive efficiency may occur because of the loss of ovarian estrogen function, but other explanations might also be valid.[23] For all of these system decrements, males also suffer in their later years, but explanatory mechanisms are not readily available as they are, at least in part, for females. A common mechanism of bone loss may exist for both elderly females and males, but hard experimental or observational data to support any postulated mechanism remain sparse.

In summary, a reduction in the efficiency of either intestinal calcium absorption or renal calcium reabsorption will have an adverse effect on calcium balance. Persistent elevations of PTH contribute to net bone loss. Furthermore, if osteoblast function declines with age, then osteoclastic function will tend to be more effective and a net loss of bone will occur, as has been observed in numerous histomorphometric studies of bone tissue, despite a slowing of the rate of bone turnover. The overall decline in bone mass tends to parallel the negative calcium balance which has been found for postmenopausal women in numerous reports. Inadequate calcium intake among the elderly generally is not accompanied by an adequate adaptation involving the vitamin D system. Therefore, any compromise of this already maladapting mechanism for absorbing and perhaps conserving calcium among elderly individuals results in the availability of less calcium for bone formation. The loss of bone mass is a continuing consequence of this maladaptation, and of other age-related maladaptations, and continuing losses eventually will lead to fractures.

VII. DIETARY RISK FACTORS FOR OSTEOPOROSIS

Many nutrients are required for normal bone development and maintenance, both of the organic matrix and the mineral phase of dynamic bone tissues. Tissue growth and development clearly need energy from the macro-nutrients and protein to support these processes; micronutrients that impinge on growth processes are also needed, but the skeleton can grow and develop very well in terms of height (length) without adequate amounts of calcium in the diet. Protein and energy are essential for the production of the organic matrix, but the avidity of the newly formed skeleton is so great for mineral ions (calcium and inorganic phosphate) that even diets low in calcium will usually supply enough calcium to mineralize the skeleton minimally for its functional roles, if not enough for a skeleton that is to retain these functions to 85 years of age or even longer for an increasing number of women. There-fore, it is very important during the years of growth to have adequate amounts of calcium, phosphorus, and other micronutrients to support the optimal min-eralization of the organic matrix of bones.

In the following sections, each nutrient known to have an important role in the support of mineralized bone tissue is briefly reviewed.

A. CALCIUM

Despite the generally held hypothesis that osteoporosis is a calcium-defi-ciency disease,[23] the intake of calcium alone, in amounts much greater than the RDA for the elderly, i.e., 800 mg/d, does not appear to be sufficient to overcome the established osteopenia *and* continuing loss of bone mass in the elderly. Several investigators have made this finding in elderly women, and, because of the relative ineffectiveness of dietary or supplemental calcium by itself, other drug modalities, such as the combination of calcium and vitamin D or the use of bisphosphonates and other drugs, need to be considered in an effort to slow the rate of bone loss of elderly subjects, both female and male.[8,25]

Several supplement studies of elderly women using calcium alone have been published, but they have not shown much benefit in skeletal measure-ments beyond 1 year of therapy. Dawson-Hughes et al.[5] measured bone mass before and after administering calcium supplements to postmenopausal women living in the Boston area. Over a 2-year period of supplementation, subjects consuming lower amounts of calcium were found to show greater improve-ments in bone mass than those whose pre-study calcium intakes were more adequate. The studies employing both calcium and vitamin D, however, have also been successful in preserving bone mass and even in increasing it. The data of Chapuy and colleagues[24] provided strong support for the efficacy of this combination of nutrients as supplements for 18 months of use. The elderly women living in Lyons, France who received a combination supplement of calcium and vitamin D for 2 years had significantly lower nonvertebral fracture rates than placebo-controlled subjects.[24] (See also sections above for additional background on calcium and bone.)

B. PHOSPHORUS

Phosphorus intakes practically always exceed those of calcium because nearly all foods contain plentiful amounts of phosphorus, but only a few contain calcium. Phosphorus deficiency then is virtually impossible to occur in adults and the elderly. The major problem with phosphorus is that our diets contain too much of this element with respect to calcium. The best diets of Americans have ratios of calcium to phosphorus in the range of 0.70: 0.75 (without any calcium supplementation), but the dietary ratios of most adult and elderly women fall below 0.60, and for many the ratio is less than 0.5.[26] Phosphorus in foods is readily removed during digestion and phosphate ions are rapidly absorbed, unlike calcium ions which are slowly absorbed.[27] The absorbed phosphate ions have a prompt lowering action on calcium in blood, which in turn stimulates PTH secretion and elevation in blood.

The low calcium-to-phosphate ratios contribute to persistent elevations in PTH,[28] which acts on bone to remove calcium and thereby homeostatically adjusts upward the depressed serum calcium concentration. The consumption of foods which contain phosphate additives by many females in the U.S. population has been increasing in recent years.[29] This increment plus the behaviors of women who avoid or reduce the consumption of the recommended number (two or more) of servings of dairy products each day are considered to be important risk factors for low bone mass and subsequent osteoporotic fractures.

C. VITAMIN D

Large numbers of elderly residents in the northern parts of the U.S. and of Europe have been shown to have depressed circulating levels of 25-hydroxyvitamin D and, in some reports, also low serum concentrations of 1,25-dihydroxyvitamin D. Seasonal differences in 25-hydroxyvitamin D have become well established in several geographic regions of the Northern Hemisphere. (See Anderson and Toverud[30] for a review of this topic.) However, 1,25-dihydroxyvitamin D insufficiency, rather than a full-scale deficiency, has only recently been documented among elderly subjects.[24,31] Because of the increasing lifespans of so many elderly, especially women, and of residence of large numbers of the elderly in nursing homes or similar facilities which permit little exposure of residents to sunlight, insufficiency of vitamin D is likely to become more common and even possibly reach epidemic proportions. The public health consequences of compromised bone tissue, including osteoporosis mixed with osteomalacia in the same individuals, and increased fracture incidence could be enormous. Thus, questions have been raised about the adequacy of the current allowance of vitamin D, i.e., 200 IU/d, for the elderly. A number of reports have recommended between 500 and 800 IU of vitamin D per day for elderly individuals, especially those from northern latitudes.

A study of postmenopausal women living in England suggests that low serum 25-hydroxyvitamin D levels *per se* may have an effect on bone tissue independent of the hormonal form of this vitamin, i.e., 1,25-dihydroxyvitamin D.[32] Furthermore, this same report provided a hypothesis that a low circulating 25-hydroxyvitamin D level can be a major contributory factor to osteoporosis beginning in women as early as menopause and the early postmenopausal period, not just among the late elderly. This attractive idea that the low 25-hydroxyvitamin D blood concentrations are in some way linked to higher concentrations of PTH in blood is not, however, generally accepted.

A recent report from Finland, where wintertime deficiencies of vitamin D among the elderly become relatively severe, demonstrated that intramuscular vitamin D injections of single yearly doses of 150,000 to 300,000 IU of ergocalciferol (vitamin D_2) maintained serum levels of 25-hydroxyvitamin D within the normal range and reduced hip fracture incidence.[33] Wintertime supplementation of elderly women in the northern latitude of the U.S., in Boston, has also been shown to result in improved 25-hydroxyvitamin D blood levels during this part of the year.[34] Similar seasonal differences in vitamin D status and bone mineral density were made of women living in northern Maine.[35]

In summary, these reports highlight significant percentages of the elderly who are insufficient or truly deficient with respect to vitamin D status. The primary reasons for deficits in vitamin D status are insufficient exposures to ultraviolet light for skin biosynthesis of the vitamin and limited intakes of vitamin D from foods, mainly fortified dairy products and fish. Supplementation of elderly individuals with vitamin D *and* calcium, at least in the winter and spring months, appears to be a practical solution to the problem of vitamin D deficiency or insufficiency among the elderly living at high latitudes in either hemisphere.

D. VITAMIN K

A new role of vitamin K has been recently discovered. Vitamin K has been demonstrated to be required for the synthesis of a bone extracellular protein known as osteocalcin or bone GLA-protein. (The GLA signifies glutamic acid residues, which are abundant in these vitamin K-dependent proteins.) This protein has similar calcium-binding GLA groups as prothrombin. It is speculated that osteocalcin may be involved in the initial step of mineralization of the collagen matrix of bone, but not of collagen in other connective tissues of the body. Osteocalcin is produced by osteoblasts in bone tissues, but not by fibroblasts or other cells in connective tissues other than bone. The synthesis of two additional bone matrix proteins also appears to be dependent on the availability of vitamin K.

Elderly subjects have been shown by different investigators to be low in vitamin K in both the diet and blood. In addition, osteocalcin is reduced in its carboxylation under conditions of vitamin K deficiency. Two reports have shown that elderly patients, especially those living in nursing homes and related institutions, have undercarboxylated levels of osteocalcin in circulating blood.[36,37] Furthermore, vitamin K replacement of elderly subjects resulted in higher carboxylation of circulating osteocalcin.[36] Vitamin K deficiency may also be associated with a deficiency of vitamin D, and therefore vitamin K deficiency is linked to osteoporosis and fractures by complex mechanisms operating in osteoblasts. In a multicenter supplement study of elderly Japanese women with 1α-hydroxyvitamin D, bone mass was shown to be increased after 24 or 48 weeks of vitamin K therapy.[38] Finally, a study of dialysis patients who had higher vitamin K status demonstrated that they also had fewer fractures compared to dialysis patients with low vitamin K status.[39] Thus, it appears that vitamin K nutriture remains important for bone health throughout life.

E. MAGNESIUM

The literature on the association of magnesium and bone mass is extremely limited. Only one prospective human trial involving magnesium supplementation has been conducted, and the results from this Israeli study are inconclusive.[40] Clearly, the magnesium-calcium-bone triad needs greater investigation. Some researchers have suggested that high intakes of calcium from supplements may inhibit or otherwise interfere with magnesium absorption, and thereby have an adverse effect on the function of magnesium in bone and other tissues. This idea has not yet been validated experimentally in humans. The ratio of calcium to magnesium in typical American diets ranges between 3:1 and 4:1, but some investigators suggest that the optimal dietary ratio should be closer to 2:1. Further long-term data are also needed in this area.

F. PROTEIN

A review of almost all studies of the effect of dietary protein on urinary calcium losses by Kerstetter and Allen[41] demonstrated that protein increases urinary calcium losses. The calciuretic effect is both acute and, if dietary practices are persistent, also chronic. Mechanistic explanations have not been satisfactory for the protein-induced hypercalciuria, but at least one report suggests that part of the explanation may relate to elevated glucagon levels induced by the absorbed load of amino acids.[42] If urinary calcium losses are chronic, bone losses would also follow. Therefore, a high protein dietary pattern would place postmenopausal women who typically have low calcium intakes at increased risk for osteoporosis.

A well-established risk factor of high animal protein consumption is the generation of excess hydrogen ions (acid) and thereby extra work for the kidneys to remove these ions in order to defend against pH lowering. The urinary pH of meat-eating omnivores are significantly lower than the pH of strict vegetarians which often are in the alkaline range. Within reasonable limits of protein intake, however, the renal and other organ adjustments to the increased hydrogen ions are sufficient to minimize the losses of calcium in the urine of meat-eaters. This conclusion is not entirely based on hard data, but the studies of lactoovovegetarians (LOVs) by Tylavsky et al.[6] and Hunt et al.[7] suggest that the measurements of BMC and BMD of elderly LOVs are not different from those of omnivorous women. In these studies, dietary protein had a positive effect on bone mass.

G. SODIUM

Sodium intake has been known for several decades to influence urinary calcium excretion. Typically high sodium intakes lead to increased urinary calcium losses, and persistent net losses of urinary calcium must ultimately be derived from the skeleton. Therefore, bone losses over extended periods of high sodium intakes could contribute to osteoporosis and fractures. Data obtained from postmenopausal women placed on a high sodium diet not only increased their urinary calcium/creatinine ratio, but also their urinary ratio of hydroxyproline/creatinine.[43] The greatest effect of sodium on urinary calcium losses has been shown to occur when calcium intakes are low, the typical situation among elderly women. Elevations in PTH and 1,25-dihydroxyvitamin D most likely accompany the sodium-induced renal losses of calcium, although this point is not yet settled. Salt restriction would, nevertheless, seem to be a logical recommendation to delay or prevent bone loss, especially among low-calcium consuming postmenopausal women.

H. FLUORIDE

At reasonable intake levels (1 ppm or somewhat higher) fluoride ions consumed in drinking water or via other sources in the diet or from consumer tooth-protective products can have positive effects on developing bone tissue (and tooth enamel) by increasing the surface hardness of the crystals in the mineral phase of the skeleton. Too much fluoride, however, can actually make the crystals more fracture-prone because of their strong chemical properties and reduce bone strength, as has been demonstrated in supplementation trials of osteoporotic patients.[44] Therefore, a narrow window exists in which fluoride ions can benefit mineralized tissues, i.e., bones and teeth. High consumption of fluoride also has adverse effects on GI function in addition to *increasing* fractures.[45]

I. OTHER MICRONUTRIENTS

A few additional trace elements and vitamins also play important roles in bone tissue, especially in relation to the activities of bone cells, e.g., formation of the matrix proteins, such as collagen.

Several other trace elements, including iron, copper, manganese, zinc, and boron, may have important roles in bone metabolism, but human experimental evidence is not sufficient to conclude that dietary deficits of these elements are so critical to bone health. One report suggests that supplementation with combinations of several of these micronutients (zinc, copper, and manganese) along with calcium (1000 mg/d) may improve spinal bone mass in postmenopausal women, compared to women who received either the trace elements or calcium alone, or placebo.[46] All three of the other groups lost spinal bone density over the 2-year trial. Little data exist on the relationships of single trace elements alone and bone mass. Therefore, it presently is not possible to make dietary micronutrient recommendations with respect to optimizing bone mass.

Iron is essential for the enzymatic posttranslational conversion of proline and lysine residues to hydroxyproline and hydroxylysine in newly formed collagen prior to secretion by osteoblasts into extracellular fluids of the nascent bone matrix. Vitamin C is also required in these same reaction steps.

Several other vitamins, notably vitamin B_6, vitamin A, folate, and vitamin B_{12}, and possibly β-carotene, also have critical roles in the metabolism of bone tissue, especially in the activities of osteoblasts that produce the organic matrix and of osteoclasts which initiate bone resorption. Relatively little is known of the direct or indirect roles of these vitamins, and the dietary amounts needed for optimal bone health are only estimated. Limited intakes of fruits and vegetables by the elderly in national food surveys suggest, however, that this segment of the population may be much more likely to have deficiencies of several micronutrients which have important roles in bone metabolism.

J. DIETARY FIBER AND OTHER NONNUTRIENT COMPONENTS OF PLANT FOODS

The effect of dietary fiber with respect to bone tissue is generally neutral. A few studies have shown significant negative effects of fiber on intestinal calcium absorption because of reduced bioavailability of calcium ions in the luminal milieu of the gut, but no long-term study has found an adverse effect of high fiber vegetarian diets on measurements of bone mass. One study of late adolescent girls (18 to 20 years) suggested that high fiber intakes led to later age of menarche, lower body weights, lower circulating estrogens, and lower bone densities at several sites.[47] Dietary fiber intakes at the recommended levels of 20 to 30 g/d, which few Americans obtain, are not likely, however, to have an adverse influence on bone mass of women during the later years of life, since bone development and growth have long been completed.

Several other molecules found in plant foods have been suggested to influence calcium metabolism or bone tissue and, hence, bone mass. It appears that sufficient amounts of these molecules are ingested by some consumers to be of concern to toxicologists. These phyto-molecules include phytoestrogens, oxalates, molecules found in caffeine/tea, and many others. Except for oxalates, little knowledge exists about these 10,000 or more natural chemicals produced by diverse species of the plant kingdom. Oxalates in spinach and rhubarb have been shown to substantially reduce calcium absorption because of their chelation or tight binding of calcium ions within the gut lumen.[48] The effects of phytoestrogens on bone cells are presently being investigated in a number of laboratories. Phytoestrogens, such as genistein, have weak agonistic effects on osteoblasts or related cells studied in tissue culture and thereby they may help to retain bone mass, somewhat like estrogenic molecules such as estradiol do. Understandings of the mechanisms of phytoestrogens and other phytomolecules on bone tissue are just beginning to unfold.[49] This area of investigation is potentially enormous and largely uncharted.

K. SUMMARY

Several nutrients considered critical for bone development and maintenance are calcium, phosphorus, and vitamin D. Vitamin K may also fall in this critical category, but more information is needed before this classification can be made. These nutrients need to be provided in optimal, but not excessive, amounts for bone health. The role of magnesium in bone tissue, though essential, has not yet been resolved. Protein and energy are nutrient variables that are absolutely essential for optimal skeletal development, but not for BMC. In addition, several other nutrients and a few nonnutrients may also be important and essential for bone, but not critical because deficiencies of these nutrients have typically relatively minor effects on bone. Finally, a few nutrients in excessive intakes can have severe deleterious effects on bone tissue; these include phosphorus, protein, vitamin D, sodium, and fluoride. Little is known of the influences on bone of non-nutrient components derived from plant sources, but phytoestrogens, such as genistein, are receiving interest by researchers because of their potential for preventing bone loss, without having adverse effects on breast and other reproductive tissues of women.

VIII. NONDIETARY RISK FACTORS FOR OSTEOPOROSIS

Several other nonnutritional risk factors considered important for osteoporosis include inheritance of bone tissue, hormonal influences on bone and other organs involved in calcium metabolism, and body size or mass, especially of the lean and fat compartment in addition to the bone compartment. A strong association exists between the lean body mass and skeletal mass in both males and females. Because females develop less bone mass *and* less muscle mass, the major contributor to lean body mass, they are typically at increased risk for fractures, especially of the hips, at the conclusion of the early life growth and consolidation phases of skeletal development, i.e., at age 30 to 35. Hereditary factors, as expressed through familial and racial/ethnic contributions, are most powerful early in life, perhaps contributing as much as 70 to 80% of the early life development compared to 20 to 30% for environmental determinants.[1] After menopause, however, environmental factors become more important and they contribute as much as 50 to 60% to the variability in bone mass of postmenopausal women. This section highlights a few of the nondietary risk factors that affect bone mass and density in late life.

The nondietary risk factors for osteoporosis are given in Table 3.

A. PHYSICAL INACTIVITY

Results of well-designed prospective trials involving regular exercises or upper-body strength activities in early postmenopausal women are typically supportive of a retention of bone mass. The effects of these exercise/strength factors only last, however, as long as the subjects continue to practice them. What has been disappointing has been the observation that the gains in bone

TABLE 3
Non-dietary Adverse Risk Factors for Osteoporosis

Risk Factor	Explanation
Hereditary	Family history, and race/ethnicity; whites and Asians are at increased risk compared to blacks; low bone mass runs in families
Hormonal status	Loss of estrogens or androgens contributes to loss of bone mass in the later years of life in both sexes
Thinness/low fat mass	Fat tissues, especially those of the buttocks, serve as protectors in falls, and in females the fat tissue can produce estrogens by peripheral conversion of adrenal androgens
Physical inactivity	Lifestyle of regular activities, such as carrying, lifting, and walking up stairs, is beneficial
Immobility	Extended bed rest, casting, and outer-space living (astronauts) contribute to bone loss
Cigarette smoking	Excessive smoking is an adverse factor, often coupled with excessive alcohol consumption
Alcohol	Excessive alcohol is deleterious for several reasons, including the increased risk of falling
OTC drugs	A number of OTC drugs adversely affect calcium or bone metabolism
Prescription Drugs	Several drugs, such as corticosteroids and anticonvulsants, can contribute to bone loss
Falls	Loss of balance from drugs, or unsafe living conditions can lead to fractures of the hips

mass quickly decay with disuse.[50] The obvious conclusion, then, is that regular activities need to be built into everyday living patterns in order to provide routinely the loads (strains) on the skeleton. These loads have to operate periodically in order to provide benefit to skeletal tissue. It is generally thought that people living in mountainous regions of the world maintain their bone mass better than in more level areas because of their hill-climbing with loads on practically a daily basis. Much more research is needed in this area of investigation because of the potential benefits of exercise in the preservation of the skeleton and in the potential for the prevention of osteoporosis, especially hip fractures.[51]

B. IMMOBILITY

Elderly individuals who can no longer ambulate without the use of mechanical aids are at increased risk for lower bone mass, greater fragility of bone tissue, and osteoporotic fractures.[8,52] Canes, crutches, wheelchairs, and other devices reduce the musculoskeletal strength of individuals and place them at greater risk of fracture from minimal trauma or other factors of daily living, such as coughing or shifting weight to another position. Space flights of astronauts or cosmonauts have demonstrated that large amounts of bone mass are lost when flights last longer than a few days. Weightlessness or near-zero gravity has severe deleterious effects on bone, and bedrest has similar though less devastating effects.

C. CIGARETTE SMOKING

Cigarette smoking has both direct adverse effects on skeletal tissues and negative indirect effects operating through suppression of food intake and the less-than-optimal nutritional intakes of heavy smokers. Reports on the adverse influence on bone of cigarette-smoking women have shown that the magnitude of the effects on bone mass is typically small, though significant.[53]

D. ALCOHOL CONSUMPTION

Excessive intake of ethanol (alcohol) in any type of beverage can be harmful to the skeleton, but moderate intake patterns (two or fewer drinks per day) apparently have little or no effect on the skeleton. (Alcohol is not considered a nutrient in this context because it has adverse effects on health, in general, and it is therefore a potentially modifiable nonnutrient life-style factor.) Because alcohol metabolism generates hydrogen ions and because bone tissue serves as an enormous buffer for these ions, bone degradation can be increased by repetitive acid-generating alcohol loads. Alcohol, which probably directly affects bone tissue, has an adverse effect on BMC and BMD when consumed in high amounts.[53]

E. OVER-THE-COUNTER DRUGS

The adverse effects of over-the-counter (OTC) drugs on bone tissue, either through direct or indirect mechanisms, have basically been ignored by researchers. Many cases of adverse drug effects, however, have been reported in the literature. Many of these reports relate more to drug-drug interactions or to drug-nutrient interactions than to damaging effects on skeletal tissues per se. With so many elderly using polypharmacy or multiple drugs, including prescription medications, these adverse interactions or effects need to be monitored more closely. For example, common laxatives taken chronically by elderly women can cause damage to the lining mucosa of the small intestine and reduce intestinal calcium absorption. Mineral oil laxatives can reduce the absorption of vitamin D, vitamin K, and other fat-soluble vitamins (see Table 4). Other examples could be given, but the point is that OTC drugs should be more closely inspected as potential contributors to low bone mass, osteomalacia, osteoporosis, and fractures.

In addition, any drugs that have appetite-suppressive actions place the elderly at increased risk of getting sufficient amounts of micronutrients accompanying their calories from the macronutrients, without supplementation. Drugs that unfavorably affect balance or equilibrium can also have additional adverse effects because of the greater likelihood of falling by elderly women (see Section VIII.G).

F. PRESCRIPTION DRUGS

Much of what was stated above about OTC drugs also applies to prescription drugs, except that prescription drugs are much more closely monitored by the medical profession for adverse effects. Classic examples of medications that adversely affect bone tissue are high doses of corticosteroids (glucocorticoids), anticonvulsant drugs, and diuretics. Corticosteroids damage bone directly through effects on bone cells and indirectly via actions on the vessels (vascular tissue) supplying bone tissue with nutrients and oxygen. This damage, i.e., low bone mass and often osteoporosis, can occur even with increased intakes of calcium and vitamin D during the period of medication.[54,55] Another example is that of anticonvulsant drugs, such as phenobarbital, which stimulate hepatic microsomal enzymes to degrade not only the drug, but also vitamin D and its metabolites.[56] Therefore, deficient amounts of 25-hydroxyvitamin D are made and hence the hormonal form, 1,25-dihydroxyvitamin D, is not sufficiently available for enhancing intestinal calcium absorption and osteoblastic bone-forming activity, both of which also tend to be depressed in the elderly. Finally, diuretics can lead to hypercalciuria as well as losses of other divalent cations. Numerous drugs can increase calcium losses and contribute to secondary osteoporosis; several of these are listed in Table 4.

TABLE 4
Commonly Used Drugs Related to Secondary
Osteoporosis: Prescription and OTC

Class	Examples
Prescription:	
Anticonvulsants	Phenytoin (Dilantin), phenobarbital, barbiturates
Corticosteroids	Prednisone
Diuretics	Furosemide, ethacrynic acid
Sedatives	Glutethimide
Thyroid hormone	Levo-thyroxine
OTC	
Laxatives	Mineral oil

G. FALLS

Any of the factors listed above may contribute to falling in the later years of life. Cummings and colleagues[57] have recently reported on the relative contributions of numerous lifestyle factors to falls. The avoidance of falls among the elderly has become increasingly important because of the high probability that a fall will result in the fracture of a hip or other bone. Therefore, any strategy that can reduce the possibility of falls will have an enormous impact on fracture reduction.

H. SUMMARY

The nonnutrient risk factors that are part of the lifestyle of individuals become increasingly important late in life when the impact of hereditary contribution to bone mass declines. The increased disease morbidity during the senescent period of life reflects on the loss of lean body mass, especially muscle tissue and strength, and thereby the loss of basal metabolism (or resting energy expenditure). When both lean body mass and metabolism decline in concert, bone mass also declines, but more slowly. It is at this stage, too often, that fractures are waiting to happen, because of little protection of bone tissue by fat in the buttocks when falls occur, and of the increasingly fragile bone tissues of the hips, wrists, ribs, upper arms, and vertebrae in late life.

IX. SECONDARY PREVENTION/TREATMENT OF OSTEOPOROSIS

The benefits and potential disadvantages of improved dietary intakes and/or nutritional supplements to postmenopausal women are minimal — really quite small — compared to the benefits from estrogens and the newer bisphosphonate drugs in preserving bone mass and density (only supplements of calcium and vitamin D in combination have been used with substantially positive results so far). None of these drugs increases bone mass, but they do have potent effects on retaining or conserving bone tissue, and therefore they can prevent osteoporotic fractures as long as they are taken.

A. DIET AND/OR SUPPLEMENTS

The investigation of Chapuy et al.[24] provided strong support for the simple use of supplements of calcium (1200 mg/d as calcium phosphate), and vitamin D (800 IU/d) to prevent or delay hip and other nonvertebral fractures in elderly French women living in and around Lyons. In addition, mean measurements of bone mass and density of these women increased slightly during the 18-month treatment period compared to women given placebos. A few other studies have provided support for the French study, but additional prospective trials are needed to demonstrate the effectiveness of simple dietary measures for the secondary prevention of hip fractures. Bone loss by postmenopausal women can also be partially prevented by calcium supplements coupled with estrogen therapy.[58]

B. DRUGS

Many drugs have been investigated in attempts to conserve or even improve bone mass. Some success has been achieved with estrogens, but estrogens have lost favor because of concerns about cancers in the reproductive organs of postmenopausal women. The newer third-generation bisphosphonate drugs hold promise because of relatively minor side effects, at far as is known at this time, and good efficacy on skeletal tissue retention.[59] The trials on a few of these drugs have been completed or are nearly done, and one or more drugs will be approved soon by the FDA for use in treating osteoporotic patients.

Other drugs, such as fluorides and parathyroid hormone, may also prove beneficial to bone mass conservation, but practical applications of these drugs are not yet available. Fluorides (see also above) act on osteoblasts directly to improve bone mass, and therefore if they could be given in doses that did not yield adverse side effects, they could stimulate bone formation, which the above-mentioned drugs cannot do. Parathyroid hormone also acts on osteoblasts to generate new bone mass when administered in an intermittent fashion, but not in a continuous way. Continuous administration of PTH causes tremendous osteoclastic activity and bone destruction, but with intermittent delivery PTH increases bone formation.

Because so many numbers of postmenopausal women are surviving into their 80s and 90s now, the emphasis on drug discovery to preserve bone mass by the pharmaceutical industry will likely continue.

X. CONCLUDING REMARKS

In spite of the existence of reasonable scientific evidence of appropriate means to prevent or delay osteoporotic hip fractures, the most devastating of all the fractures, this information has not been adequately put into action by any society. Furthermore, national health services administrators have not yet begun to appreciate the enormity of the problem of hip fractures over the next several decades. Although hospital repair and treatment of hip fracture patients are good, rehabilitative services are currently not adequate and nursing home beds and facilities also are not sufficient for the projected needs early in the 21st century. Preventive strategies for the reduction of hip fractures, including dietary changes and moderate lifestyle modifications, are available for application at the present time,[60] but no major national effort has been mounted nor has planning for preventive approaches been initiated. Since osteoporosis is a multifactorial disease, various approaches must also be taken in order to try to lessen the consequences of the disease.

Recommendations of nutrient intakes by women over the period from menopause to late life are given in Table 5 along with the current RDAs.[61] These guidelines are subject to change as new information becomes available. A good diet, in general, with optimal amounts of calcium and these other nutrients supports good bone health, whereas typically low-calcium diets are associated with less than optimal intakes of most micronutrients.[62] Other life-style factors, in addition to nutritional ones, must also be considered when assessing the potentially modifiable contributors to bone health and osteoporosis.

TABLE 5
Recommended Nutrient Intakes for Postmenopausal Women Compared to the Current RDAs (1989)[61]

Nutrient	Recommendation	RDA (1989)
Calcium	800–1000 mg/d	800 mg/d
Phosphorus	None	800 mg/d
Vitamin D	600–800 IU/d	200 IU/d
	(15–20 μg/d)	(5 μg/d)
Vitamin K	>100 μg/d	65 μg/d
Magnesium	350–400 mg/d	280 mg/d

Note: RDAs are from the Recommended Dietary Allowances, 1989.[61]

REFERENCES

1. Pollitzer, W. A. and Anderson, J. J. B., Ethnic and genetic differences in bone mass: a review with an hereditary vs. environmental perspective, *Am. J. Clin. Nutr.*, 50, 1244, 1989.
2. Riggs, B. L. and Melton, L. J., III, Involutional osteoporosis, *N. Engl. J. Med.*, 314, 1676, 1986.
3. WHO Technical Report Series No. 843, *Assessment of Fracture Risk and Its Application to Screening for Postmenopausal Osteoporosis*, report of a World Health Organization Study Group, World Health Organization, Geneva, 1994.
4. Melton, L. J., III, Hip fractures: a world-wide problem today and tomorrow, *Bone*, 14(Suppl. 1), S1, 1993.
5. Dawson-Hughes, B., Dallal, G. E., Krall, E. A., Sadowski, L., Sahyoun, N., and Tannenbaum, S., A controlled trial of the effect of calcium supplementation on bone density in postmenopausal women, *N. Engl. J. Med.*, 323, 878, 1990.
6. Tylavsky, F. A. and Anderson, J. J. B., Dietary factors in bone health of elderly lactoovovegetarian and omnivorous women, *Am. J. Clin. Nutr.*, 48, 842, 1988.
7. Hunt, I. F., Murphy, M. J., Henderson, C., Clark, V. A., Jacobs, R. M., Johnson, P. K., and Coulston, A. H., Bone mineral content in postmenopausal women: comparison of omnivores and vegetarians, *Am. J. Clin. Nutr.*, 50, 517, 1989.
8. Reed, J. A., Anderson, J. J. B., Tylavsky, F. A., and Gallagher, P. N., Jr., Comparative changes of radial bone density of elderly female lactoovovegetarians and omnivores, *Am. J. Clin. Nutr.*, 59 (Suppl.), 1197s, 1994.
9. Wilkinson, R., Absorption of calcium, phosphorus and magnesium, in *Calcium, Phosphorus and Magnesium Metabolism*, Nordin, B. E. C., Ed., Churchill Livingstone, Edinburgh, 1976, 36.
10. Heaney, R. P., Recker, R. R., Stegman, M. R., and Moy, A. J., Calcium absorption in women: relationships to calcium intake, estrogen status, and age, *J. Bone Miner. Res.*, 4, 469, 1989.
11. Recker, R. R., Calcium absorption and achlorhydria, *N. Engl. J. Med.*, 313, 70, 1985.

12. Avioli, L. V., McDonald, J. E., and Lee, S. W., The influence of age on the intestinal absorption of ^{47}Ca in women and its relation to ^{47}Ca absorption in postmenopausal osteoporosis, *J. Clin. Invest.*, 44, 1960, 1965.

13. Bullamore, J. R., Wilkinson, R., Gallagher, J. C., Nordin, B. E. C., and Marshall, D. H., Effect of age on calcium absorption, *Lancet*, 2, 535, 1970.

14. Gallagher, J. C., Riggs, B. L., Eisman, J., Hamstra, A., Arnaud, S. B., and DeLuca, H. F., Intestinal absorption and vitamin D metabolites in normal subjects and osteoporotic patients: effect of age and dietary calcium, *J. Clin. Invest.*, 64, 729, 1979.

15. Ireland, P. and Fordtran, J. S., Effect of dietary calcium and age on jejunal calcium absorption in humans studied by intestinal perfusion, *J. Clin. Invest.*, 52, 2672, 1973.

16. Eastell, R., Yergey, A. L., Vieira, N. E., Cedel, S. L., Kumar, R., and Riggs, B. L., Interrelationship among vitamin D metabolism, true calcium absorption, parathyroid function, and age in women: evidence of an age-related intestinal resistance to 1,25-dihydroxyvitamin D action, *J. Bone Miner. Res.*, 6, 125, 1991.

17. Wiske, P.S., Epstein, S., Bell, N.H., Queener, S.F., Edmonsen, J., and Johnston, C.C., Jr., Increases in immunoreactive parathyroid hormone with age, *N. Engl. J. Med.*, 300, 1419, 1979.

18. Gallagher, J. C., Riggs, B. L., Jerpbak, C. M., and Arnaud, C. D., The effect of age on serum immunoreactive parathyroid hormone in normal and osteoporotic women, *J. Lab. Clin. Med.*, 95, 373, 1980.

19. Marcus, R., Madvig, P., and Young, G., Age-related changes in parathyroid hormone action in normal humans, *J. Clin. Endocrinol. Metab.*, 58, 223, 1984.

20. Orwoll, E. S. and Meier, D. E., Alterations in calcium, vitamin D, and parathyroid hormone physiology in normal men with aging: relationship to the development of senile osteoporosis, *J. Clin. Endocrinol. Metab.*, 63, 1262, 1986.

21. Epstein, S., Bryce, G., Hinman, J. W., Miller, O. N., Riggs, B. L., Hui, S. L., and Johnston, C. C., Jr., The influence of age on bone mineral regulating hormones, *Bone*, 7, 421, 1986.

22. Forero, M. S., Klein, R. F., Nissenson, R. A., Nelson, K., Heath, H., III, Arnaud, C. D., and Riggs, B. L., Effect of age on circulating immunoreactive and bioactive parathyroid hormone levels in women, *J. Bone Miner. Res.*, 2, 363, 1987.

23. Nordin, B. E. C. and Morris, H. A., The calcium deficiency model for osteoporosis, *Nutr. Rev.*, 47, 65, 1989.

24. Chapuy, M. C., Arlot, M. E., Duboeuf, F., Brun, J., Crouzet, B., Arnaud, S., Delmas, P. D., and Meunier, P. J., Vitamin D_3 and calcium to prevent hip fractures in elderly women, *N. Engl. J. Med.*, 327, 1637, 1992.

25. van Beresteijn, E. C. H., Dekker, P. R., van der Heiden-Winkeldermaat, H. J., van Schaik, M., Visser, R. M., and de Waard, H. E., The habitual calcium intake from milk products and its significance for bone health: a longitudinal study, in *Nutritional Aspects of Osteoporosis*, Burckhardt, P. and Heaney, R. P., Eds., Raven Press, New York, 1991, 206.

26. Anderson, J. J. B. and Barrett, C. J. H., Dietary phosphorus: the benefits and the problems, *Nutr. Today*, 20(2), 29, 1994.

27. Anderson, J. J. B. Nutritional biochemistry of calcium and phosphorus, *J. Nutr. Biochem.*, 2, 300, 1991.

28. Calvo, M. S., Kumar, R., and Heath, H., III, Persistently elevated parathyroid hormone secretion and action in young women after four weeks of ingesting high phosphorus low calcium diets, *J. Clin. Endocrinol. Metab.*, 70, 1334, 1990.

29. Calvo, M. S., Dietary phosphorus, calcium metabolism, and bone, *J. Nutr.*, 123, 1627, 1993.

30. Anderson, J. J. B. and Toverud, S. U., Diet and vitamin D: a review with emphasis on human function, *J. Nutr. Biochem.*, 5, 58, 1994.

31. Sherman, S. S., Hollis, B. W., and Tobin, J. D., Vitamin D status and related parameters in a healthy population: the effects of age, sex, and season, *J. Clin. Endocrinol. Metab.*, 71, 405, 1990.

32. Khaw, K.-T., Sneyd, M.-J., and Compston, J., Bone density, parathyroid hormone and 25-hydroxyvitamin D concentrations in middle aged women, *Br. Med. J.*, 305, 273, 1992.

33. Heikinheimo, R. J., Inkovaara, J. A., Harju, E. J., Haavisto, M. V., Kaarela, R. H., Kataja, J. M., Kokko, A. M. L., Kolho, L.A., and Rajala, S. A., Annual injection of vitamin D and fractures of aged bones, *Calcif. Tissue Int.*, 51, 105, 1992.

34. Dawson-Hughes, B., Dallal, G. E., Krall, E. A., Harris, S., Sokoll, L. J., and Falconer, G., Effect of vitamin D supplementation on wintertime and overall bone loss in healthy postmenopausal women, *Ann. Intern. Med.*, 115, 505, 1991.

35. Rosen, C. J., Morrison, A., Zhou, H., Storm, D., Hunter, S. J., Musgrave, K., Chen, T., Wen-Wei, and Holick, M. F., Elderly women in northern New England exhibit seasonal changes in bone mineral density and calciotropic hormones, *Bone Miner.*, 25, 83, 1994.

36. Plantalech, L., Guillaumont, M., Leclercq, M., and Delmas, P. D., Impaired carboxylation of serum osteocalcin in elderly women, *J. Bone Miner. Res.*, 6, 1211, 1991.

37. Szulc, P., Chapuy, M. C., Meunier, P. J., and Delmas, P. D., Serum undercarboxylated osteocalcin is a marker of the risk of hip fracture in elderly women, *J. Clin. Invest.*, 91, 1769, 1993.

38. Orimo, H., Shiraki, M., Fujita, T., Inoue, T., and Kushida, K., Clinical evaluation of menatetrenone in the treatment of involutional osteoporosis, *J. Bone Miner. Res.*, 7 (Suppl. 1), (Abstr.) S122, 1992.

39. Kohlmeier, M., Saupe, J., and Shearer, M. J., Risk of bone fracture in hemodialysis patients is related to vitamin K status, *J. Bone Miner. Res.*, 10, 5361, 1995.

40. Stendig-Lindberg, G., Tepper, R., and Leichter, I., Trabecular bone density in a two year controlled trial of peroral magnesium in osteoporosis, *Magnesium Res.*, 6, 155, 1993.

41. Kerstetter, J. E. and Allen, L. H., Dietary calcium increases urinary calcium, *J. Nutr.*, 120, 134, 1990.

42. Anderson, J. J. B., Thomsen, K., and Christiansen, C., High protein meals, insular hormones and urinary calcium excretion in human subjects, in *Osteoporosis 1987*, Christiansen, C., Johansen, J. S., and Riis, B. J., Eds., Osteopress ApS, Copenhagen, 1987, 240.

43. Nordin, B. E. C. and Need, A. G., The effect of sodium on calcium requirement, in *Nutrition and Osteoporosis*, Vol. 9, *Advances in Nutritional Research*, Draper, H. H., Ed., Plenum Press, New York, 1994, 209.

44. Klerekoper, M., Peterson, E., Phillips, D., Nelson, D., Tilley, B., and Parfitt, A. M., Continuous sodium fluoride therapy does not reduce vertebral fracture rate in postmenopausal osteoporosis, *J. Bone Miner. Res.*, 4 (Suppl. 1) (Abstr.) s376, 1989.

45. Riggs, B. L., Hodgson, S. F., O'Fallon, W. M., Chao, E. Y. S., Wahner, H. W., Muhs, J. M., Cedel, S. L., and Melton, L. J., III, Effect of fluoride treatment on the fracture rate in postmenopausal women with osteoporosis, *N. Engl. J. Med.*, 322, 802, 1990.

46. Strause, L., Saltman, P., Smith, K. T., Bracker, M., and Andon, M.B., Spinal bone loss in postmenopausal women supplemented with calcium and trace minerals, *J. Nutr.*, 124, 1060, 1994.

47. Dhuper, S., Warren, M. P., Brooks-Gunn, J., and Fox, R., Effects of hormonal status on bone density in adolescent girls, *J. Clin. Endocrinol. Metab.*, 71, 1083, 1990.

48. Weaver, C. M., Martin, B. R., and Heaney, R. P., Calcium absorption from foods, in *Nutritional Aspects of Osteoporosis*, Serono Symp. No. 85, Burckhardt, P. and Heaney, R. P., Eds., Raven Press, New York, 1991, 133.

49. Anderson, J. J. B., Ambrose, W. W., and Garner, S. C., Orally dosed genistein from soy and prevention of cancellous bone loss in two ovariectomized rat modes, *J. Nutr.*, 125, (Abstr.), 799s, 1995.

50. Dalsky, G. P., Stocke, K. S., Ehsani, A. A., Slatopolsky, E., Lee, W. C., and Birge, S. J., Jr., Weight-bearing exercise training and lumbar bone mineral content in postmenopausal women, *Ann. Intern. Med.*, 108, 824, 1988.

51. Smith, E. L., Gilligan, C., Shea, M. M., Ensign, P., and Smith, P. E., Exercise reduces bone involution in middle-aged women, *Calcif. Tissue Int.*, 44, 312, 1989.

52. Ooms, M. E., Lips, P., Van Lingen, A., and Valkenburg, H. A., Determinants of bone mineral density and risk factors for osteoporosis in healthy elderly women, *J. Bone Miner. Res.*, 8, 669, 1993.
53. Lau, E., Donnan, D., Barker, D., and Cooper, C., Physical activity and calcium intake in fracture of the proximal femur in Hong Kong, *Br. Med. J.*, 296, 1441, 1988.
54. Baylink, D. J., Glucocorticoid-induced osteoporosis, *N. Engl. J. Med.*, 309, 306, 1983.
55. Reid, I. R., Steroid osteoporosis, *Calcif. Tissue Int.*, 45, 63, 1989.
56. Hahn, T. J., Drug-induced disorders of vitamin D and mineral metabolism, *Clin. Endocrinol. Metab.*, 9, 107, 1980.
57. Cummings, S. R., Nevitt, M. C., Browner, W. S., Stone, K., Fox, K. M., Ensrud, K. F., Cauley, J., Black, D., and Vogt, T. M., Risk factors for hip fractures in white women, *N. Engl. J. Med.*, 332, 767, 1995.
58. Aloia, J. F., Vaswani, A., Yeh, J. K., Ross, P. L., Flaster, E., and Dalmanian, F. A., Calcium supplementation with and without hormone replacement therapy to prevent postmenopausal bone loss, *Ann. Intern. Med.*, 120, 97, 1994.
59. Fleisch, H., Editorial: prospective use of bisphosphonates in osteoporosis, *J. Clin. Endocrinol. Metab.*, 76, 1397, 1993.
60. Anderson, J. J. B. and Metz, J. A., Contributions of dietary calcium and physical activity to primary prevention of osteoporosis in females, *J. Am. Coll. Nutr.*, 12, 378, 1993.
61. 10th ed., Subcommittee on Dietary Allowances, Food and Nutrition Board, National Research Council, *Recommended Dietary Allowances,* National Academy Press, Washington, D.C., 1989.
62. Barger-Lux, M. J., Heaney, R. P., Packard, P. T., Lappe, J. M., and Recker, R. R., Nutritional correlates of a low calcium diet, *Clin. Appl. Nutr.*, 2(4), 39, 1992.

Chapter 5

NUTRITIONAL ANEMIAS

Kelley S. Scanlon and Ray Yip

CONTENTS

I. INTRODUCTION

Anemia, defined as a hemoglobin concentration or hematocrit lower than the reference cutoff value, is a nonspecific finding that can be caused by a number of conditions. Although iron deficiency plays a major role in the occurrence of anemia in both the developing and developed regions of the world, other nutritional deficiencies and nonnutritional diseases and hereditary disorders also cause anemia.[1]

Anemia is common throughout the world, with the highest rates occurring in developing countries and among persons of lower socioeconomic status (Table 1).[2,3] Among adults, anemia disproportionately affects women of child-bearing age, especially pregnant women, primarily because women are more likely to have iron deficiency. Overall, anemia affects nearly 50% of women in the developing regions of the world and 11% of women from the developed regions. In the U.S., an estimated 3% of women and 10% of pregnant women are anemic.[5] During late pregnancy, as many as one third of low-income U.S. women who attend public assistance programs show evidence of anemia.[6]

TABLE 1
Estimates of the Prevalence (%) of
Anemia (*circa* 1980) in Adults

		Females	
	Males	**Pregnant**	**All**[a]
Africa	20	63	44
North America	4	—	8
Latin America	13	30	17
East Asia	11	20	18
South Asia	32	65	58
Europe	2	14	12
Oceana	7	25	19
Developed regions	3	14	11
Developing regions	26	59	47
World	18	51	35

[a] Includes pregnant and nonpregnant women.

From MacPhail, P. and Bothwell, T.H., *Nutritional Anemias*, Vol. 30, Raven Press, New York, 1992, 2. With permission.

Data from De Maeyer, E. and Adiels-Tegman, M., *World Health Stat. Q.*, 38, 302, 1985.

Anemia is caused by decreased production of red blood cells and hemo-globin, increased destruction of red blood cells (hemolysis), and excessive blood loss. It occurs when the hemoglobin in the red blood cells falls below normal, which is traditionally defined as more than two standard deviations below the median hemoglobin observed in a reference population of healthy individuals of the same gender and age.

Mild anemia, defined as a hemoglobin concentration 1 to 2 g/dl below the reference cutoff, has little clinical consequence. The underlying deficiency or disease is of greater concern and contributes to the more critical clinical manifestations. For example, in vitamin B-12 deficiency anemia, the neurologic consequences of the deficiency are far more serious than the associated anemia. In severe anemia (hemoglobin <7 g/dl) from any cause, however, there are definite cardiovascular consequences related to reduced oxygen transport to tissues. In extreme cases, very severe anemia (hemoglobin <4.0 g/dl) contributes to or directly causes childhood and maternal mortality.

To properly treat and prevent anemia, it is critical to determine the underlying cause. If the cause is nutritional, assessment is performed to identify the nutrient or nutrients involved. Nutritional anemias can be caused by any nutrient essential to the production of hemoglobin;[7] however, they are most commonly caused by a deficiency in iron. Folate and vitamin B-12 deficiency anemias are the second and third most common nutritional anemias, but they are much less prevalent than iron deficiency.

This chapter will focus on the main nutritional anemia found in adult U.S. women: iron deficiency anemia. A brief summary of the megaloblastic anemias caused by folate and vitamin B-12 deficiencies is also included. Folate and vitamin B-12 deficiency anemias are rare in the U.S., but the associated deficiencies do occur among specific groups of women. Women of low socioeconomic status who are pregnant are at greatest risk for folate deficiency and women with impaired absorption of vitamin B-12 and strict vegetarian women who consume no animal products are at greatest risk for vitamin B-12 deficiency.

The nutritional anemia represents a late stage of the nutrient deficiency, when the deficiency is severe enough to result in a subnormal concentration of hemoglobin in the blood. When using anemia to estimate the prevalence of a nutritional deficiency in the population, one can safely assume that the actual rates of deficiency of the nutrient are higher.

In this chapter, we will discuss the stages of nutrient deficiency that lead to anemia and the main factors that contribute to the underlying nutrient deficiencies. We will also provide a brief summary of the main parameters used to diagnose iron, folate, and vitamin B-12 deficiency anemia and the recommendations for prevention of each condition.

II. IRON DEFICIENCY ANEMIA

A. INTRODUCTION

Iron deficiency is one of the most common nutrient deficiencies in the world and the single most common cause of nutritional anemia.[8] In countries where the prevalence of anemia is greater than 20%, the majority of cases are associated with a primary iron deficiency or iron deficiency in combination with other conditions. Because iron deficiency without anemia is equally common, an even greater proportion of women have some degree of iron deficiency. Iron deficiency is not restricted to women in developing countries. In the U.S., an estimated 5 to 10% of women 20 to 44 years of age have some level of iron deficiency.[5,9] The prevalence is believed to be highest among pregnant women due to increased physiologic demands; however, national estimates for pregnant women are not available. Data from national surveys and special studies suggest that the prevalence of iron deficiency is higher among women of lower socioeconomic status, African American and Hispanic women, women with high parity, women with a history of heavy menses and poor dietary intake, and women who donate blood more than three times per year.[10]

B. IRON AND ANEMIA

Iron is an essential component of several body compounds. The approximate amount of iron present in the body of an average 55-kg woman is 2300 mg (Table 2). Approximately 88% of this iron is found in functional iron compounds and 12% is found in iron transport and storage compounds. Hemoglobin, the oxygen-carrying pigment of the red blood cell, is the main functional iron compound, comprising approximately 85% of the functional iron in the body. The remaining 15% of functional iron is accounted for by myoglobin, the red iron-containing protein of muscle, and the heme and nonheme enzymes.

TABLE 2
Iron-Containing Compounds in a
55-kg Woman (Approximate)

Functional	Hemoglobin	1700 mg
	Myoglobin	222 mg
	Heme enzymes	50 mg
	Nonheme enzymes	55 mg
Transport	Transferrin	3 mg
Storage	Ferritin	200 mg
	Hemosiderin	70 mg

Modified from Bothwell, T.H. and Charlton, R.W., *Iron Deficiency in Women*, report of the International Nutritional Anemia Consultative Group (INACG), Nutrition Foundation, Washington, D.C., 1981, 2. With permission.

Of the 12% of body iron that is not contained in functional compounds, less than 1% is found in transport iron as transferrin and close to 12% is found in the storage compounds: ferritin and hemosiderin. Iron is stored primarily in the liver, spleen, and bone marrow. The stored iron is used for the production of essential iron compounds and for maintaining iron homeostasis by regulating iron absorption from the diet.[11]

Hemoglobin is made up of iron, protoporphyrin, and globin, with iron comprising one third the weight. In iron deficiency, the supply of iron is insufficient for normal hemoglobin synthesis. Thus, the production of red blood cells is reduced and the cells that are produced are microcytic and hypochromic.

The stages of iron deficiency that lead to anemia are summarized in Table 3. In general, the iron depletion stage is characterized by a reduction in iron stores, primarily reflected by a decrease in serum levels of ferritin. No loss in function occurs at this stage, but iron absorption increases as a result of a lower body iron content. As the deficiency progresses to iron deficient erythropoiesis, the iron stores are exhausted and the production of hemoglobin and other iron compounds is impaired. Although a hemoglobin concentration above the cutoff that defines anemia is maintained, the second stage is characterized by a decrease in the percentage of transferrin saturation, indicating that there is an insufficient amount of iron being supplied to the bone marrow. This stage is also reflected by an increased free erythrocyte protoporphyrin concentration, marking the accumulation of protoporphyrin that occurs due to a lack of iron to form hemoglobin. Anemia occurs in the final stage of iron deficiency, characterized by a hemoglobin concentration (or hematocrit level) below the normal range.[12]

TABLE 3
Stages of Iron Deficiency

	Iron overload	Normal	Iron depletion	Iron-deficient erythropoiesis	Iron deficiency anemia
Serum ferritin	Elevated	Normal	Low	Low	Low
Transferrin saturation (%)	Elevated	Normal	Normal	Low	Low
Free erythrocyte protoporphyrin	Normal	Normal	Normal	Elevated	Elevated
Erythrocytes	Normal	Normal	Normal	Normal	Microcytic/ hypochromic
Mean cell volume	Normal	Normal	Normal	Normal	Low

From Herbert, V., *Am. J. Clin. Nutr.*, 46, 387, 1987. With permission.

C. CONSEQUENCES OF IRON DEFICIENCY ANEMIA

The consequences of iron deficiency anemia among women are related to the deficiency of iron and to the anemia. The consequences of greatest concern include the potential effects on pregnancy outcome and work capacity.

Very severe anemia (hemoglobin <4 g/dl) is associated with increased maternal mortality.[3] Deaths associated with severe anemia generally occur at times of increased physiologic stress, such as the peripartum period when oxygen delivery and cardiovascular function are further compromised by worsening hemoglobin.

Large observational studies in the U.S. have indicated an association between less severe anemia and the occurrence of premature births, low birth weight, or fetal death. However, a lack of statistical adjustment for factors known to be associated both with anemia and with pregnancy outcome have made it difficult to draw definite conclusions select studies.[6,13-15] The detailed study by Scholl and co-workers[16] was designed to take into account these factors. Scholl et al.[16] measured serum ferritin concentrations in addition to hematologic measures to examine specifically the association of iron deficiency anemia and pregnancy outcome. After adjusting for a number of potential confounders, Scholl and co-workers[16] found a threefold increase in low birth weight and a twofold increase in preterm delivery among women with iron deficiency anemia, but not among women with other types of anemia. The results of this study provided stronger evidence that iron deficiency anemia is associated with adverse birth outcome.

It is well established that iron deficiency anemia reduces work performance. A classic study by Viteri and Torun[17] demonstrated a linear dose-response relationship between hemoglobin level and the Harvard step-test performance. Similarly, studies in Africa report poorer cardiovascular fitness among anemic compared to nonanemic workers.[18] The effect of iron deficiency on work performance or energy expenditure appears to be mediated through a decreased oxygen-carrying capacity from the anemia and impaired muscle function related to the iron deficit. Studies report increased productivity when anemic workers are supplemented with iron.[19,20]

Additional consequences of iron deficiency anemia include impaired body temperature regulation in cold climates[21,22] and increased risk of lead poisoning that is related to increased lead absorption when iron is deficient.[23-26] Interestingly, evidence is lacking to support the commonly held belief of increased tiredness and fatigue among anemic women.[27]

Iron deficiency anemia among children is associated with altered behavior and impaired intellectual performance.[28] Although, behavior effects among iron-deficient women have not been adequately studied, one study suggests that iron-deficient adults have impaired attention span and short-term memory.[29]

D. FACTORS CONTRIBUTING TO IRON DEFICIENCY

The major causes of iron deficiency anemia among women are inadequate iron intake, increased physiologic requirements, and excessive blood loss. Anemia caused by these factors occurs more rapidly when iron stores are inadequate to compensate for increased need. Women of childbearing age are one of the highest risk groups for anemia because they may not have adequate amounts of iron intake or stores relative to iron needs and losses. Among these women, those with excessive blood loss during menstruation and pregnant women are at highest risk. Postmenopausal women are less likely to develop iron deficiency anemia. When women in this age group are affected, gastrointestinal blood loss is usually the cause.

On average, women lose approximately 30 ml of blood per month in menses. However, data from Sweden and Britain indicate that approximately 10% of women lose more than 80 ml/month (Figure 2).[53-56] This excessive blood loss can contribute to the development of iron deficiency anemia because increased iron absorption cannot compensate for such high losses. Also, women generally do not have adequate stored iron to compensate for the iron lost in heavy menses.

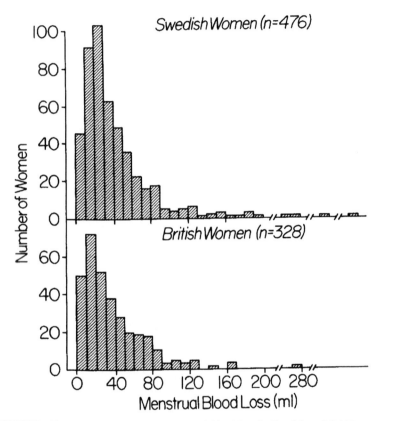

FIGURE 2. Frequency distribution of menstrual blood loss in Swedish and British women. (From Bothwell, T. H., Charlton, R. W., Cook, J. D., Finch, C. A., *Iron Metabolism in Man*, Blackwell Scientific, Oxford, 1979, 251. With permission.) (Data from Hallberg et al.,[54] and Cole et al.,[55] and Göltner.[56])

The amount of iron lost through menstruation also varies with the type of contraception used. Intrauterine devices can cause a twofold increase in blood loss, whereas the contraceptive pill can reduce blood loss by one half.[11]

Pathological blood loss from parasitic infection and gastrointestinal lesions can also be significant and contribute to iron deficiency anemia. Hookworm infestation is extremely rare in the U.S., but it is a significant burden for women in developing countries. Although iron deficiency anemia is relatively

1. Inadequate Intake

The main sources of iron in the American diet are meat, poultry and fish, eggs, vegetables, and whole, iron-enriched, and iron-fortified grain products. National survey data indicate that women of childbearing age obtain approximately 10 to 11 mg of iron daily from food.[30] Preliminary data from the first phase of the Third National Health and Nutrition Examination Survey (NHANES III) do indicate that average iron intakes have increased to approximately 12 to 13 mg/d.[31] However, this is still less than the 15 mg of daily iron recommended for women of childbearing age.[32] Supplemental iron (alone or in combination with other nutrients) is taken daily by approximately 20% of women.[33]

The adequacy of iron intake from the diet is associated with the consumption of foods rich in iron, but is also strongly affected by the variation in absorption of iron.[34] Iron absorption varies with physiologic need: absorption increases when iron status is reduced and decreases when iron status is adequate. Iron absorption is also associated with the type of iron consumed and factors in the diet that enhance or inhibit absorption.

The type of iron consumed is far more important than the quantity of iron in the diet.[34,35] Heme iron, from the hemoglobin and myoglobin of animals, is generally well absorbed and unaffected by factors that inhibit iron absorption. The high absorbability is related to the fact that heme iron is taken up by the mucosal cell intact within the porphyrin ring, protecting the iron from ingredients in the diet that inhibit iron absorption. Nonheme iron, which makes up about 90% of the iron in the diet, is found in nonmeat food sources, including grains, vegetables, fruits, eggs, the nonheme iron of animals, and iron supplements. Although nonheme iron is found in a variety of foods and contributes significantly to the iron ingested, it is not well absorbed. In addition, the bioavailability of nonheme iron is generally affected by several factors, factors that enhance or inhibit absorption. The effect of these factors is less pronounced when the entire composition of a diverse diet is considered. For example, Cook and colleagues found a 5.9 fold difference (13.5 vs. 2.3%) in iron absorption rates between a single iron absorption-enhancing meal and a single iron absorption-inhibitory meal, respectively, but only a 2.5 fold difference (8.0 vs. 3.2%) in iron absorption when an iron absorption-enhancing diet and an iron absorption-inhibitory diet were consumed for two consecutive weeks.[35]

The main inhibitors of nonheme iron absorption are phytates and polyphenols.[36-39] Phytates are found primarily in cereal grains, nuts, legumes, and some vegetables (e.g., spinach and beet greens). Polyphenols are found in tea, vegetables, and legumes. The high rates of anemia in many regions of the world are commonly attributed to dependence on a cereal- and legume-based diet.[4] In some countries, the common practice of drinking tea with a meal may also have a negative effect on iron nutriture. However, meals that contain nonheme iron along with phytates and polyphenols can still contribute an important source of absorbable iron if the meal also contains an enhancer of iron absorption, such as ascorbic acid.[39]

The effects of factors that inhibit iron absorption from the diet can be overcome by factors that enhance absorption. The main enhancers of nonheme iron absorption are ascorbic acid and the "meat factor" found in fish, poultry, and beef.[39-41] These factors are relatively high in the diet of most Americans. Other organic acids (e.g., lactic acid) and alcohol are less powerful enhancers of iron absorption.[4]

2. Increased Requirement

The recommended dietary allowance (RDA) for iron for women of child-bearing age, which assumes an overall 10 to 15% rate of absorption, is 15 mg/d for nonpregnant and lactating women and 30 mg/d for pregnant women.[32] The requirement is not increased in lactation because the amount of iron lost through breast milk is less than the iron lost in menstruation, which is often absent during lactation.[42,43]

The iron requirement is increased in pregnancy to meet the iron demands of an increased blood volume, to provide iron to the fetus and placenta, and to compensate for blood loss during delivery (Table 4).[10,11,44] Iron deficiency anemia in pregnancy occurs when iron intake and stores are not adequate to meet these increased needs, which average about 1000 mg during the course of pregnancy.[11,44] Most women do not have this level of iron in stores. In fact, less than 5% of women have more than 400 mg of stored iron.[5] Increased iron absorption during the second half of pregnancy helps to make up the increased requirement, but the high iron requirement of 3 to 5 mg/d during this period cannot be easily met by increased absorption alone (Figure 1). Increased intake and mobilization from stores are necessary. Because women generally begin pregnancy with low iron stores and because food intake will unlikely supply the iron needed, iron supplementation during pregnancy is often recommended to prevent the onset of iron deficiency. Several studies have shown an association between iron supplementation and increased hemoglobin levels in the third trimester of pregnancy.[46-52] However, there is no clear evidence that iron supplementation during pregnancy improves the clinical outcome of pregnancy.[27] Part of the reason for the lack of strong evidence that better iron status is associated with better clinical outcomes is related to the fact that physicians routinely prescribe supplements with iron to women during pregnancy. Thus, it would be difficult to conduct a proper evaluation of clinical outcomes with a control group not receiving iron.

3. Blood Loss

Blood loss can occur from trauma, disease, or blood donation. Among women, physiologic blood loss occurs through menstruation. The effect of this loss on iron status depends on the quantity of blood lost and the iron stores of the individual.

TABLE 4
Iron Losses during Pregnancy in a 55-kg Iron Replete Woman[a]

		Amount of iron (mg)
Gross Losses		
Fetus		280
Umbilical cord and placenta		90
Maternal blood loss		150
Obligatory losses from gut, etc. during gestation		230
Expansion of material red cell mass		
	Gross total	1200
Net Losses		
Contraction of maternal red cell mass after delivery		450
	Total	750

[a] These represent average values. Considerable individual variations have been reported different studies.

From Bothwell, T.H. and Charlton, R.W., Iron Deficiency in Women, report of the Internation Nutritional Anemia Consultative Group (INACG), Nutrition Foundation, Washington, D.C., 19 8. With permission.

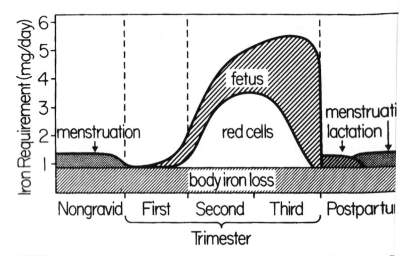

FIGURE 1. Daily iron requirements during pregnancy. (From Bothwell, T. H., Charlton, R Cook, J. D., and Finch, C. A., *Iron Metabolism in Man*, Blackwell Scientific, Oxford, 197 With permission.)

1. Inadequate Intake

The main sources of iron in the American diet are meat, poultry and fish, eggs, vegetables, and whole, iron-enriched, and iron-fortified grain products. National survey data indicate that women of childbearing age obtain approximately 10 to 11 mg of iron daily from food.[30] Preliminary data from the first phase of the Third National Health and Nutrition Examination Survey (NHANES III) do indicate that average iron intakes have increased to approximately 12 to 13 mg/d.[31] However, this is still less than the 15 mg of daily iron recommended for women of childbearing age.[32] Supplemental iron (alone or in combination with other nutrients) is taken daily by approximately 20% of women.[33]

The adequacy of iron intake from the diet is associated with the consumption of foods rich in iron, but is also strongly affected by the variation in absorption of iron.[34] Iron absorption varies with physiologic need: absorption increases when iron status is reduced and decreases when iron status is adequate. Iron absorption is also associated with the type of iron consumed and factors in the diet that enhance or inhibit absorption.

The type of iron consumed is far more important than the quantity of iron in the diet.[34,35] Heme iron, from the hemoglobin and myoglobin of animals, is generally well absorbed and unaffected by factors that inhibit iron absorption. The high absorbability is related to the fact that heme iron is taken up by the mucosal cell intact within the porphyrin ring, protecting the iron from ingredients in the diet that inhibit iron absorption. Nonheme iron, which makes up about 90% of the iron in the diet, is found in nonmeat food sources, including grains, vegetables, fruits, eggs, the nonheme iron of animals, and iron supplements. Although nonheme iron is found in a variety of foods and contributes significantly to the iron ingested, it is not well absorbed. In addition, the bioavailability of nonheme iron is generally affected by several factors, factors that enhance or inhibit absorption. The effect of these factors is less pronounced when the entire composition of a diverse diet is considered. For example, Cook and colleagues found a 5.9 fold difference (13.5 vs. 2.3%) in iron absorption rates between a single iron absorption-enhancing meal and a single iron absorption-inhibitory meal, respectively, but only a 2.5 fold difference (8.0 vs. 3.2%) in iron absorption when an iron absorption-enhancing diet and an iron absorption-inhibitory diet were consumed for two consecutive weeks.[35]

The main inhibitors of nonheme iron absorption are phytates and polyphenols.[36-39] Phytates are found primarily in cereal grains, nuts, legumes, and some vegetables (e.g., spinach and beet greens). Polyphenols are found in tea, vegetables, and legumes. The high rates of anemia in many regions of the world are commonly attributed to dependence on a cereal- and legume-based diet.[4] In some countries, the common practice of drinking tea with a meal may also have a negative effect on iron nutriture. However, meals that contain nonheme iron along with phytates and polyphenols can still contribute an important source of absorbable iron if the meal also contains an enhancer of iron absorption, such as ascorbic acid.[39]

The effects of factors that inhibit iron absorption from the diet can be overcome by factors that enhance absorption. The main enhancers of nonheme iron absorption are ascorbic acid and the "meat factor" found in fish, poultry, and beef.[39-41] These factors are relatively high in the diet of most Americans. Other organic acids (e.g., lactic acid) and alcohol are less powerful enhancers of iron absorption.[4]

2. Increased Requirement

The recommended dietary allowance (RDA) for iron for women of child-bearing age, which assumes an overall 10 to 15% rate of absorption, is 15 mg/d for nonpregnant and lactating women and 30 mg/d for pregnant women.[32] The requirement is not increased in lactation because the amount of iron lost through breast milk is less than the iron lost in menstruation, which is often absent during lactation.[42,43]

The iron requirement is increased in pregnancy to meet the iron demands of an increased blood volume, to provide iron to the fetus and placenta, and to compensate for blood loss during delivery (Table 4).[10,11,44] Iron deficiency anemia in pregnancy occurs when iron intake and stores are not adequate to meet these increased needs, which average about 1000 mg during the course of pregnancy.[11,44] Most women do not have this level of iron in stores. In fact, less than 5% of women have more than 400 mg of stored iron.[5] Increased iron absorption during the second half of pregnancy helps to make up the increased requirement, but the high iron requirement of 3 to 5 mg/d during this period cannot be easily met by increased absorption alone (Figure 1). Increased intake and mobilization from stores are necessary. Because women generally begin pregnancy with low iron stores and because food intake will unlikely supply the iron needed, iron supplementation during pregnancy is often recommended to prevent the onset of iron deficiency. Several studies have shown an association between iron supplementation and increased hemoglobin levels in the third trimester of pregnancy.[46-52] However, there is no clear evidence that iron supplementation during pregnancy improves the clinical outcome of pregnancy.[27] Part of the reason for the lack of strong evidence that better iron status is associated with better clinical outcomes is related to the fact that physicians routinely prescribe supplements with iron to women during pregnancy. Thus, it would be difficult to conduct a proper evaluation of clinical outcomes with a control group not receiving iron.

3. Blood Loss

Blood loss can occur from trauma, disease, or blood donation. Among women, physiologic blood loss occurs through menstruation. The effect of this loss on iron status depends on the quantity of blood lost and the iron stores of the individual.

TABLE 4
Iron Losses during Pregnancy in a 55-kg Iron Replete Woman[a]

		Amount of iron (mg)
Gross Losses		
Fetus		280
Umbilical cord and placenta		90
Maternal blood loss		150
Obligatory losses from gut, etc. during gestation		230
Expansion of material red cell mass		
	Gross total	1200
Net Losses		
Contraction of maternal red cell mass after delivery		450
	Total	750

[a] These represent average values. Considerable individual variations have been reported in different studies.

From Bothwell, T.H. and Charlton, R.W., Iron Deficiency in Women, report of the International Nutritional Anemia Consultative Group (INACG), Nutrition Foundation, Washington, D.C., 1981, 8. With permission.

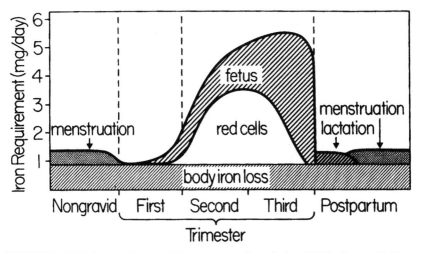

FIGURE 1. Daily iron requirements during pregnancy. (From Bothwell, T. H., Charlton, R. W., Cook, J. D., and Finch, C. A., *Iron Metabolism in Man,* Blackwell Scientific, Oxford, 1979, 21. With permission.)

On average, women lose approximately 30 ml of blood per month in menses. However, data from Sweden and Britain indicate that approximately 10% of women lose more than 80 ml/month (Figure 2).[53-56] This excessive blood loss can contribute to the development of iron deficiency anemia because increased iron absorption cannot compensate for such high losses. Also, women generally do not have adequate stored iron to compensate for the iron lost in heavy menses.

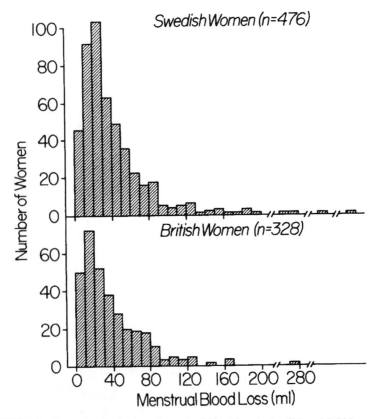

FIGURE 2. Frequency distribution of menstrual blood loss in Swedish and British women. (From Bothwell, T. H., Charlton, R. W., Cook, J. D., Finch, C. A., *Iron Metabolism in Man*, Blackwell Scientific, Oxford, 1979, 251. With permission.) (Data from Hallberg et al.,[54] and Cole et al.,[55] and Göltner.[56])

The amount of iron lost through menstruation also varies with the type of contraception used. Intrauterine devices can cause a twofold increase in blood loss, whereas the contraceptive pill can reduce blood loss by one half.[11]

Pathological blood loss from parasitic infection and gastrointestinal lesions can also be significant and contribute to iron deficiency anemia. Hookworm infestation is extremely rare in the U.S., but it is a significant burden for women in developing countries. Although iron deficiency anemia is relatively uncommon among postmenopausal women, when detected, it is most often due to gastrointestinal blood loss associated with lesions of the gastrointesinal tract.[57] Gastritis, ulcers, colonic carcinoma, and colonic polyps are among the common lesions. Increased blood loss can also result from the ingestion of certain medications. For example, adrenocorticosteroids or nonsteroidal anti-inflammatory agents may cause some gastrointestinal bleeding, and aspirin, particularly when taken with ethanol, may also cause hemorrhage, gastritis, and subsequent blood loss. Unexplained iron deficiency in a postmenopausal woman requires a thorough investigation to identify a cause.

Blood donation is a nonpathological reason for significant blood loss. Iron deficiency as a result of blood donation is not a concern when donations are made infrequently or when the donor has adequate iron stores that can easily be replenished. However, because women generally have low stores of iron, donating blood more than three times per year increases a woman's risk for iron deficiency if she does not regularly take iron supplements.[10]

E. DIAGNOSIS OF IRON DEFICIENCY ANEMIA

Because iron deficiency is the most common cause of anemia in women, a diagnosis of anemia alone has often been used as the screening test for iron deficiency anemia. Anemia is commonly diagnosed on the basis of a hemoglobin concentration or hematocrit level that is below a specific cutoff value for the population under study. The anemia criteria for women of childbearing age proposed by the Centers for Disease Control and Prevention are based on population data from the Second National Health and Nutrition Examination Survey (NHANES II, 1987–1988) (Table 5). To assess whether iron deficiency is the cause of the anemia, the most common follow-up tests are hemoglobin response to iron supplementation and abnormal results on laboratory measures of iron status.

TABLE 5
Anemia Criteria for U.S. Women

	Hemoglobin (g/dl)	Hematocrit (%)
Nonpregnant	<12.0	36.0
Pregnant		
1st trimester	<11.0	33.0
2nd trimester	<10.5	32.0
3rd trimester	<11.0	33.0

From Centers for Disease Control and Prevention, *Morbid. Mortal. Wkly. Rep.*, 38, 400, 1989.

Observing an individual's response to iron therapy is one of the more specific tests to confirm iron deficiency as the cause of anemia. If hemoglobin levels increase at least 1.0 g/dl after 1 month of iron treatment, then iron deficiency is the most likely etiology of the anemia. Iron supplementation can also be done at the population level. The hemoglobin distribution for the population is then compared for presupplementation and postsupplementation. Supplementation of the population may be preferred over individual supplementation when the prevalence of anemia is high and it can be assumed that most persons in the population have some level of iron deficiency.[59]

When confirmation of iron deficiency is based on measures of iron status, the common measures taken and calculated include mean corpuscular volume (MCV), serum ferritin, percent transferrin saturation, and free erythrocyte protoporphyrin (Table 6). A diagnosis of anemia accompanied by abnormal results on at least two of the iron status measures is an established method of confirming iron deficiency anemia for population-based assessment.[60] For individual-based assessment, a single test other than hemoglobin or hematocrit is helpful in the confirmation of iron deficiency. However, other common causes of mild anemia can interfere with the test results. For example, in addition to indicating iron deficiency anemia, a low MCV can also be the result of infection, chronic inflammatory conditions, or mild hereditary anemia such as α- or β-thalassemia traits. Inflammatory conditions can also cause depressed transferrin saturation and elevated erythrocyte protoporphyrin levels. Among the battery of common iron tests listed in Table 6, serum ferritin appears to be the most specific indicator of iron deficiency when levels are low. However, serum ferritin is an acute reactant and becomes elevated with infection and chronic inflammatory conditions. Therefore, the absence of a low serum ferritin level does not rule out iron deficiency. Recently, transferrin receptor concentration has been shown to be a measure that correlates well with iron status and is not affected by inflammatory conditions.[61]

F. PREVENTION AND TREATMENT
1. Prevention

Iron deficiency anemia is prevented by maintaining a balance between iron intake and iron requirement and loss. The amount of iron necessary varies from one woman to another depending on her reproductive history and the quantity of blood lost during menstruation.

To prevent iron deficiency anemia caused by increased blood loss it is important to clinically evaluate possible sources of gastrointestinal blood loss that may be due to lesions or infectious agents and to avoid medications and contraceptive practices that increase blood loss.

Increasing iron intake to meet iron requirements is accomplished through improved dietary choices. A diet that provides adequate iron should emphasize the consumption of foods that contain heme iron and foods that contain factors that enhance the absorption of nonheme iron, while minimizing the consumption of foods that contain factors that inhibit absorption.

TABLE 6
Common Measures Taken To Confirm Iron Deficiency Anemia

Measure	Meaning of the Test	Common Cutoffs Used for Identifying Iron Deficiency in Adult Women	Comments
Mean cell volume (MCV)	Reflects the average size of the red blood cell	<80 fl	Decreased in iron deficiency anemia, may also decrease in the anemias of infection, chronic inflammatory disease, thalassemia minor, and lead poisoning
Serum ferritin	Reflects the amount of iron in storage	<12 ng/ml	Decreased during the early stage of iron depletion. Increased by several factors, including infection and chronic inflammatory diseases, acute and chronic liver disease, leukemia, Hodgkin's disease, and the decreased erythropoiesis associated with vitamin B-12 and folate deficiency
% transferrin saturation	Reflects the amount of iron in transit from the reticuloendothelial system to the bone marrow, percent transferrin saturation = serum iron/total iron binding capacity (TIBC)	<16%	Decreased in iron deficiency, as serum iron decreases and TIBC increases, in chronic inflammatory disease, serum iron and TIBC decrease, which results in a low normal percent transferrin saturation
Free erythrocyte protoporphyrin	Reflects the accumulation of protoporphyrin in the RBC that results from decreased heme synthesis	>70 μg/dl RBC	Increased in early iron deficiency, also increased in chronic inflammatory disease and lead poisoning

If the iron requirement is too high for normal dietary intake, then iron intake can be improved by taking iron supplements. Supplementation may be especially important as a strategy to prevent iron deficiency among high-risk women, particularly pregnant women. However, iron supplementation as a strategy to increase iron intake can only be successful if the individual complies with daily supplement use. There are many factors that contribute to poor compliance, from personal difficulty in remembering to take the supplement each day to financial difficulty in purchasing the supplements on a regular basis. A major factor attributed to poor compliance with iron supplement is the occurrence of unpleasant side effects from the iron, specifically, gastrointestinal disturbances. A recently developed capsule made by packing iron sulfate with a compound called "gastric delivery system" appears to improve tolerance for iron supplements by minimizing these adverse gastrointestinal effects.[62] The new capsule also appears to improve iron absorption from supplement pills. Other strategies to improve compliance with iron supplementation include educating women on the importance of supplements and providing advice on the common side effects experienced.[63]

Iron fortification of cereal and grain products continues to be an inexpensive strategy for improving the iron intake of the population. However, in the U.S., grain products are only partially fortified. The impact of this program on the iron status of women has not been formally evaluated. In Sweden, where highly fortified grain products contribute up to 40% of dietary iron,[64] the fortification program has contributed significantly to the decline in iron deficiency among women of childbearing age.[65]

There has been strong opposition to increasing the amount of iron added to grain products in the U.S. diet because of concern that higher levels of iron in the diet will increase the risk for iron overload and related illness among persons with undiagnosed hemochromatosis. Although this concern is valid, universal screening for hemochromatosis might be an effective strategy to identify persons with this disorder for proper treatment and prevention of illness and to enable increasing iron fortification to take place so that rates of iron deficiency decline. Recent studies indicate that screening for hemochromatosis is cost effective.[66]

2. Selective Treatment with Screening

Routine evaluation of high-risk women for iron deficiency anemia is important. Women at risk should be counseled on dietary strategies to prevent anemia and should be treated and followed up if anemia presents during evaluation. Women with iron deficiency anemia should be treated with oral supplements and parenteral iron should be administered if higher doses are needed to compensate for high losses.

Recently, the Food and Nutrition Board of the Institute of Medicine[67] proposed that all nonpregnant women be screened for anemia between 15 and 25 years of age, with follow-up screening every 5 to 10 years if there are no risk factors for anemia, and more frequently if medical or social risk factors are present (e.g., high parity, frequent blood donation, high menstrual blood loss, previous diagnosis of iron deficiency anemia, poverty, or recent immigration). Women with severe anemia (defined by the Institute of Medicine as a hemoglobin concentration more than 2 g/dl below normal) should be followed up with additional laboratory tests and physical exams. Women with mild anemia should be treated with a therapeutic iron dose, counseled on dietary intake, and followed up in 1 to $1^1/_2$ months to determine the response to therapy or the need to consider other causes of anemia.

In the 1993 report, the Institute of Medicine (IOM) recommends that pregnant women be screened at least once during each trimester of pregnancy (Table 7). High-risk women should also be screened at the 4 to 6-week postpartum visit. For the first two thirds of pregnancy, the IOM recommends the determination of serum ferritin in addition to hemoglobin concentration and suggests supplementation if a lower than normal serum ferritin level accompanies the anemia. The committee recommends that all women be supplemented with iron during the third trimester of pregnancy: nonanemic women with 30 mg/d and anemic women with 60 to 120 mg/d. Severely anemic women would undergo additional medical evaluation.

TABLE 7
Recommended Guidelines for Selective Treatment
with Iron Status Screening during Pregnancy

Action	Trimester		
	First	Second	Third
Screening	Hemoglobin, g/dl (Hgb) Serum ferritin, μ/l(SF)	Hemoglobin Serum ferritin	Hemoglobin
No treatment	Hgb ≥11.0 and SF >20	SF >20, regardless of Hgb	
Treat with 30 mg iron/day	Hgb 9.0–10.9 and SF 12–20 or Hgb ≥11.0 and SF ≤20	Hgb ≥10.5 and SF ≤20	Hgb ≥11.0
Treat with 60–120 mg iron/day	Hgb 9.0–10.9 and SF <12	Hgb 9.0–10.4 and SF <12	Hgb 9.0–10.9
Further medical evaluation	Hgb <9.0 or Hgb 9.0–10.9 and SF >30 or No response to iron supplement	Hgb <9.0 or No response to iron supplement	Hgb <9.0 or No response to iron supplement

Note: African American women may normally have hemoglobin levels 0.8 g/dL less than those of other races. Cutoff hemoglobin values for African American women should therefore be set at 0.8 g/dL lower than the hemoglobin values given above.

The recommended guidelines are published by the Institute of Medicine, *Iron Deficiency Anemia: Recommended Guidelines for the Prevention, Detection, and Management among U.S. Children and Women of Childbearing Age,* Earl, R. and Woteki, C. E., Eds., National Academy Press, Washington, D.C., 1993, 1.

III. FOLATE AND VITAMIN B-12 DEFICIENCY ANEMIA

A. INTRODUCTION

Nutritional megaloblastic anemia is associated with advanced folate and vitamin B-12 deficiencies. Folate deficiency anemia is the second most common nutritional anemia in the world; however, its magnitude is still quite small compared to iron deficiency anemia. In developing countries, folate deficiency anemia occurs among pregnant and lactating women. However, in industrialized countries, less severe folate deficiencies are more likely. Although data on the prevalence of folate deficiency anemia in the U.S. are unavailable, data from the second National Health and Nutrition Examination Survey indicate that 13% of women 20 to 44 years of age have low red blood cell folate levels and 6% of women have both low red blood cell and low serum folate levels.[68] Data from small studies suggest that, among women, those at increased risk include low-income pregnant women, particularly adolescents, and women who abuse alcohol.[69-71]

National data on the extent of vitamin B-12 deficiency anemia in the population are also lacking, but it is considered relatively rare, occurring primarily in elderly persons who have inadequate levels of the factor (intrinsic factor) necessary for the intestinal absorption of vitamin B-12, a condition referred to as pernicious anemia. The prevalence of pernicious anemia is highest among persons over 50 years of age and increases with increasing age. Among all persons over 60 years of age, the estimated prevalence of pernicious anemia is 1%.[72] Vitamin B-12 deficiency without anemia is more common among the elderly, affecting between 10 and 15% of elderly persons.[73,74]

At least one study reports a slightly increased occurrence of pernicious anemia among younger African American women compared to younger women of other racial and ethnic backgrounds; however, these data are limited and further study is warranted.[75] Among vegetarians who consume no animal products, a group at risk for vitamin B-12 depletion, the advanced stage of vitamin B-12 deficiency that characterizes megaloblastic anemia is extremely rare.

B. THE B VITAMINS AND ANEMIA

The hematologic manifestations of folate and vitamin B-12 deficiencies are indistinguishable because both vitamins are involved in DNA synthesis. Specifically, vitamin B-12 is an essential coenzyme in the transfer of a methyl group from methyl folate to homocysteine, an important step in regenerating tetrahydrofolic acid and the 5,10-methylene THFA involved in thymidylate and thus DNA synthesis. In folate deficiency, there is an inadequate supply of folate for conversion to tetrahydrofolic acid. In vitamin B-12 deficiency, folate is "trapped" as metabolically inactive methyl folate. In both deficiencies, DNA synthesis is impaired, leading to abnormal cell replication, hypersegmentation of neutrophils, macrocytosis, and megaloblastosis.

In addition to the essential role the two vitamins play in DNA synthesis, vitamin B-12 is also essential to myelin synthesis. Thus deficiency of vitamin

B-12, but not folate, can lead to impaired nerve function. The neurologic abnormalities of vitamin B-12 deficiency include paresthesias, impaired vibration sense, impaired touch or pain perception, ataxia, abnormal gait, memory loss, decreased reflexes and muscle strength, psychiatric disorders, disorientation, spasticity, and decreased vision or optic atrophy.[76,77] It is therefore of critical importance to determine the nutritional cause of the megaloblastic anemia before initiating treatment. Inappropriate treatment of a vitamin B-12 deficiency anemia with folic acid can mask the megaloblastic anemia. Masking of the anemia will interfere with the diagnosis of the vitamin B-12 deficiency, thus allowing neurologic manifestations to progress unnoticed. This is of much concern, especially because some of the neurologic manifestations can lead to permanent neurologic damage.[76,77]

The stages of folate deficiency leading to folate deficiency anemia are summarized in Table 8. Initially, serum folate levels begin to drop. This can occur after only 2 to 3 weeks of negative folate balance. As the deficiency progresses, red blood cell folate levels also fall, indicating folate depletion. Folate deficient erythropoiesis is characterized by an abnormal diagnostic deoxyuridine (dU) suppression test corrected *in vitro* by folates, which indicates of defective DNA synthesis, by decreased liver stores (<1.2 μg/g), and by hypersegmentation of the neutrophils (lobe average >3.5). When stores are severely depleted, folate deficiency anemia is observed. At this final stage of deficiency, macrocytic red blood cells can be observed in the circulating blood, MCV is elevated, hemoglobin is decreased, and megaloblasts are observed in the bone marrow. The anemia may occur months after the initial folate depletion. In a severe folate deficiency of very short duration, the anemia may occur sooner, even before red blood cell folate levels have a chance to decrease.

TABLE 8
Stages of Folate Deficiency

	Normal	Negative folate balance	Folate depletion	Folate deficient erythro-poiesis	Folate deficiency anemia
Serum folate	Normal	Low	Low	Low	Low
RBC folate	Normal	Normal	Low	Low	Low
dU suppression	Normal	Normal	Normal	Abnormal	Abnormal
Hypersegmentation	No	No	No	Yes	Yes
Liver folate	Normal	Normal	Low normal	Low	Low
Erythrocytes	Normal	Normal	Normal	Normal	Macroovalocytic
Mean cell volume	Normal	Normal	Normal	Normal	Elevated
Hemoglobin	Normal	Normal	Normal	Normal	Low

Modified from Herbert, V., *Am. J. Clin. Nutr.*, 46, 387, 1987. With permission.

The stages of vitamin B-12 deficiency that lead to anemia are summarized in Table 9. Initially, there is a decrease in the amount of vitamin B-12 absorbed, resulting in a decreased level of the vitamin B-12 transport protein transcobalamin (TC) II with attached vitamin B-12 (holotranscobalamin II) and a reduced percentage saturation of TC II. If the negative balance continues, serum vitamin B-12 levels are depressed and indicate vitamin B-12 depletion. The third stage of deficiency, vitamin B-12-deficient erythropoiesis, is marked by further reductions in the vitamin B-12 transport protein measures and serum vitamin B-12, an abnormal dU suppression test, and hypersegmentation of the neutrophils. Because of vitamin B-12's role in the transport and uptake of folate by the cells, red blood cell folate is also decreased during this stage. The final stage of deficiency is characterized by the presence of megaloblastic anemia.

TABLE 9
Stages of Vitamin B-12 Deficiency

	Normal	Negative vitamin B-12 balance	Vitamin B-12 depletion	Vitamin B-12 deficient erythropoiesis	Vitamin B-12 deficiency anemia
HoloTC II	Normal	Low	Low	Low	Low
TC II % saturation	Normal	Low	Low	Low	Low
Serum vitamin B-12	Normal	Normal	Normal	Low	Low
dU suppression	Normal	Normal	Normal	Abnormal	Abnormal
Hypersegmentation	No	No	No	Yes	Yes
RBC folate	Normal	Normal	Normal	Low	Low
Erythrocytes	Normal	Normal	Normal	Normal	Macroovalocytic
Mean cell volume	Normal	Normal	Normal	Normal	Elevated
Hemoglobin	Normal	Normal	Normal	Normal	Low

Modified from Herbert, V., *Am. J. Clin. Nutr.*, 46, 387, 1987. With permission.

C. FACTORS CONTRIBUTING TO FOLATE DEFICIENCY ANEMIA

The main cause of folate deficiency among U.S. women is inadequate dietary intake of the vitamin. Additional important causes include poor absorption of dietary folate and increased physiologic requirement for the nutrient. Less common causes of folate deficiency, including folate antagonists (e.g., methotrexate) and congenital or acquired enzyme deficiencies (inadequate folate utilization), renal dialysis (increased folate loss), and specific disease states and drugs, are discussed elsewhere.[78-80]

1. Inadequate Intake

Naturally occurring folate is widely distributed in food, the main sources being liver, yeast, fresh leafy vegetables and some fresh fruits, and legumes. Synthetic folic acid (pteroylglutamic acid) is also present in the food supply, primarily as an additive to breakfast cereals, some breakfast beverages, and dietary supplements. National food consumption surveys indicate that the average folate intake of U.S. women is approximately 200 μg/d.[81] Preliminary data from the third National Health and Nutrition Examination Survey indicate that average folate intakes are slightly increased to approximately 220 to 240 μg/d, with slightly higher intakes among Mexican American women.[31] Therefore, on average, folate intake is adequate to meet the 180 μg/d recommended for nonpregnant women,[82] but many women still do not consume enough folate to meet this level. In addition to poor food choices, overprocessing of foods contributes to inadequate folate ingestion. Approximately 50 to 95% of the folate in food may be destroyed by food processing and cooking.[78]

2. Poor Absorption

Folate is ingested in both the polyglutamate and monoglutamate form. Approximately 75% of naturally occurring folates in a typical U.S. diet are in the polyglutamate form.[82] These excess glutamic acid residues are split off by enzyme conjugases (pteroylpolyglutamate hydrolase) present in the brush border of the intestine. The formed monoglutamates are absorbed primarily through the jejunum by an energy-dependent, carrier-mediated process. The monoglutamate form of synthetic folic acid does not require hydrolysis and can be absorbed intact and more efficiently.[83]

The bioavailability of food folate is compromised by specific factors in the foods. For example, a factor in yeast and legumes inhibits the action of the intestinal enzyme conjugases. Overall, it is estimated that the bioavailability of food folate is approximately 50% that of crystalline folic acid, which is thought to be close to 100% bioavailable.[84] In formulating the RDA for folate, a 50% bioavailability of the food folate was considered.[82]

In general, folate malabsorption occurs under conditions that create an acidic pH of the intestinal environment, which inhibits the action of conjugase. Folate absorption is also impaired in malabsorption syndromes such as gluten-induced enteropathy and tropical sprue and as a result of ingestion of certain drugs, including salicylazosulfapyridine and diphenylhydantoin, and alcohol.[83]

3. Increased Requirement

The RDA for folate for U.S. women is 180 μg/d. Recommended intake is increased to 400 μg/d in pregnancy and to 280 μg/d during the first 6 months of lactation to provide the folate needed for normal fetal development and human milk production.[82] Needs are highest during the third trimester of pregnancy. It is possible to meet these increased requirements through diet, however, a high consumption of fresh fruits and vegetables and other folate-rich foods, including fortified breakfast cereals, would have to be included in the diet each day. This is not always practical. Oral folate supplements are recommended for those at high risk for deficiency, particularly pregnant women.

Folate requirements are also increased by infection, the growth of malignant tumors, and increased hematopoiesis. Alcohol consumption increases folate requirements through its interference with folate utilization.[78]

D. FACTORS CONTRIBUTING TO VITAMIN B-12 DEFICIENCY ANEMIA

The main cause of vitamin B-12 deficiency anemia in the U.S. is impaired absorption of the nutrient. To better understand impaired absorption of vitamin B-12 and its effects, the main aspects of absorption are briefly outlined below.

Initially, gastric acid and gastric and intestinal enzymes work to release the ingested vitamin B-12 from polypeptide linkages in food. The vitamin B-12 then binds to salivary R binder polypeptides (nonintrinsic factor), a linkage that is later broken when the R binders are destroyed in the intestine by pancreatic trypsin acting at an alkaline pH. This separation allows the free vitamin B-12 to combine with intrinsic factor (IF), a protein produced by normal gastric parietal cells. The vitamin B-12 intrinsic factor complex is then absorbed through the wall of the ileum in the presence of calcium and at a pH greater than 6.[78,85]

Vitamin B-12 absorption is impaired under conditions that affect the function of intrinsic factor and under conditions that alter the conditions of the ileum. Pancreatic disease also affects the conditions for absorption. Specific drugs, including para-aminosalicylic acid, colchicine, neomycin, ethanol, and metformin, also decrease vitamin B-12 absorption. Oral contraceptive agents may also impair absorption of the vitamin. Deficiency as a result of poor absorption can occur 3 to 6 years after absorption is impaired.[85]

In addition to vitamin B-12 deficiency resulting from poor absorption, a deficiency of the vitamin itself can also produce poor absorption. Specifically, the megaloblastosis that occurs in vitamin B-12 and folate deficiencies affects all cells, including those of the intestinal lumen, causing atrophy of the intestinal absorptive cells.[85]

Vitamin B-12 deficiency anemia due to poor absorption as a result of insufficient secretion of intrinsic factor is specifically referred to as pernicious anemia. Approximately half of all adult cases of pernicious anemia result from acquired gastric atrophy as an end result of inflammatory gastritis.[78]

Pernicious anemia is diagnosed with the Schilling test.[86,87] If the first part of the test indicates vitamin B-12 malabsorption, which is corrected by the addition of intrinsic factor in the follow-up test, pernicious anemia is indicated. If the malabsorption is not corrected, other etiologies of the malabsorption are suspected, such as an ileal or pancreatic defect or parasitic infestation (e.g., fish tapeworm). For the elderly, who lose their ability to split vitamin B-12 off from food as they age, it is important to perform the first part of the test with food rather than crystalline vitamin B-12.

Vitamin B-12 deficiency caused by inadequate intake of the nutrient is very rare but can occur in strict vegetarians who consume no foods of animal origin and no supplemental source of vitamin B-12.[88,89] Among persons consuming no animal products, vitamin B-12 depletion occurs slowly because the body recycles any vitamin B-12 that is ingested, including the small amount found in foods contaminated by microorganisms.

Much less common causes of vitamin B-12 deficiency, including vitamin B-12 antagonists, congenital or acquired enzyme deficiencies or deletions, abnormalities in the binding proteins, and specific diseases and drugs, are reviewed elsewhere.[78-80]

E. ASSESSING THE ETIOLOGY OF NUTRITIONAL MEGALOBLASTIC ANEMIA

When it is apparent from initial studies of cell morphology or other laboratory measures that the observed anemia is not due to iron deficiency, an inquiry into other possible causes of anemia should be undertaken. Inquiry into other possible causes should also be done in the presence of iron deficiency because the macrocytosis of folate and vitamin B-12 deficiency could be masked by a concurrent iron deficiency.

If abnormally large red blood cells or if hypersegmentation of neutrophils are observed on the peripheral blood smear, folate or vitamin B-12 deficiency anemia is suspected. The evaluation of neutrophil hypersegmentation is useful (in nonpregnant women) because it is apparent even if the macrocytosis is masked by iron deficiency. If it is known that the diet of the individual or the population contains no animal foods, vitamin B-12 deficiency would be suspected. However, because a concurrent folate deficiency could also be present, diagnostic tests for both deficiencies should still be undertaken.

The presence of macrocytosis is confirmed by measuring MCV, which is reviewed in Table 6. If the red cell measure is elevated, a bone marrow biopsy may be performed to confirm the presence of megaloblasts (abnormally large red cell precursors) in the bone marrow. Once megaloblastic anemia is confirmed, additional laboratory tests are performed to determine whether the etiology of the anemia is folate or vitamin B-12 deficiency.[90]

Serum and RBC folate and serum vitamin B-12 are routinely measured as a battery to differentiate between folate and vitamin B-12 deficiency as the nutritional cause of the megaloblastic anemia (Table 10). In general, serum folate levels are low (usually <3.0 ng/ml) in folate deficiency anemia, but can also be low in the absence of deficiency because serum levels of folate are very sensitive to recent changes in folate intake and metabolism.[91] Serum folate is also lowered as a result of alcohol consumption[92] and cigarette smoking.[90] Studies on the effect of oral contraceptive use on serum folate levels have had inconsistent findings.[93]

TABLE 10
Three Common Assays Used in Differentiating Folate
and Vitamin B-12 Deficiency Anemia

Clinical situation	Serum folate	Red cell folate	Serum Vitamin B-12
Folate deficiency anemia	Low	Low	Generally normal, but may be low
Vitamin B-12 deficiency anemia	Generally normal, but may be high	Low	Low
Folate and vitamin B-12 deficiency anemia	Low	Low	Low

Modified from Herbert, V., *Clinical Nutrition*, 2nd ed., Paige, D., Ed., C. V. Mosby, St. Louis, 1988, 593. With permission.

Red blood cell folate concentration, a more stable measure that reflects liver stores of the nutrient, is usually low (generally <100 ng/ml) in folate deficiency anemia,[78,91] unless the progression was very rapid, which may occur in the megaloblastic anemia of pregnancy. In addition, red blood cell folate concentrations are depressed in vitamin B-12 deficiency because vitamin B-12 is involved in the transport and storage of folate in cells.[94,95]

A low serum vitamin B-12 alone is insufficient evidence to conclude that a megaloblastic anemia is due to vitamin B-12 deficiency alone. A normal vitamin B-12 level (>100 pg/ml) in the presence of low serum or red blood cell folate concentrations suggests a primary folate deficiency; however, low levels on all three vitamin assays do not rule out a primary folate deficiency. Approximately one third of individuals with megaloblastic anemia due to primary folate deficiency have low serum vitamin B-12 levels that are restored in 7 to 10 d of folate treatment. The reason for this finding is unknown.[86]

The *in vitro* dU suppression test is a more precise test to distinguish between folate and vitamin B-12-deficient anemia.[85,91,96] The test is designed to assess defective DNA synthesis in cultured bone marrow cells. The general principle of the test is based on the fact that normal folate metabolism is necessary in the methylation of dU to thymidine. Folate or vitamin B-12 is added to separate cell cultures to determine which vitamin corrects the test results. Although the addition of folate corrects the test results for folate and vitamin B-12-deficient cultures, the addition of vitamin B-12 partially corrects the results in the vitamin B-12 deficiency culture and does not correct the results in the folate-deficient culture. An advantage of this test is that the results are not affected by a concurrent iron deficiency or other confounding disease states; however, the difficulty of the test makes it impractical for routine use.

The measurement of serum (or urinary) methylmalonic acid (MMA) is particularly useful in determining the cause of megaloblastic anemia because the test is specific to vitamin B-12 deficiency. A vitamin B-12-containing coenzyme is essential for the conversion of methylmalonyl-coenzyme A to succinyl-coenzyme A. Thus, an inadequate supply of vitamin B-12 results in the accumulation of MMA in the serum. It is estimated that an elevated serum MMA is found in over 90% of persons with vitamin B-12 deficiency.[73,97,98] A disadvantage of the test is that, like the dU suppression test, the laboratory procedures involved are difficult and not practical for all settings.

Additional laboratory measures of interest in assessing folate and vitamin B-12 deficiency include the FIGLU test, which measures urinary excretion of formiminoglutamic acid (FIGLU) and serum homocysteine levels.[97,98] However, these measures are of limited use in differentiating between the two vitamin deficiencies that cause megaloblastic anemia, because levels of both metabolites are elevated in both folate and vitamin B-12 deficiency.

F. PREVENTION AND TREATMENT

Folate deficiency and folate deficiency anemia are prevented by providing adequate dietary folate to meet requirements. This is accomplished through a choice of folate-rich foods and minimal processing of the foods before consumption. Dietary folates should come from a variety of sources, not solely from folate-rich foods that contain conjugase inhibitors. High-risk women, specifically pregnant women, should be counseled on how to improve their folate intake through diet and supplements. More comprehensive and aggressive intervention is required to prevent and treat folate deficiency among alcoholics. Although improved dietary intake is important, the first priority should be to treat the alcohol addiction.

In the 1970s, fortification of the food supply with folic acid had been suggested to improve the folate status of the U.S. population;[100] however, to date there is no general food fortification program. Currently, individual foods, such as breakfast cereals and some breakfast beverages, are fortified with up to 400 µg of folic acid per serving. Recently, folic acid fortification of the U.S. cereal grain supply has been proposed to reduce a woman's risk of having a neural tube defect-affected pregnancy.[101,102] While the main purpose of this program is to reduce a woman's risk of a neural tube defect-affected pregnancy, it may also benefit women in terms of improving their folate status.

Among women who absorb adequate amounts of vitamin B-12, deficiency is avoided by the consumption of foods of animal origin, including meat, fish, poultry, and milk. Women who consume no animal products should be advised to take supplemental vitamin B-12. This is especially important for pregnant and lactating women. Women who do not absorb adequate amounts of vitamin B-12 should receive periodic injections of the vitamin.

Treatment for megaloblastic anemia due to folate and vitamin B-12 deficiencies will vary according to the cause of the underlying deficiency and to the presence of concurrent illnesses and nutrient deficiencies. The appropriate treatment should be administered under the care of a clinician.

REFERENCES

1. Beutler, E., The common anemias, *J.A.M.A*, 259, 2433, 1988.
2. De Maeyer, E. and Adiels-Tegman, M., The prevalence of anaemia in the world, *World Health Stat. Q.*, 38, 302, 1985.
3. World Health Organization, *The Prevalence of Anaemia in Women: A Tabulation of Available Information*, 2nd Ed., WHO, Geneva, Switzerland, 1992, 1.
4. MacPhail, P. and Bothwell, T. H., The prevalence and causes of nutritional iron deficiency anemia, in *Nutritional Anemias*, Fomon, S. J. and Zlotkin, S., Eds., Nestle Nutrition Workshop Series, Vol. 30, Raven Press, New York, 1992, 1.
5. Cook, J. D., Skikne, B. S., and Reussner, M. E., Estimates of iron sufficiency in the US population, *Blood*, 68, 726, 1986.
6. Kim, I., Hungerford, D. W., Yip, R., Kuester, S. A., Zyrkowski, C., and Trowbridge, F. L., Pregnancy nutrition surveillance system — United States, 1979-1990, CDC surveillance summaries, *Morbid. Mortal. Wkly. Rep.*, 41, 26, 1992.
7. Oski, F. A., Anemia related to nutritional deficiencies other than vitamin B_{12} and folic acid, in *Hematology*, 3rd Ed., Willams, W. J., Beutler, E., Erslev, A. J., and Lichtman, M. A., Eds., McGraw-Hill, New York, 1983, chap. 53.
8. United Nations ACC/SCN, *Second Report on the World Nutrition Situation, Vol 1: Global and Regional Results*, ACC/SCN, Geneva, 1992.
9. Pilch, S. M. and Senti, F. R., Eds., *Assessment of the Iron Nutritional Status of the U.S. Population Based on Data Collected in the Second National Health and Nutrition Examination Survey, 1976–1980*, Life Sciences Research Office, Federation of American Societies for Experimental Biology, Bethesda, 1984, 1.
10. Institute of Medicine, *Nutrition During Pregnancy*, National Academy Press, Washington, D.C., 1990, 272.
11. Bothwell, T. H. and Charlton, R. W., *Iron deficiency in women*, report of the International Nutritional Anemia Consultative Group (INACG), Nutrition Foundation, Washington, D.C., 1981.
12. Herbert, V., The 1986 Herman Award Lecture. Nutrition science as a continually unfolding story: the folate and vitamin B-12 paradigm, *Am. J. Clin. Nutr.*, 46, 387, 1987.
13. Lieberman, E., Ryan, K. J., Monsen, R. R., and Schoenbaum, S. C., Association of maternal hematocrit with premature labor, *Am. J. Obstet. Gynecol.*, 159, 107, 1988.
14. Garn, S. M., Ridella, S. A., Petzold, A. S., and Falkner, F., Maternal hematological levels and pregnancy outcomes, *Semin. Perinatol.*, 5, 155, 1981.
15. Klebanoff, M. A., Shiono, P. H., Selby, J. V., Trachtenberg, A. I., and Graubard, B. I., Anemia and spontaneous preterm birth, *Am. J. Obstet. Gynecol.*, 164, 59, 1991.
16. Scholl, T. O., Hediger, M. L., Fischer, R. L., and Shearer, J. W., Anemia vs. iron deficiency: increased risk of preterm delivery in a prospective study, *Am. J. Clin. Nutr.*, 55, 985, 1992.
17. Viteri, F. E. and Torun, B., Anemia and physical work capacity, in *Clinics in Hematology*, Vol. 3, Garby, L., Ed., W. B. Saunders, London, 1974, 609.
18. Davies, C. T. M., Chukweumeka, A. C., and van Haaren, J. P. M., Iron-deficiency anemia: its effect on maximum aerobic power and responses to exercise in African males aged 17–40 years, *Clin. Sci.*, 44, 555, 1973.
19. Basta, S. S., Soekirman, M., Karayadi, D., and Scrimshaw, N. S., Iron deficiency anemia and the productivity of adult males in Indonesia, *Am. J. Clin. Nutr.*, 32, 916, 1979.
20. Bradley, D. J., Rahmathullah, L., and Narayan, R., The tea plantation as a research ecosystem, in *Capacity for Work in the Tropics*, Collin, K. J. and Roberts, D. F., Eds., University Press, New York, 1988, 277.
21. Dillman, E., Mackler, B., Johnson, D., Brengelman, G., Green, W., Gale, C., Martin, J., Layrisse, M., Martinez-Torres, C., and Finch, C., Effect of iron deficiency on catecholamine metabolism and body temperature regulation, in Iron Deficiency: Brain Biochemistry and Behaviour, Pollitt, E. and Leibel, R. L., Eds., Raven Press, New York, 1982, 57.

22. Martinez-Tores, C., Cubeddu, L., Dillman, E., Brengelman, G. L., Leets, I., Layrisse, M., Johnson, D. G., and Finch, C., Effective exposure to low temperature on normal and iron deficient subjects, *Am. J. Physiol.*, 246, R380, 1984.

23. Clark, M., Royal, J., and Seeler, R., Interaction of iron deficiency and lead and hematologic findings in children with severe lead poisoning, *Pediatrics*, 81, 247, 1988.

24. Dallman, P. R., Siimes, M. A., and Stekel, A., Iron deficiency in infancy and childhood, *Am. J. Clin. Nutr.*, 33, 86, 1980.

25. Watson, W. S., Hume, R. M., and Moore, M. R., Oral absorption of lead and iron, *Lancet*, ii, 236, 1980.

26. Yip, R., Multiple interactions between childhood iron deficiency and lead poisoning: evidence that childhood lead poisoning is an adverse consequence of iron deficiency, in *Recent Knowledge on Iron and Folate Deficiencies in the World*, Vol. 197, Hercberg, S., Galan, P., and Dupin, H., Eds., Colloque INSERM, Paris, 1990, 523.

27. U.S. Preventive Task Force, Routine iron supplementation during pregnancy: policy statement, *J.A.M.A.*, 270, 2846, 1993.

28. Politt, E. and Metallinos-Katsaras, E., Iron deficiency and behavior: constructs, methods, and validity of the findings, *Nutr. Brain*, 8, 101, 1990.

29. Groner, J. A., Holtzman, E., Charney, E., and Mellits, D. E., A randomized trial of oral iron on tests of short-term memory and attention span in young pregnant women, *J. Adolescent Health Care*, 7, 44, 1986.

30. Life Sciences Research Office, Federation of American Societies for Experimental Biology, Nutrition Monitoring in the United States — An Update Report on Nutrition Monitoring, DHHS Publication No. (PHS) 89-1255, Public Health Service, U.S. Government Printing Office, Washington, D.C., 1989, 62.

31. Alaimo, K., McDowell, M. A., Briefel, R. R., Bischof, A. M., Caughman, C. R., Loria, C. M., and Johnson, C. L., Dietary Intake of Vitamins, Minerals, and Fiber of Persons Ages 2 Months and Over in the United States: Third National Health and Nutrition Examination Survey, Phase 1, 1988–91, Advance Data from Vital and Health Statistics, No. 258, National Center for Health Statistics, Hyattsville, 1994.

32. National Research Council, *Recommended Dietary Allowances*, 10th ed., National Academy Press, Washington, D.C., 1989, chap. 10.

33. Moss, A. J., Levy, A. S., Kim, I., and Park, Y. K., Use of Vitamin and Mineral Supplements in the United States: Current Users, Types of Products, and Nutrients, Advance Data from Vital and Health Statistics, No. 174, National Center for Health Statistics, Hyattsville, 1989.

34. Bothwell, T. H., Baynes, R. D., MacFarlane, B. J., and MacPhail, A. P., Nutritional iron requirements and food iron absorption, *J. Int. Med.*, 226, 357, 1989.

35. Cook, J. D., Dassenki, S. A., and Lynch, S. R., Assessment of the role of non-heme iron availability in iron balance, *Am. J. Clin. Nutr.*, 54, 717, 1991.

36. Hallberg, L., Brune, M., and Rossander, L., Iron absorption in man: ascorbic acid and dose-dependent inhibition by phytate, *Am. J. Clin. Nutr.*, 49, 140, 1989.

37. Morck, T. A. and Cook, J. D., Factors affecting the bioavailability of dietary iron, *Cereal Foods World*, 26, 667, 1981.

38. Gillooly, M., Bothwell, T. H., Torrance, J. D., MacPhail, A. P., Derman, D. P., Bezwoda, W. R., Mills, W., and Charlton, R. W., The effects of organic acids, phytates, and polyphenols on the absorption of iron from vegetables, *Br. J. Nutr.*, 49, 331, 1983.

39. Siegenberg, D., Baynes, R. D., Bothwell, T. H., Macfarlane, B. J., Lamparelli, R. D., Car, N. G., MacPhail, P., Schmidt, U., Tal, A., and Mayet, F., Ascorbic acid prevents the dose-dependent inhibitory effects of phenols and phytates on non-heme iron absorption, *Am. J. Clin. Nutr.*, 53, 537, 1991.

40. Hallberg, L., Brune, M., and Rossander, L., Effect of ascorbic acid on iron absorption from different types of meals. Studies with ascorbic acid given in different amounts with different meals, *Ann. Nutr. Appl. Nutr.*, 40A, 97, 1986.

41. Charlton, R. W. and Bothwell, T. H., Iron absorption, *Annu. Rev. Med.*, 34, 55, 1983.
42. Lönnerdal, B., Keen, C. L., and Hurley, L. S., Iron, copper, zinc, and manganese in milk, *Annu. Rev. Nutr.*, 1, 149, 1981.
43. Habicht, J. P., DaVanzo, J., Butz, W. P., and Meyers, L., The contraceptive role of breastfeeding, *Popul. Stud.*, 39, 213, 1985.
44. Hallberg, L., Iron balance in pregnancy, in *Vitamins and Minerals in Pregnancy and Lactation*, Berger, H., Ed., Raven Press, New York, 1988, 115.
45. Bothwell, T. H., Charlton, R. W., Cook, J. D., and Finch, C. A., *Iron Metabolism in Man*, Blackwell Scientific, Oxford, 1979, 21.
46. Chanarin, I. and Rothman, D., Further observations on the relation between iron and folate status in pregnancy, Br. Med. J., 2, 81, 1971.
47. Svanberg, B., Arvidsson, B., Norrby, A., Rybo, G., and Sölvell, L., Absorption of supplemental iron during pregnancy — a longitudinal study with repeated bone-marrow studies and absorption measurements, *Acta Obstet. Gynecol. Scand. Suppl.*, 48, 87, 1976.
48. Puolakka, J., Jänne, O., Pakarinen, A., and Vihko, R., Serum ferritin as a measure of stores during and after normal pregnancy with and without iron supplements, *Acta Obstet. Gynecol. Scand. Suppl.*, 95, 43, 1980.
49. Taylor, D. J., Mallen, C., McDougall, N., and Lind, T., Effect of iron supplementation on serum ferritin levels during and after pregnancy, *Br. J. Obstet. Gynecol.*, 89, 1011, 1982.
50. Romslo, I., Haram, K., Sagen, N., and Augensen, K., Iron requirements in normal pregnancy as assessed by serum ferritin, serum transferrin saturation, and erythrocyte protoporphyrin determinations, *Br. J. Obstet. Gynecol.*, 90, 101, 1983.
51. Wallenburg, H. C. S. and van Eijk, H. G., Effect of oral iron supplementation during pregnancy on maternal and fetal iron status, *J. Perinat. Med.*, 12, 7, 1984.
52. Dawson, E. B. and McGanity, W. J., Protection of maternal iron stores in pregnancy, *J. Reprod. Med.*, 32, 478, 1987.
53. Bothwell, T. H., Charlton, R. W., Cook, J. D., and Finch, C. A., *Iron Metabolism in Man*, Blackwell Scientific, Oxford, 1979, 251.
54. Hallberg, L., Högdahl, A. M., Nilsson, L., and Rybo, G., Menstrual blood loss — a population study. Variation at different ages and attempts to define normality, *Acta Obstet. Gynecol. Scand.*, 45, 320, 1966.
55. Cole, S. K., Billewicz, W. Z., and Thompson, A. M., Sources of variation in blood loss, *J. Obstet. Gynaecol. Br. Commonw.*, 78, 933, 1971.
56. Göltner, E., Iron requirement and deficiency in menstruating and pregnant women, in *Iron Metabolism and Its Disorders*, Kief, H., Ed., Exerpta Medica, Amsterdam, 1975, 159.
57. Rockey, D. C. and Cello, J. P., Evaluation of the gastrointestinal tract in patients with iron-deficiency anemia, *N. Engl. J. Med.*, 329, 1691, 1993.
58. Centers for Disease Control, CDC criteria for anemia in children and childbearing-aged women, *Morbid. Mortal. Wkly. Rep.*, 38, 400, 1989.
59. Binkin, N. and Yip, R., When is anemia screening of value in detecting iron deficiency?, in *Recent Knowledge on Iron Deficiency and Folate Deficiencies in the World*, Vol. 197, Hercberg, S., Galan, P., and Dupin, H., Eds., Colloque INSERM, Paris, 1990, 137.
60. Cook, J. D. and Finch, C. A., Assessing iron status of a population, *Am. J. Clin. Nutr.*, 32, 2115, 1979.
61. Ferguson, B. J., Skigne, B. S., Simpson, K. M., Baynes, R. D., and Cook, J. D., Serum transferrin receptor distinguishes the anemia of chronic disease from iron deficiency anemia, *J. Lab. Clin. Med.*, 119, 385, 1992.
62. Cook, J. D., Garriaga, M., Kahn, S. G., Schalch, W., and Skikne, B., Gastric delivery system for iron supplementation, *Lancet*, 335, 1136, 1990.
63. Galloway, R., *Supplies, Side Effects or Psychology? Determinants of Compliance with Iron Supplementation in Pregnancy*, World Bank, Washington, D.C., 1991, 1.

64. Hallberg, L., Iron balance in pregnancy and lactation, in *Nutritional Anemias*, Fomon, S. J. and Zlotkin, S., Eds., Nestle Nutrition Workshop Series, Vol. 30, Raven Press, New York, 1992, 13.

65. Hurrell, R. F., Prospects for improving the iron fortification of foods, in *Nutritional Anemias*, Forman, S. J. and Zlotkin, S., Eds., Raven Press, New York, 1992, 193.

66. Phatak, P. D., Guzman, G., Woll, J. E., Robeson, A., and Phelps, C. E., Cost-effectiveness of screening for hereditary hemochromatosis, *Arch. Intern. Med.*, 154, 769, 1994.

67. Institute of Medicine, *Iron Deficiency Anemia: Recommended Guidelines for the Prevention, Detection, and Management among U.S. Children and Women of Childbearing Age*, Earl, R. and Woteki, C. E., Eds., National Academy Press, Washington, D.C., 1993, 1.

68. Senti, F. R. and Pilch, S. M., Eds., *Assessment of the Folate Nutritional Status of the U.S. Population Based on Data Collected in the Second National Health and Nutrition Examination Survey, 1976–1980*, Life Sciences Research Office, Federation of American Societies for Experimental Biology, Bethesda, 1984, 1.

69. Shojania, A. M., Folic acid and vitamin B-12 deficiency in pregnancy and in the neonatal period, *Clin. Perinatol.*, 11, 433, 1984.

70. Bailey, L. B., Mahan, C. S., and Dimperio, D., Folacin and iron status in low-income pregnant adolescent and mature women, *Am. J. Clin. Nutr.*, 33, 1997, 1980.

71. Savage, D. and Lindenbaum, J., Anemia in alcoholics, *Medicine*, 65, 322, 1986.

72. Chanarin, I., *The Megaloblastic Anemias*, 3rd ed., Blackwell Scientific, Oxford, 1990, chap. 10.

73. Lindenbaum, J., Rosenberg, I. H., Wilson, P. W. F., Stabler, S. P., and Allen, R. H., Prevalence of cobalamin deficiency in the Framingham elderly population, *Am. J. Clin. Nutr.*, 60, 2, 1994.

74. Pennypacker, L. C., Alen, R. H., Kelly, J. P., Matthews, L. M., Grigsby, J., Kaye, K., Lindenbaum, J., and Stabler, S. P., High prevalence of cobalamin deficiency in elderly outpatients, *J. Am. Geriatr. Soc.*, 40, 1197, 1992.

75. Carmel, R. and Johnson, C. S., Racial patterns in pernicious anemia: early age at onset and increased frequency of intrinsic-factor antibody in black women, *N. Engl. J. Med.*, 298, 647, 1978.

76. Lindenbaum, J., Healton, E. B., Savage, D. G., Brust, J. C. M., Garrett, T. J., Podell, E. R., Marcell, P. D., Stabler, S. P., and Allen, R. H., Neuropsychiatric disorders caused by cobalamin deficiency in the absence of anemia or macrocytosis, *N. Engl. J. Med.*, 318, 1720, 1988.

77. Healton, E. B., Savage, D. G., Brust, J. C. M., Garrett, T. J., and Lindenbaum, J., Neurologic aspects of cobalamin deficiency, *Medicine*, 70, 229, 1991.

78. Herbert, V. and Das, K. C., Folic acid and vitamin B-12, in *Modern Nutrition in Health and Disease*, 8th ed., Shils, M. E., Olson, J. A., and Shike, M., Eds., Lea & Febiger, Philadelphia, 1994, 402.

79. Chanarin, I., *The Megaloblastic Anemias*, 3rd ed., Blackwell Scientific, Oxford, 1990, 1.

80. Beck, W. S., Megaloblastic anemias, in *Cecil Textbook of Medicine*, 18th ed., Wyngaarden, J. B. and Smith, L. H., Eds., W. B. Saunders, Philadelphia, 1988, 900.

81. Subar, A. F., Block, G., and James, L. D., Folate intake and food sources in the U.S. population, *Am. J. Clin. Nutr.*, 50, 508, 1989.

82. National Research Council, *Recommended Dietary Allowances*, 10th ed., National Academy Press, Washington, D.C., 1989, chap. 8.

83. Halsted, C. H., Intestinal absorption of dietary folates, in *Folic Acid Metabolism in Health and Disease*, Picciano, M. F., Stokstad, E. L. R., and Gregory, J. F., III, Eds., Wiley-Liss, New York, 1990, 23.

84. Sauberlich, H. E., Kretsch, M. J., Skala, J. H., Johnson, H. L., and Taylor, P. C., Folate requirement and metabolism in nonpregnant women, *Am. J. Clin. Nutr.*, 46, 1016, 1987.

85. Herbert, V. Anemias, in *Clinical Nutrition*, 2nd Edition, Paige, D., Ed., C. V. Mosby, St. Louis, 1988, 593.

86. Chanarin, I., *The Megaloblastic Anemias*, 3rd ed., Blackwell Scientific, Oxford, 1990, chap. 4.

87. Schilling, R. F., Intrinsic factor studies. II. The effect of gastric juice on the urinary excretion of radioactivity after oral administration of radioactive vitamin B-12, *J. Lab. Clin. Med.*, 42, 860, 1953.

88. Rose, M., Vitamin B-12 deficiency in Asian immigrants [letter], *Lancet*, 2, 681, 1976.

89. Chanarin, I., Malkowska, V., O'Hea, A.-M., Rinsler, M. G., and Price, A. B., Megaloblastic anemia in a vegetarian Hindu community, *Lancet*, ii, 1168, 1985.

90. Gibson, R. S., *Principles of Nutritional Assessment*, Oxford University Press, New York, 1990, chap. 22.

91. Herbert, V., Making sense of laboratory tests of folate status: folate requirements to sustain normality, *Am. J. Hematol.*, 26, 199, 1987.

92. Hillman, R. S., McGuffin, R., and Campbell, C., Alcohol interference with the folate enterohepatic cycle, *Trans. Assoc. Am. Physicians*, 90, 145, 1977.

93. Chanarin, I., *The Megaloblastic Anemias*, 3rd ed., Blackwell Scientific, Oxford, 1990, chap. 22.

94. Tisman, G. and Herbert, V., B-12 dependence of cell uptake of serum folate: an explanation for high serum folate and cell folate depletion in B-12 deficiency, *Blood*, 41, 465, 1973.

95. Allen, R. H., Human vitamin B-12 transport proteins, *Prog. Hematol.*, 9, 57, 1975.

96. Das, K. C. and Herbert, V., In vitro DNA synthesis by megaloblastic bone marrow, effect of folates and cobalamin on thymidine incorporation and de novo thymidylate synthesis, *Am. J. Hematol.*, 31, 11, 1989.

97. Allen, R. H., Stabler, S. P., Savage, D. G., and Lindenbaum, J., Diagnosis of cobalamin deficiency. I. Usefulness of serum methylmalonic acid and total homocysteine concentrations, *Am. J. Hematol.*, 34, 90, 1990.

98. Lindenbaum, J., Savage, D. G., Stabler, S. P., and Allen, R. H., Diagnosis of cobalamin deficiency. II. Sensitivity of serum cobalamin, methylmalonic acid, and total homocysteine concentrations, *Am. J. Hematol.*, 34, 99, 1990.

99. Stabler, S. P., Allen, R. H., Savage, D. G., and Lindenbaum, J., Clinical spectrum and diagnosis of cobalamin deficiency, *Blood*, 76, 871, 1990.

100. Food and Nutrition Board, NAS, *Proposed Fortification Policy for Cereal-Grain Products*, National Academy of Sciences, Washington, D.C., 1974, 1.

101. Food and Drug Administration, Food standards: amendment to the standards of identity for enriched grain products to require addition of folic acid (Docket No. 91N-100S), *Fed. Reg.*, 58, 53305, 1993.

102. Centers for Disease Control, Recommendations for the use of folic acid to reduce the number of cases of spina bifida and other neural tube defects, *Morbid. Mortal. Wkly. Rep.*, 41, 1, 1992.

Chapter 6

OBESITY AND EVALUATION OF WEIGHT CONTROL PROGRAMS

Judith S. Stern and Paul R. Thomas

CONTENTS

I. INTRODUCTION

Obesity is a disease that is a particular burden for women. Compared to men, nonobese women are fatter, a greater percentage of women are overweight, and women bear a greater psychological burden with respect to the social pressures to be thin and social consequences of obesity.

We are in the midst of an obesity epidemic in the U.S. with 35% of adult women and 31% of adult men aged 20 years and older considered obese.[1] Obesity is a disease linked to increased morbidity and mortality.[2] For 1990, it was estimated that there were from 309,000 to 582,000 diet/activity related deaths per year.[3] The economic cost of obesity in the U.S. in terms of health costs and money spent on weight-reduction products is estimated to be $100 billion/year.[2]

Given the costs of obesity it is surprising that there are not uniform standards used to develop and to evaluate weight management programs. New York City, the state of Michigan, and the National Institutes of Health (NIH) have independently developed standards, but these have not been accepted widely by programs or clients.[4-8] The Federal Trade Commission (FTC) has focused on advertising claims and the Federal Drug Administration (FDA) in January 1995 was in the process of reviewing guidance for development and use of prescription drugs in the treatment of obesity.[9,10] The Institute of Medicine (IOM) has issued a report, *Weighing The Options*, which contains uniform criteria for evaluating weight management programs that can be applied by clients, programs, and regulatory agencies (e.g., FTC, FDA).[2] This chapter summarizes these efforts.

II. OBESITY: DEFINITION AND ASSESSMENT

Obesity and overweight are two terms that are often used interchangeably.[2] *Obesity* is defined as an excess of body fat. In contrast, the term *overweight* refers to an excess of total body weight with respect to height. It is possible for some individuals to be overweight but not obese (e.g., athletes with increased muscle mass) or obese and not overweight (e.g., very sedentary people and some elderly with decreased muscle mass). For practical reasons, many researchers and clinicians use obesity and overweight interchangeably.

One of the more common techiques for assessing overweight is to use the body mass index (BMI). BMI is calculated by dividing weight in kilograms by height in meters squared (BMI = kg/m^2). Table 1 expresses BMI in terms of weight in pounds and height in inches.

The National Center for Health Statistics (NCHS) has identified the *cutting edge* for overweight by using the extremes of the distribution of BMI for young adults aged 20 to 29 years. Data for these cut points were collected as a result of the National Health and Nutrition Examination Survey conducted during 1976 to 1980 (NHANES II). Overweight corresponds to the sex-specific 85th percentile and severe overweight corresponds to the 95th percentile for BMI (27.3 and 32.3 for females; 27.8 and 31.1 for males, respectively). Also using BMI, the NIH National Task Force on Prevention and Treatment of Obesity stated that adults are obese if BMI is 25 for younger adults (through age 34) and 27 for older adults (greater than age 34).[8]

TABLE 1

Body Mass Index According to Height (in Inches) and Weight (in Pounds)

Height (in.)	Body mass index													
	20	21	22	23	24	25	26	27	28	29	30	35	40	45	50
	Body weight (lb)														
58	95	100	105	110	114	119	124	129	133	138	143	167	191	214	238
59	99	104	109	114	119	124	129	134	139	144	149	174	198	223	248
60	102	107	112	117	122	127	132	138	143	148	153	178	204	229	255
61	106	111	117	122	127	132	138	143	148	154	159	185	212	238	265
62	109	114	120	125	130	136	141	147	152	158	163	190	217	245	272
63	113	119	124	130	135	141	147	152	158	164	169	198	226	254	282
64	117	123	129	135	141	146	152	158	164	170	176	205	234	264	293
65	120	126	132	138	144	150	156	162	168	174	180	210	240	270	300
66	124	131	137	143	149	156	162	168	174	180	187	218	249	280	311
67	127	134	140	147	153	159	166	172	178	185	191	223	255	287	319
68	132	139	145	152	158	165	172	178	185	191	198	231	264	297	330
69	135	142	149	155	162	169	176	182	189	196	203	236	270	304	338
70	140	147	154	161	168	175	182	189	196	203	210	244	279	314	349
71	143	150	157	164	171	179	186	193	200	207	214	250	286	321	357
72	148	155	162	170	177	185	192	199	207	214	221	258	295	332	369
73	151	158	166	174	181	189	196	204	211	219	226	264	302	340	377
74	156	164	171	179	187	195	203	210	218	226	234	273	312	351	390
75	159	167	175	183	191	199	207	215	223	231	239	279	318	358	398
76	164	172	181	189	197	205	214	222	230	238	246	287	328	370	411

Note: BMI is calculated by dividing weight in kilograms by height in meters squared (BMI = kg/m^2).

Modified from Reference 2.

Using NCHS cut point of 27.3 for overweight, data from the most recent governmental nationwide survey (NHANES III, 1988 to 1991) established that in adult women percent overweight increases with age, peaks at ages 55 to 64 years, and decreases at ages 65 to 74 years (Figure 1). This represents an increase in prevalence from the two previous NHANES surveys. Clearly, the U.S. is moving farther away from the year 2000 goal proposed by the federal government that no more than 20% of adults aged 20 years and over be overweight.[11] Prevalence of obesity also varies by race. In comparison to white-nonhispanic females (32.1%), the prevalence of obesity is higher in black and Mexican American females (48.5 and 47.2%, respectively) (Figure 2).[2] For women in developed countries, there is a strong inverse relationship between socioeconomic status (SES) and obesity.[12] Women with the lowest SES tend to be more obese than women with the highest SES. The relationship is reversed in developing countries.[12]

There is much speculation as to why the 20th century has seen a sharp increase in the prevalence of obesity, especially in women. Throughout most of human history, food has been relatively scarce. It has been speculated that genetic traits that cause fatness would be selected in times of food scarcity

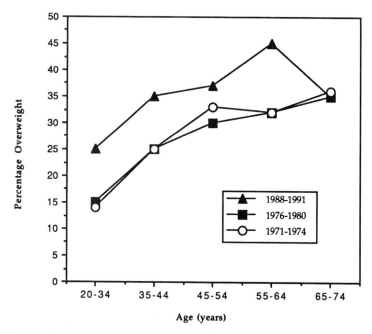

FIGURE 1.   Percentage of overweight women 20 to 74 years of age from NHANES I (1971 to 1974), II (1976 to 1980), and III (1988 to 1991). Overweight women are those at or above the 85th percentile for persons 20 to 29 years, age and gender specific, in NHANES II. (From Institute of Medicine, *Weighing the Options: Criteria for Evaluation of Weight Management Programs,* Thomas P. R., Ed., Copyright 1995 by the National Academy of Sciences. Courtesy of the National Academy Press, Washington, D.C.)

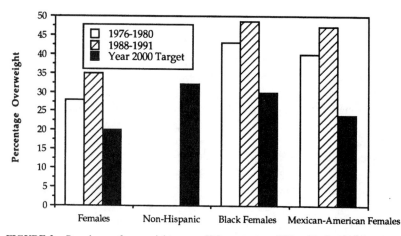

FIGURE 2.   Prevalence of overweight among U.S. women aged 20 to 74. Overweight women are those at or above the 85th percentile for persons 20 to 29 years, age and gender specific, in NHANES II. Target goals are from *Healthy People 2000*.[2,11]

especially in pregnant and nursing women.[13] Kissebah and Krakower speculated that lower body fat distribution in females (which does not favor lipolysis)
had survival value for energy storage which could then be mobilized during
lactation.[13] Furthermore, upper body fat distribution in males (which favors
lipolysis) could also have had survival value providing rapidly available energy
stores during activity.

III. IMPACT ON WOMEN'S HEALTH

A. BODY MASS INDEX

The health risks associated with obesity are related to the amount of body
fat and its distribution.[13] Obesity or increased BMI is associated in women
and men with increased risk for certain diseases including noninsulin-depen-
dent diabetes mellitus (NIDDM), coronary heart disease, stroke, hypertension,
gall bladder disease, gout, sleep apnea, osteoarthritis of weight-bearing joints
and in women with polycystic disease of the ovaries, menstrual irregularities,
ovulatory failure, and certain cancers (e.g., breast, cervix, endometrium, ovary,
gallbladder), and in men with colorectal and prostate cancer.[2,14] Small weight
losses, as little as 10 to 15%, result in improvements of some of these obesity-
related comorbidities and may prevent the appearance of these disorders.[2] In
a large-scale clinical trial using healthy severely obese individuals, gastric
reduction surgery (experimental) resulted in significant weight loss compared
to the standard treatment of using nutrition counseling, exercise, and behavior
change (control).[15] The percentage of individuals developing NIDDM within
2 years was lower in the surgical group (0.5%) than in the control group (7.8%).

Both BMI and weight gain as an adult are associated with increased risk
for coronary heart disease. In a 14-year follow-up study of 115,818 female
registered nurses, higher levels of body weight within the "normal" range
(BMI, 18 to 25), as well as modest weight gains, were associated with
increased risks for coronary heart disease in middle-aged women.[16] As seen
in Table 2, there was an increase in relative risk (RR) with BMIs of 23 to 24.9
(RR = 1.46) and an even sharper increase with BMIs of 25 to 28.9 (RR =
2.06). Relative risk also increased as the amount of weight gain increased.
Women who gained from 5 to 7.9 kg had a relative risk of 1.25, whereas
women who gained more than 20 kg had a relative risk of 2.65. These data
raise a concern that the aforementioned 1990 U.S. weight guideline which
increased BMI to 27 for men and women aged over 34 years is too liberal
with respect to coronary heart disease risk.

Some obesity-related health hazards are less for women than for men.[13]
For both men and women, deaths from coronary heart disease increase with
age. At comparable age and body weight, women experience lower morbidity
and mortality from coronary heart disease than do men.[17] It is estimated that
women lag behind men by almost 10 years.[13] These differences are related,
in part, to differences in risk factors such as blood pressure, dyslipidemia,

TABLE 2
Weight and Weight Change and Coronary Heart Disease Risk in 115,818 Female Nurses

BMI	Relative risk	Weight gain	Relative risk
<21	1.00	<5.0 kg	1.00
21–22.9	1.19	5–7.9	1.25
23.0–24.9	1.46	8.0–10.9	1.64
25–28.9	2.06	11.0–19.9	1.92
≥29.0	3.56	≥20.0	2.65

Note: The data were collected during 14 years follow-up where incidence of coronary heart disease was defined as non-fatal myocardial infarction or fatal coronary infarction. The reference woman for BMI had a BMI less than 21; the reference woman for weight gain gained less than 5.0 kg. BMI = body mass index.

Data from Willet, W. C., Manson, J. E., Stampfer, J. J., Colditz, G. A., Rosner, B., Speizer, F. E., and Hennekens, C. H., *J.A.M.A.,* 273, 461, 1995.

glucose intolerance, hyperinsulinemia, and insulin sensitivity and may reflect differences in body fat distribution.[13,18-20]

B. BODY FAT DISTRIBUTION

In 1956, Vague first hypothesized that lower body obesity or gynecoid obesity (commonly seen in women) was "benign".[21] Upper body obesity or android obesity (commonly seen in men) was associated with greater health risk for diseases such as diabetes, atherosclerosis, and gout.[21] In these studies, android obesity was assessed by averaging two ratios, brachial-to-femoral and adipose to-muscle.

Body fat distribution is crudely assessed by a variety of measures including brachial-to-femoral fat-to-muscle ratios, skinfold thickness, waist-to-hip ratio (WHR), waist circumference, and waist-to-thigh ratio.[13] Computed tomography scanning (CT), magnetic resonance imaging (MRI), and ultrasound are more precise and are strong predictors of health risk. Currently, limitations of the use of these techniques with large numbers of individuals include cost, time, availability, and exposure to ionizing radiation (i.e., CT).[13] The IOM report recommended using WHR as a simple, inexpensive way to assess upper body or abdominal fat distribution.[2] WHR is calculated by dividing circumference of the waist by circumference of the hips. A WHR greater than 0.8 in women and 1.0 in men suggests upper body fat distribution.[2]

Numerous investigators using a variety of other techniques to assess body fat distribution have amplified the original findings of Vague[21] and reported that abdominal body obesity is a risk factor for NIDDM in a number of different ethnic groups including Caucasian Americans, Japanese Americans, Mexican Americans, Native Americans, Micronesian Nauruans, Asian Indians, and Chinese and Creoles in Mauritius.[13]

Health risks are increased in women with abdominal obesity (i.e., a male-type obesity pattern).[13] In one study of over 15,000 Caucasian women, the frequency of NIDDM increased tenfold with increasing WHR.[22] However, with comparable fat distribution, as assessed by WHR, men and women had comparable levels of lipids, lipoproteins, and insulin.[13] Even more powerful are the results from the Gothenburg study[23] where the strong difference in cardiovascular disease morbidity between men and women disappeared after correcting for body fat distribution.[13]

Thus, abdominal body fat distribution, in particular visceral fat, is associated with increased morbidity and mortality.[13] This is reviewed in great detail in a comprehensive article on body fat distribution and morbidity written by Kissebah and Krakower.[13] To quote from this review, " Abdominal obesity and its associated insulin resistance are predictive of a myriad of disorders, including glucose intolerance, NIDDM, salt-sensitive hypertension, hyperapobetalipoproteinemia, hypoalphalipoproteinemia, and coronary heart disease."[13]

The work of Rebuffe-Scrive and colleagues[24] clearly demonstrates regional differences in adipose tissue metabolism that are gender specific and related to sex hormones. They have reported shifts in triglyceride storage in regional adipose tissue in pregnancy, lactation, and postmenopause associated with changes in activity of lipoprotein lipase.[24,25]

How does excess abdominal/visceral fat increase disease risk? Kissebah and Krakower[13] have postulated that one of the ways that abdominal body obesity may increase glucose intolerance is related to the increased lipolytic activity of enlarged fat cells in the abdominal region. The resultant enhanced release of free fatty acids into the circulation is postulated to inhibit glucose utilization by peripheral tissues and to increase insulin resistance as indicated by increased fasting and glucose-stimulated blood glucose and insulin.

Additional mechanisms include genetic linkage between body fat distribution and metabolic variables and/or a neuroendocrine maladjustment relative to over- reaction to stress and sex hormone imbalance.[13]

To summarize, upper body fat distribution in women is increased with: increasing age, the degree of obesity, smoking, alcohol intake, and increases in androgenic activity.[13,26,27] Some conditions in women such as polycystic ovary syndrome, idiopathic hirsutism, and ingestion of glucocorticoids (for therapeutic reasons) can also lead to abdominal obesity and its complications.[28,29]

C. SOCIAL AND PSYCHOLOGICAL FACTORS

Although harder to assess, there is concensus that there are economic, social, and psychological consequences of being obese. In a 7-year prospective study of over 10,000 individuals ranging in age from 16 to 24 years, overweight women completed fewer years of schooling, were less likely to be married, and had lower household incomes.[30] The authors concluded that "discrimination against overweight persons may account for these results." There is evidence that discrimination is also seen in relatively young children. In one study, children, by the time they reached the first grade, preferred other *disabilities* over obesity.[31]

Undoubtedly a driving current emphasis on thinness in the U.S. and other affluent nations, especially among females, influences weight-related attitudes of all.[32] Wadden and Stunkard have postulated that adolescent girls, obese women, and the morbidly obese suffer the most from society's negative attitudes toward the obese.[33] Obese individuals also reflect society's negative attitudes. In a subsequent study Wadden and Stunkard[34] reported that dissatisfaction with body weight was common among adolescent girls and was more severe in obese girls. Obese children have problems with self-esteem and may suffer from depression.[35,36]

IV. TYPES OF WEIGHT-CONTROL PROGRAMS

Many women in the U.S. want to lose weight to improve their appearance, increase self-esteem, and to improve health.[2] The National Health Interview Survey conducted in 1990 concluded that 44 million adults (40.1% of women and 23.3% of men) were trying to lose weight by eating less, increasing physical activity, or both.[37] These estimates excluded people who were told to lose weight by their physicians. Other methods used to lose weight included use of commercial meal replacements (used by 15% of adult females and 13% of adult males), use of over-the-counter and prescription weight-loss pills (used by 14% of adult females and 7% of adult males), and participating in organized weight-loss programs (13% of adult females and 5% of adult males).[38] Other popular weight-loss approaches include cutting down on high-calorie and high-fat foods, using low-fat and low-calorie foods and drinks, and skipping meals.[39]

The vast majority of weight-control programs use one or more of the following approaches: diet, physical activity, behavior modification, drug therapy, and gastric surgery. Organizing the programs that exist into a small number of types or categories is somewhat arbitrary and could be based on many defining factors, including intensity of treatment, cost, nature of the intervention(s), and degree of involvement of health-care providers. The IOM report, *Weighing The Options*, organized the plethora of weight-control programs into three major categories: (1) do-it-yourself programs, (2) nonclinical programs, and (3) clinical programs.[2]

A. DO-IT-YOURSELF

These programs are the most varied because they are individually formulated. This category includes any effort by an individual to lose weight by herself or with a group of like-minded others, through programs such as Overeaters Anonymous and TOPS (Take Off Pounds Sensibly) or community-based and work-site programs. The individual judgments, books, products, and group therapies that comprise this category dispense good or bad advice. The common denominator of programs in this category is that outside resources are not used in a personalized or individualized manner.

B. NONCLINICAL

These programs are often commercially franchised, and include well-known programs such as Weight Watchers® and Jenny Craig®. Programs in this category typically have a structure created by a parent company and often use instructional and guidance materials prepared in consultation with health-care providers. These programs rely on variably trained counselors (who are not health-care providers) to provide services to clients, but they are often managed or advised by qualified and licensed health-care providers. Many popular programs offer regular classes or meetings where topics such as nutrition, physical activity, and behavior modification are discussed, and some sell prepared foods, meal replacement, and other products to their clients.

C. CLINICAL

These programs provide services through trained and licensed health-care providers who may or may not have received special training to treat obese patients. Some are part of a commercial franchise system (e.g., Optifast® and Medifast®). There are two subgroups within this category. One is the program where a provider (e.g., physician, psychologist, or dietitian) works alone, though s/he refers patients as appropriate for special consultations. The other subgroup is a program that includes a multidisiplinary group of professional providers working together and coordinating their efforts, records, and patient base.

V. CRITERIA FOR EVALUATION OF WEIGHT-CONTROL PROGRAMS

Weight loss for the purposes of improved health and appearance supports an industry worth billions of dollars in products and service. To provide consumers protection against any excesses of this industry, efforts have been made by regulatory agencies and health-care providers to influence and regulate industry practices and advertising claims and the care given by providers.

This section briefly reviews criteria for evaluation of weight-loss programs established by the New York City Department of Consumer Affairs (DCA), the Michigan Task Force to Establish Weight Loss Guidelines, and the NIH; actions by the FTC to regulate deceptive claims by weight-loss programs; attitudes towards the use of antiobesity drugs by the FDA and state medical practice review boards; and criteria for the conduct of weight-loss programs proposed in the report *Weighing The Options*, published by the IOM in 1995.[2,4-,10]

A. NEW YORK CITY DEPARTMENT OF CONSUMER AFFAIRS

In 1991, the New York City DCA investigated some of the deceptive practices used by rapid-weight-loss centers in New York City by having several staff members, posing as potential clients, visit 14 weight-loss centers.[4] These investigators reported that most centers did not discuss the potential risks of weight loss, even when asked to do so. Furthermore, some centers made false and misleading statements, counseled underweight individuals to lose weight, and engaged in practices deemed to be quackery. DCA defined rapid weight loss as weight loss of more than 1 to 2 lb or 1% of body weight per week.

As a result of its investigation, DCA issued the nation's first "Truth-in-Dieting" regulation on May 17, 1992. Rapid weight-loss centers are required to post a "Weight-Loss-Consumer Bill of Rights" sign and provide potential clients a "palm-size" copy, as well as disclose up front all the costs of the program (including products to purchase and laboratory tests) and its duration. The required "Bill of Rights" sign is to state:

1. WARNING: Rapid weight loss may cause serious health problems. (Rapid weight loss is weight loss of more than 1.5 to 2 lb/week or weight loss of more than 1% of body weight per week after the second week of participation in a weight-loss program.)
2. Only permanent life-style changes — such as making healthful food choices and increasing physical activity — promote long-term weight loss.
3. Consult your personal physician before starting any weight-loss program.
4. Qualifications of this provider's staff are available on request.
5. You have a right to
    *   Ask questions about the potential health risks of this program, its nutritional content, and its psychological-support and educational components
    *   Know the price of treatment, including the price of extra products, services, supplements, and laboratory tests
    *   Know the program duration that is being recommended for you

B. MICHIGAN DEPARTMENT OF PUBLIC HEALTH

In 1990, a task force of the Michigan Department of Public Health developed guidelines for the conduct of adult weight-loss programs in that state.[5,6] The guidelines, provided in Table 3, are quite detailed and apply to both nonclinical and clinical programs. They call for providers to screen prospective clients to assess their level of health risk and, depending on results, recommend appropriate individualized and multidisciplinary weight-loss approaches that include nutrition, exercise, and behavior modification. The Michigan guidelines attempted to forge a match between program and client dictated by the client's health needs. They call for clinics being staffed by qualified professionals capable of delivering appropriate levels of health care and that potential clients be screened for health risks prior to beginning a calorie-restricted diet. The task force hoped that its guidelines would be adopted as legally enforceable standards of health care in weight-loss programs throughout Michigan, but this has not happened to date.

C. NATIONAL INSTITUTES OF HEALTH

Guidelines for evaluating weight-loss methods and programs were developed by the NIH as a result of an NIH Technology Assessment Conference on methods of voluntary weight loss and control.[7] These guidelines encouraged full disclosure of program characteristics (e.g., amount and kind of counseling, flexibility of food choices) to the potential client of a program's "track record" by standardizing the type of data to be obtained and the statistics to be provided by weight-loss programs. Additional guidelines were issued by the NIH Obesity Task Force to help consumers choose a safe and successful weight-loss program.[8] Five common features of a safe and successful weight-loss program were identified (e.g., diet should be safe and include all of the recommended dietary allowances; clients should be provided with a detailed list of fees and cost of additional items).

D. FEDERAL TRADE COMMISSION

The FTC efforts in regard to the weight-loss industry address and challenge specific, allegedly deceptive advertising claims that companies have made to promote their programs and diet aids. The FTC actions seek to place the companies under an order designed to remedy those allegedly deceptive claims.[9] By December 1993, the FTC has either begun litigation or settled complaints it has issued against 11 commercial weight-loss companies.[55]

In each of the settled complaints the FTC's order requires that any statements made about participants succeeding at weight loss or maintaining weight control be based on representative data from all participants or a clearly defined subset.[55] When a claim is made that participants in a program successfully maintain lost weight, the order requires in most instances that the claim be accompanied by data that reflect the actual experience of program participants and a general statement about the temporary nature of most weight loss. An example given by FTC of "acceptable disclosure" is "participants maintain an average of 60% of weight loss 22 months after active weight loss (includes 18 months on maintenance program)." For many dieters weight loss is temporary.[9]

E. FOOD AND DRUG ADMINISTRATION

The FDA is the government agency responsible for approving drugs for use in the U.S. Prescription drugs must be found by FDA to be both effective and reasonably safe for their intended use. However, while there is increased interest in the use of medications to treat obesity, few antiobesity drugs are available to physicians, and no new drugs have been approved to treat obesity

TABLE 3

Detailed Weight-Loss Guidelines Issued by the State Of Michigan[2,5,6]

Screening of client
  Verify that there are no medical or psychological conditions which could make weight loss
    inappropriate
  Identify level of health risk: low, moderate, or high
Level of care
  Provide level of care appropriate to client's level of health risk: levels of care 1, 2, or 3
Individualized treatment plan
  Identify factors that contribute to client's weight status which should serve as bases for each
    client's individualized weight-loss plan; these may include weight goal, and plans for
    nutrition, exercise, behavioral change, medical monitoring or supervision, and health
    supervision
Staffing
  Providers should be trained adequately for level of health risk of client
Full disclosure
  Client should give informed consent after informed of potential risks from weight loss and
    regain, likely long-term success of program, full costs, and credentials of weight-loss
    providers
Reasonable weight goal
  Base weight goal on personal and family weight history, not exclusively on height and weight charts
Rate of weight loss
  Energy level should be adjusted so that client can achieve but not exceed recommended rate
    of weight loss; energy intake should not be lower than 1000 kcal at level 1; 800 kcal at level
    2; and 600 kcal at level 3; if daily energy level is below 800 kcal, additional safeguards
    should be in place
Diet Composition
  Protein: 0.8–1.5 g protein per kilogram goal body weight, no more than 100 g/d
  Fat: 10–30% of energy
  Carbohydrate: at least 100 g/d for level 1; 50 g/d for level 2
  Fluid: at least 1 qt of water daily
Nutritional adequacy
  Client to obtain 100% of the client's RDA; if nutrition supplements are used, nutrient levels
    should not greatly exceed 100% of the RDA
Nutrition education
  Encourage permanent healthful eating patterns
Formula Products
  Food plan to consist of a variety of foods available from the conventional food supply
  Formula products not recommended for treatment of moderate obesity, and should not be used
    at low-calorie formulations without specialized medical supervision
Exercise component
  Include exercise that is safe and appropriate for individual client
  Screen client for conditions which would make medical clearance before exercise appropriate
  Instruct client to recognize and deal with potentially dangerous physical responses to exercise
  Work toward 30–60 min of continuous exercise five to seven times/week, with gradual increases
    in intensity and duration
Psychological component
  Teach behavior modification techniques appropriate for the specific client
Appetite suppressants
  Not recommended and should not take the place of changes in diet, exercise, and behavior
Weight maintenance
  Include in treatment program

since 1973.[40] This country has lagged behind other countries in the approval and use of antiobesity drugs. For example, *d*-fenfluramine, approved in Europe and much of the rest of the world for years, is still pending approval in the U.S. In November 1995, FDA's Endocrinologic and Metabolic Advisory Committee narrowly voted to approve *d*-fenfluramine. In addition, fluoxetine, approved here to treat depression and obsessive-compulsive disorder, has been under FDA consideration for the treatment of obesity for more than 6 years.[56]

The "drug lag" in obesity treatment has taken on added importance in light of the growing prevalence of obesity in the country and increasing evidence that antiobesity drugs can help some obese individuals to lose weight and control weight gain.[41] A NIH workshop on the pharmacological treatment of obesity concluded that "obesity drugs produce short-term weight loss and may remain effective for extended periods of time in some patients."[40] In three major studies of longer-term drug therapy, antiobesity drugs helped some subjects maintain lower weights, and there is some indication that the drugs may help change behavior.[42-46] Weintraub has reported that a combination of two types of drugs may be more effective for long-term weight loss and weight maintenance than either used alone.[45,46] Drugs either approved or in development for treating obesity may decrease energy intake (e.g., serotonin uptake inhibitors, peptide-based appetite suppressants), increase energy expenditure or thermogenesis (e.g., beta-adrenergic receptor agonists), stimulate lipolysis (e.g., alpha-adrenergic receptor antagonists), or decrease fat or other macronutrient absorption (e.g., pancreatic lipase inhibitors).[41,47]

The reluctance of many health-care providers and government regulators to look favorably upon the use and encourage the development of antiobesity drugs has several causes. Perhaps most importantly, there is a common view that obesity is not a disease, but a disorder of willful misconduct — eating too much and exercising too little. In addition, fears exist about the abuse or misuse potential of these medications and previous indiscriminate prescription of antiobesity drugs by some physicians.[40] Atkinson and Hubbard conclude that "obesity drugs are held to higher standards than drugs used for other diseases...obesity drugs are limited to short-term use ...typically no longer than 3 months..." "Physicians who prescribe obesity drugs for longer periods are subject to scrutiny by state medical review boards and may face loss of licensure."[40] In contrast to current medical practice, Stallone and Stunkard[48] recommend that appetite-suppressant medication be used on a long-term basis or not at all.

With the growing acceptance of obesity as a chronic degenerative disease that contributes substantially to the burden of disease and death in the U.S., current standards for antiobesity drugs appear unreasonable. Drugs used for treating other chronic diseases or disease processes, such as hypertension and diabetes, are approved with the understanding that they will be used for long periods of time, and that treatment effectiveness may require continued use of medication. Candidates most appropriate for drug therapy for obesity include those with comorbidities (e.g., hypertension, hypercholesterolemia, asthma, schizophrenia, and diabetes). Such a view is needed toward obesity and the use of antiobesity drugs as adjuncts to treatment along with diet, activity, and behavior modification in carefully selected individuals.

The FDA is reevaluating "guidance" for development, approval, and use of antiobesity drugs. FDA's Endocrinologic and Metabolic Drugs Advisory Committee, in a meeting for January 1995, decided that "weight loss alone was an appropriate end point in clinical trials for products that will be used in long-term therapy for obesity."[10] Furthermore, seven out of ten committee members agreed that a 5% weight loss from baseline which was maintained for 1 year was sufficient for approval of an antiobesity drug. In subsequent meetings, the committee modified this definition of effectiveness to be 5% difference from placebo. The "placebo", in this case, refers to diet, exercise, and behavior modification, clearly not a "placebo". While the committee's recommendations are not binding, FDA Deputy Director of Metabolism and Endocrine Drug Products noted that the division has "every intention of accepting the committee's advice."[10] If these recommendations are approved, they would not be consistant with recommendations made by other organizations (e.g., North American Association for the Study of Obesity, IOM).

F. INSTITUTE OF MEDICINE REPORT

In December 1994, the IOM released a report that proposed criteria for evaluating weight-control programs in a consistent and comprehensive manner.[2] Among its major recommendations was that weight-*control* and weight-*loss* programs evolve into weight-*management* programs, focusing more on the overall health of participants than on weight loss and its maintenance alone. The report emphasizes that weight management requires a lifelong plan with the individual at the center of decision making about how to proceed.

The report is organized around a simple conceptual overview of decision making, where an individual makes a decision about a weight-management option and then experiences and evaluates it. Figure 3 illustrates the model and the committee's three major criteria for program evaluation. Each criterion (pertaining to matching programs and consumers, ensuring the safety and soundness of programs, and evaluating program outcomes) is described from the point of view of the program and the consumer. The program is expected to provide a high quality program and service with documented effectiveness, and the consumer is expected to ask questions and otherwise make sure that the program meets these standards. The report's three criteria are briefly described below from the perspective of the individual making a choice, followed by its recommendations for the data needed to ensure comprehensive and consistent program evaluations.

1. Criterion 1: "Match" between Program and Consumer

As shown in Figure 3, three sets of factors influence an individual's choice of programs: (1) personal, situational, and global factors (e.g., age, gender, motivation, readiness to change, views about weight and appearance, and the

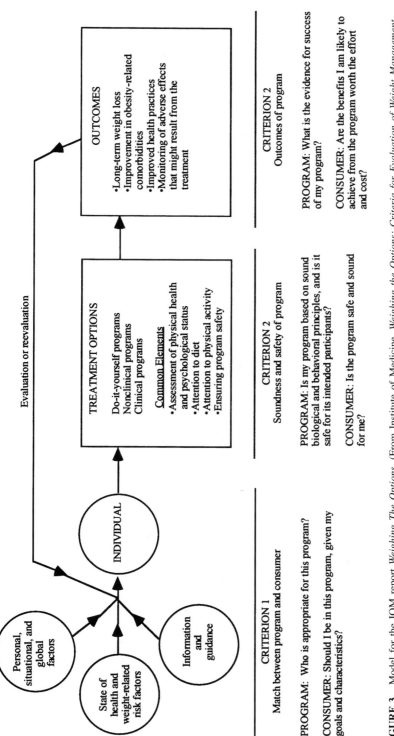

FIGURE 3. Model for the IOM report *Weighing The Options*. (From Institute of Medicine, *Weighing the Options: Criteria for Evaluation of Weight Management Programs*, Thomas, P.R., Ed., Copyright 1995 by the National Academy of Sciences. Courtesy of the National Academy Press, Washington, D.C.)

cost and ready availability of a program); (2) health status and weight-related risk factors (e.g., presence or absence of hypertension, dyslipidemias, and diabetes, and family history of these or other comorbidities); and (3) information and guidance (e.g., from family, friends, books, magazines, advertising, and health-care professionals). Consumers choose a program based on some combination of these factors. Unfortunately, the ability of consumers and health-care providers to make successful matches is limited at present. Several factors, however, appear to be consistently associated with success at weight loss and maintenance of that loss. These include reasonable and nutritious eating patterns, continued self-monitoring of diet and exercise, a positive problem-solving attitude toward life's stressors, and positive changes in physiological factors that are often adversely affected by obesity.[49-54]

In relation to this criterion, a woman should be asking: "Should I be in this program, given my goals and characteristics?" To decide, the IOM report recommends the following:

- Consider carefully your weight-loss goals and whether you are an appropriate candidate for weight loss.
- Decide whether the time is right to be able to devote the considerable attention and effort required to succeed at weight loss.
- Be evaluated by a health-care provider (or have been in the recent past) before undertaking a do-it-yourself or nonclinical program. Discuss the program or product with a health-care provider.
- Expect that programs will provide sufficient information so you can assess whether you are appropriate or inappropriate as a candidate.

2. Criterion 2: Soundness and Safety of Program

Weight-management programs should be based on sound biological and behavioral principles. Four critical areas were identified as needs for all programs to address: (1) assessment of physical health and psychological status, (2) attention to diet, (3) attention to physical activity, and (4) ensuring program safety. In relation to these criteria, a woman should ask, "Is the program safe and sound for me?" To decide, the IOM recommends the following:

- Have a good understanding of the program and what to expect from it through the treatment and maintenance phase.
- Monitor weight weekly and continue to assess (or have assessed) your diet and physical activity patterns at 6-month intervals or more frequently after the weight-loss phase of the program.
- Expect that the program will be a safe and sound one.
- Expect that do-it-yourself programs will provide the credentials and qualifications of the author/originator. Nonclinical and clinical programs will make available information about the qualifications and training of staff.

3. Criterion 3: Program Outcomes

The IOM report recommends that weight-control programs be judged by how well individuals do in four areas: (1) long-term weight loss (defined as a loss of at least 5% of body weight or a reduction in BMI by one or more units for 1 year or more), (2) improvements in obesity-related comorbidities, (3) improved health practices (in terms of improved eating patterns, obtaining regular exercise, and improved well-being), and (4) monitoring of adverse effects that might result from the program. In relation to this criterion, a woman should ask, "Are the benefits I am likely to achieve from the program worth the effort and cost?" To decide, the IOM report recommends the following:

- Remember that you and the program have joint responsibilities for your final outcome.
- Have realistic expectations of the program and be willing to devote the time and effort required.
- Choose a program in light of your own short- and long-term goals for weight management. Reevaluate your goals every 3 to 6 months.
- Choose programs that focus on long-term weight management; provide instruction in healthful eating, increasing activity, and improving self-esteem; and explain thoroughly the potential health risks from weight loss.
- Look for programs that devote considerable effort to helping people change their behaviors through information, guidance, and skill training.
- For do-it-yourself programs, look through the program literature for evidence (beyond testimonials or other anecdotal evidence) that the program is successful.
- If you are in a do-it-yourself and nonclinical program, be in touch with a health-care provider who can monitor any changes in your health.
- Expect that at 3- to 6-month intervals, the program will evaluate whether you are meeting your goals and whether the goals or treatment should be modified.

Ultimately, what is critical to making comparisons of effectiveness among weight-control programs is information obtained in a systematic, scientific fashion. The IOM report recommended that weight-control programs making claims of success collect the data summarized in Table 4. It is difficult at present to compare different programs, in part, because of differences in the clients selected and in the data collected and reported. Instead, many companies provide testimonials, often from prominent people, to show a program's success at achieving weight loss.

TABLE 4
Collection of Data by Weight Management Programs[2]

The number of people attending the first treatment session (this is the group of potential clients
  and those who will become actual clients)
Number of clients attending their first two treatment sessions (a gauge of those who have really
  begun a program) and percentage continuing to participate in the program at 1, 3, 6, and 12
  months (these time points seem reasonable but are selected somewhat arbitrarily, for while there
  is no set of ideal time points, it is important to have a set for standardization and comparison
  among programs; programs may, of course, use additional time points)
Average weight, height, BMI, and waist-to-hip ratio of clients attending the first two sessions and
  appropriate measures of change in these variables at 1, 3, 6, and 12 months in the program
  (these data should be assembled by gender and, if possible, by race, age, and starting weight or
  BMI
The percentage of actual clients who complete each of the stages of the treatment program; this
  means either the number of clients that complete the program's prescribed number of sessions
  (e.g., 8 weeks for an 8-week program) or the number of clients in treatment at 3 months
The percentage of actual clients who re-enroll in the same program for further treatment (this
  figure should not necessarily be interpreted as a measure of client failure in a program; it may
  indicate satisfaction with the program)

VI. CONCLUSIONS

Obesity is one of the most important nutrition-related diseases in the U.S.
It is associated with increased morbidity and mortality as well as psychosocial
burdens that even involve discrimination. This has important consequences for
the funding of research by government, foundations, and private agencies, for
health-care, and for oversight of the weight-loss industry by regulatory agencies.

A more aggressive policy is required to inform the public and health-care
providers about the nature of obesity, the difficulties inherent in treating this
disease and achieving permanent weight management, and the need for susceptible individuals to take steps to prevent its occurrence or minimize its
development. Health-care providers, in particular, should learn more about
obesity and its treatment. For the individual woman, it means becoming aware
of periods of high risk for permanent weight gain such as pregnancy and peri-
and postmenopause. It also means becoming aware of individual risks such
as abdominal obesity and the environmental factors such as smoking that
maximize abdominal fat deposition.

Unfortunately, the lay public, health-care providers, and regulatory agencies often view obesity as a problem of willful misconduct — eating too much
and exercising too little. Obesity is a remarkable disease in terms of the effort
required by an individual for its management and the extent of discrimination
its victims suffer. Women bear an extra burden with respect to discrimination.

Obesity is a complex, multifactorial disease involving biological as well
as environmental, psychosocial, and cultural factors. We now have many of
the research tools to make major advances in understanding the basic biology
of obesity. There must be increased recognition and support for research into

the genetic, molecular, and cellular endeavors that will aid our understanding of the causes of obesity and its associated comorbidities. There also must be more research into the identification of individuals at risk for developing comorbidities (e.g., not all obese individuals develop NIDDM). This should aid in the design of maximally successful means to more effectively prevent and treat obesity.

REFERENCES

1. Kuczmarski, R. S., Flegal, K. M., Campbell, S. M., and Johnson, C. L., Increasing prevalence of overweight among U.S. adults: the National Health and Nutrition Examination Surveys, 1960 to 1991, *J.A.M.A.*, 272, 205, 1994.
2. Institute of Medicine, *Weighing the Options: Criteria for Evaluation of Weight Management Programs*, Thomas, P.R., Ed., National Academy of Sciences Press, Washington, D.C., 1995.
3. McGinnis, J. M. and Foege, W. H., Actual causes of death in the United States, *J.A.M.A.*, 270, 2207, 1993.
4. Winner, K., *A Weighty Issue: Dangers and Deceptions of the Weight Loss Industry*, Department of Consumer Affairs, New York, 1991.
5. Drewnowski, A., Toward safe weight loss: recommendations for adult weight loss programs in Michigan, in *Final Report of Task Force to Establish Weight Loss Guidelines*, Petersmark, K.A., Ed., Michigan Health Council, East Lansing, MI, 1990.
6. Petersmarck, K. A., The Michigan approach: building consensus for safe weight loss, *J. Am. Diet. Assoc.*, 92, 679, 1992.
7. N.I.H., Methods for voluntary weight loss and control: technology assessment conference statement, *Ann. Intern. Med.*, 119, 764, 1993.
8. N.I.D.D.K. (National Institute of Digestive, Diabetes, and Kidney Diseases), Choosing a Safe and Successful Weight-Loss Program. *National Institutes of Health Publ. No. 94-3700, National Institutes of Health*, Rockville, MD, 1993.
9. F.T.C. (Federal Trade Commission), Nutri/System, Inc.: proposed consent agreement with analysis to aid public comment, *Fed. Reg.*, 58, 52769, 1993.
10. F.D.C. Reports, Weight loss appropriate as primary endpoint in obesity studies, in *The Pink Sheets*, Warble, W., January 23, 1995.
11. DHHS (U.S. Department of Health and Human Services), *Health People 2000: National Health Promotion and Disease Prevention Objectives*, DHHS (PHS) Publ., No. 91-50212, Public Health Service, U.S. Department of Health and Human Services, U.S. Government Printing Office, Washington, D.C., 1991.
12. Sobal, J. and Stunkard, A. J., Socioeconomic status and obesity: a review of the literature, *Psychol. Bull.*, 105, 260, 1989.
13. Kissebah, A. H. and Krakower, G. R., Regional adiposity and morbidity, *Physiol. Rev.*, 74, 761, 1994.
14. Office of Health Economics, *Obesity*, BSC Print, London, 1994, 6.
15. Sjostrom, C. D., Hakangard, A. C., Lissner, L., and Sjostrom, L., Relationships between cardiovascular risk factors and visceral and subcutaneous adipose tissue (AT) distribution. *Int. J. Obesity*, 18(Suppl. 2), 14, 1994.
16. Willett, W. C., Manson, J. E., Stampfer, J. J., Colditz, G. A., Rosner, B., Speizer, F. E., and Hennekens, C. H., Weight change and coronary heart disease in women, *J.A.M.A.*, 273, 461, 1995.

17. Lerner, D. J. and Kannel, W. B., Patterns of coronary heart disease morbidity and mortality in the sexes: a 26-year follow-up of the Framingham population, *Am. Heart J.*, 111, 383, 1986.

18. Evans, D. J., Hoffmann, R. G., Kalkhoff, R. K., and Kissebah, A. H., Relationship of androgenic activity to body fat topography, fat cell morphology, and metabolic aberrations in premenopausal women, *J. Clin. Endocrinol. Metab.*, 57, 304, 1983.

19. Freedman, D. S., Jacobsen, S. K., Barboriak, J. J., Sobocinski, K. A., Andersen, A. J., Kissebah, A. H., Sasse, E. A., and Gruchow, H. W., Body fat distribution and male/female differences in lipids and lipoproteins, *Circulation*, 81, 1498, 1990.

20. Godsland, I. F., Wynn, V., Crook, D., and Miller, N. E., Sex, plasma lipoproteins, and atherosclerosis: prevailing assumptions and outstanding questions, *Am. Heart J.*, 114, 1467, 1987.

21. Vague, J., The degree of masculine differentiation of obesities: a factor determining predisposition to diabetes, atherosclerosis, gout, and uric calculous disease, *Am. J. Clin. Nutr.*, 4, 20, 1956.

22. Hartz, A. J., Rupley, D. C., Kalkhoff, R. K., and Rimm, A. A., Relationship of obesity to diabetes: influence of obesity level and body-fat distribution, *Prev. Med.*, 12, 351, 1983.

23. Lapidus, L., Bengtsson, C., Hallstrom, T., and Bjorntorp, P., Obesity, adipose tissue distribution and health results from a population study in Gothenburg, Sweden, *Appetite*, 12, 25, 1989.

24. Rebuffe-Scrive, M., Lonnroth, P., Marin, P., Wesslau, C., Bjorntorp, P., and Smith, U., Regional adipose tissue metabolism in men and postmenopausal women, *Int. J. Obesity*, 11, 347, 1987.

25. Rebuffe-Scrive, M., Enk, L., Crona, N., Lonnroth, P., Abrahamsson, L., Smith, U., and Bjorntorp, P., Fat cell metabolism in different regions in women: effects of menstrual cycle, pregnancy and lactation, *J. Clin. Invest.*, 75, 1973, 1985.

26. Enzi, G., Gasparo, M., Biondetti, P. F., Fiore, D., Semisa, M., and Zurlo, F., Subcutaneous and visceral fat distribution according to sex, age and overweight, evaluated by computed tomography, *Am. J. Clin. Nutr.*, 44, 739, 1986.

27. Haffner, S. M., Stern, M. P., Hazuda, H. P., Pugh, J., Patterson, J. K., and Malina, R., Upper-body and centralized adiposity in Mexican Americans and non-Hispanic whites: retationship to body mass index and other behavioral and demographic variables, *Int. J. Obesity*, 10, 493, 1986.

28. Yen, S. S. C., The polycystic ovary syndrome, *Clin. Endocrinol.*, 12, 17, 1980.

29. Evans, D. J., Body Fat Distribution and Metabolic Complications, M.D. thesis, University of Cardiff, Cardiff, U.K., 1986.

30. Gortmaker, S. I., Must, A., Perrin, J. M., Sobol, A. M., and Dietz, W. H., Social and economic consequences of overweight in adolescence and young adulthood. *N. Engl. J. Med.*, 329, 1008, 1993.

31. Richardson, S. A., Goodman, N., and Hastorf, A. H., Cultural uniformity in reaction to physical disabilities, *Am. Sociol. Rev.*, 26, 241, 1967.

32. Rodin, J., Cultural and psychosocial determinants of weight concerns, *Ann. Intern. Med.*, 119, 643, 1993.

33. Wadden, T. H. and Stunkard, A. J., Social and psychological consequences of obesity, *Ann. Intern. Med.*, 103, 1062, 1985.

34. Wadden, T. H. and Stunkard, A. J., Psychosocial consequences of obesity and dieting: research and clinical findings, in *Obesity: Theory and Therapy,* 2nd ed., Wadden, T.A. and Stunkard, A.J., Eds., Raven Press, New York, 1993, 163.

35. Sallade, J., A comparison of the psychological adjustment of obese vs. non-obese children, *J. Psychosom. Res.*, 17, 89, 1973.

36. Sheslow, D., Hassnink, S., Wallace, W., and DeLancey, E., The relationship between self-esteem and depression in obese children. in *Prevention and Treatment of Childhood Obesity*, Williams, L. and Kimm, S.Y.S., Eds., Ann. NY Acad. Sci., vol. 699, 1993.

37. Horm, J. and Anderson, K., Who in America is trying to lose weight?, *Ann. Intern. Med.*, 119, 672, 1993.
38. Levy, A. S. and Heaton, A. W., Weight control practices of U.S. adults trying to lose weight. *Ann. Intern. Med.*, 119, 661, 1993.
39. Calorie Control Council, One out of every two women believe they are overweight, *Calorie Control Commentary*, 15, 5, 1993.
40. Atkinson, R. L. and Hubbard, V. S., Report on the NIH Workshop on Pharmacologic Treatment of Obesity, *Am. J. Clin. Nutr.*, 60, 153, 1994.
41. Goldstein, D. J. and Potvin, J. H., Long-term weight loss: the effect of pharmacologic agents, *Am. J. Clin. Nutr.*, 60, 647, 1994.
42. Darga, L. L., Carroll-Michals, L., Botsford, S. J., and Lucas, C. P., Fluoxetine's effects on weight loss in obese subjects, *Am. J. Clin. Nutr.*, 54, 321, 1991.
43. Marcus, M. D., Wing, R. R., Ewing, L., and Kern, E., a double-blind placebo-controlled trial of fluoxetine plus behavior modification in the treatment of obese binge-eaters and non-binge-eaters, *Am. J. Psychiatry*, 147, 876, 1990.
44. McDermott, M. and Gooding, W., A double-blind placebo-controlled trial of fluoxetine plus behavior modification in the treatment of obese binge-eaters and non-binge-eaters, *Am. J. Psychiatry,* 147, 876, 1990.
45. Weintraub, M., Long-term weight control study: conclusions, *Clin. Pharmacol. Ther.*, 51, 642, 1992.
46. Weintraub, M., Long-term weight control: the National Heart, Lung, and Blood Institute funded multimodal intervention study, *Clin. Pharmacol. Ther.*, 51, 581, 1992.
47. Bray, G. A., Use and abuse of appetite-suppressant drugs in the treatment of obesity, *Ann. Intern. Med.*, 119, 707, 1993.
48. Stallone, D. D. and Stunkard, A. J., Long-term use of appetite suppressant medication: rationale and recommendations, *Drug Development Res.*, 26, 1, 1992.
49. Brownell, K. D. and Wadden, T. A., Etiology and treatment of obesity: understanding a serious, prevalent, and refractory disorder, *J. Consult. Clin. Psychol.*, 60, 505, 1992.
50. Foreyt, J. P. and Goodrick, G. K., Factors common to successful therapy for the obese patient, *Med. Sci. Sports Exerc.*, 23, 292, 1991.
51. O'Neil, P. M. and Jarrell, M. P., Psychological aspects of obesity and dieting, in *Treatment of the Seriously Obese Patient*, Wadden, T. A. and VanItallie, T. B., Eds., Guilford, New York, 1992, 252.
52. Perri, M. G., Nezu, A. M., and Viegener, B. J., *Improving the Long-Term Management of Obesity: Theory, Research, and Clinical Guidelines*, John Wiley & Sons, New York, 1992.
53. Rossner, S., Factors determining the long-term outcome of obesity treatment, in *Obesity*, Bjorntorp, P. and Brodoff, B. N., Eds., Lippincott, Philadelphia, 1992, 712.
54. Wadden, T. J. and Letizia, K. A., Predictors of attrition and weight loss in patients treated by moderate and severe calorie restriction, in *Treatment of the Seriously Obese Patient*, Wadden, T. A. and VanItallie, T. B., Eds., Guilford, New York, 1992, 383.
55. Kelly, R. F., Assistant Director for the Division of Service Industry Practices, Federal Trade Commission, personal communication.
56. Atkinson, R. L., personal communication.

Chapter 7

EATING DISORDERS IN WOMEN

**Kelly K. Hill, Craig J. McClain, Lisa Gaetke,
and Antoinette Saddler**

CONTENTS

I. INTRODUCTION

Eating disorders are a major public health problem in the U.S. and in other industrialized countries.[1] These disorders affect large numbers of persons, with 90 to 95% occurring in adolescent and young adult females.[2] These illnesses regularly receive widespread public attention via television, newspapers, and fashion magazines. In fact, the media actually has inadvertently glamorized these disturbances. Unfortunately these disorders carry high morbidity rates and the highest mortality rates of any category of psychiatric illness. This chapter will review the diagnostic criteria, epidemiology, characteristics, medical complications, and nutritional complications/nutritional treatment of the two major classifications of eating disorders, anorexia nervosa (AN) and bulimia nervosa (BN).

II. DEFINITION OF EATING DISORDERS

A. DIAGNOSTIC CRITERIA FOR ANOREXIA NERVOSA

The essential features an individual must have to be diagnosed with AN include:[3]

1. Refusal to maintain a minimally normal body weight for age and height or failure to make expected gains during periods of growth, if a child or adolescent
2. Intense fear of gaining weight or becoming fat, even though not overweight
3. Disturbance of body image
4. The absence of at least three consecutive menstrual cycles in premenopausal women

By definition, the AN patient is malnourished, weighing below a minimally normal level for age and height. If the disease occurs in childhood or adolescence, there may not be weight loss, but the individual fails to gain weight while continuing to grow in height.

The first criterion defines a threshold for determining if the person is underweight, using 85% of that weight considered normal for age and height as the cutoff. The Metropolitan Life Insurance tables or pediatric growth charts are commonly used. A more rigorous definition is a body mass index (BMI) (calculated as weight in kilograms/(height in meters)^2) equal to or less than 17.5 kg/m^2. The person's body build and weight history also should be considered with these general guidelines.

These patients usually accomplish weight loss by drastically reducing their daily intake, restricting their diet to only a few very low calorie foods. For example, a typical daily intake for such an individual might include: breakfast consisting of 8 oz of coffee (black), followed by 8 oz of diet cola; lunch would be skipped; afternoon refreshment of two glasses of water; dinner consisting of chicken broth and tossed salad without dressing.

Many engage in purging behaviors (self-induced vomiting, abuse of laxatives and diuretics) and/or compulsive and excessive exercise regimens to counter the few calories that are eaten.

The fear of fatness seen in this population is irrational. These individuals fear being fat even though they are in an emaciated state. They are not reassured with weight loss, and the fear often intensifies with continued weight loss.

The disturbance in body image also has an irrational quality. Frequently, the patient with AN is focused on a particular body part such as hips, thighs, or stomach. The rigorous exercise schedules commonly practiced by this population often are an attempt to "fix" the unacceptable areas. The self-worth of these individuals is very dependent on their body weight and shape. Weight loss is experienced as an esteemed achievement and demonstrates superior self-discipline, whereas weight gain is experienced as an unacceptable failure.

Amenorrhea is generally thought to be caused by diminished estrogen secretion that results from inadequate pituitary secretion of follicle-stimulating hormone and luteinizing hormone. This generally occurs after the person is in a malnourished state. However, in some individuals, amenorrhea precedes weight loss. In children and young adolescents, menarche may be delayed by the disorder.

B. DIAGNOSTIC CRITERIA FOR BULIMIA NERVOSA

The criteria for the diagnosis of BN include:[3]

1. Recurrent episodes of binge eating
2. Recurrent abnormal behavior to prevent weight gain from binging
3. The binging and compensatory activities occur at least twice a week for 3 months
4. Self-worth is overly influenced by body shape and weight

Binge eating is defined as consuming large amounts of food (significantly more than most people would eat) in a discrete period of time (within 2 h). During the binge, the person feels she/he has no control over eating. A single binge episode is not restricted to one location; for example, the binge may begin in a restaurant, continue in a grocery store, and finish at home. However, a true binge is completed in a limited time period; therefore, continuous snacking throughout the day is not binging. Binge eating involves consuming abnormal amounts of food rather than craving a particular nutrient such as carbohydrates. However, common binge items include calorie-dense, sweet foods, such as cookies and ice cream. Although during binging a person with BN consumes more calories than someone who is not bulimic, the fractions of calories derived from carbohydrates, fats, and proteins usually do not differ to any major degree. A typical day in a bulimic patient's food diary might be for breakfast, one apple, two cups of coffee, morning snack of a diet cola; lunch, diet cola, tuna sandwich; afternoon snack of diet cola and rice cake; and dinner of hamburger, potato chips, and a diet cola. The binge follows dinner and consists of 1 qt of ice cream, one loaf of white bread, a package of Girl Scout cookies, 1 qt of milk, and four cups of fettucine alfredo.

Binging usually occurs in secret. Binge "triggers" include interpersonal stressors, dysphoria, anxiety, intense hunger following dietary restraint, or feelings about body weight, shape, and food.

The second criterion for diagnosing BN is the recurrent use of inappropriate compensatory behaviors to avoid weight gain. Of persons with BN who present for treatment at eating disorder clinics, 80 to 90% admit to self-induced vomiting after a binge. This immediately reduces fear of gaining weight and provides physical relief from the massive overeating. Sometimes, the act of vomiting becomes the primary goal, and the individual will binge to vomit or vomit after eating small or normal amounts of food. Methods used to induce vomiting include use of fingers or objects to stimulate the gag reflex and, more rarely, syrup of ipecac. Laxatives, diuretics, and enemas are other purgatives employed by this population to counter the effects of binging.

Other compensatory behaviors include excessive exercise and restricting nutrient intake when not binging or even fasting between binges. Inappropriate use of thyroid hormone may be observed in unusual situations.

Similar to the person with AN, the person with BN fears gaining weight, wants to lose weight, and is dissatisfied with her/his body because self-value is tied to how she/he perceives body shape and weight. BN should not be diagnosed when the disturbance occurs only during episodes of AN, thus further distinguishing BN from a patient with anorexia who also binges and purges.

III. EPIDEMIOLOGY

The prevalence of eating disorders is reported to be increasing, ranging from 1 to 4% of adolescent and young adult women.[4,5] A larger percentage of young women may be subclinical, since the national chapters of Anorexia Nervosa and Related Eating Disorders, Inc. (ANRED) and Anorexia Nervosa and Associated Disorders (ANAD) estimate that in females 12 to 30 years of age, 20% suffer from eating disorder symptoms.[6] BN is more common than AN. Although not nearly as common, increasing numbers of cases are being seen in men (homosexuals having an increased risk over heterosexuals),[7] minorities, and women of all ages.[8] Some experts report that these diseases are also increasing in preadolescent children.[2] There are other patterns of disturbed eating such as fad dieting and compulsive eating which affect an important portion of the population. These would be categorized as eating disorders, not otherwise specified (EDNOS), and these are not reviewed in this chapter.

IV. CHARACTERISTICS

Persons suffering from these disorders routinely oscillate from predominately anorexic symptoms to primarily bulimic symptoms.[2] The newest version of the diagnostic manual of mental disorders divides AN into restricting and binge-eating/purging subtypes.[3] Fifty percent of persons with AN develop bulimic symptoms. Significant numbers of bulimic patients develop anorexic symptoms. Some experts consider these disorders to occur along a continuum.[2]

Confirmed histories of sexual and physical abuse are rampant among patients with eating disorders. Data from the C.F. Menninger Memorial Hospital mesh well with reports in the literature that indicate a history of sexual abuse in 35 to 65% of these patients.[9] Frequently, there is a history of medical and surgical illnesses, family separations and deaths, and behavioral disturbances. Whether the prevalence is higher than that found in other forms of psychopathology is not well studied.[2]

These disorders have high rates of psychiatric comorbidity. Of individuals with AN, 50 to 70% suffer from major depression and/or dysthymia.[10] Of these patients, 10 to 15% suffer from obsessive-compulsive disorder.[10] In individuals with BN, 43% suffer from anxiety, 49% from addictive diseases,[11] 12% from bipolar disorder,[12] and 50 to 75% from personality disturbances.[13-15] Many bulimics have impulsive behaviors that include shopping sprees, promiscuity, self-mutilation, and shoplifting.[16-19]

V. SELECTED MEDICAL COMPLICATIONS

The eating disorders are unique among psychiatric illnesses because of the severe medical complications that result from the abnormal eating behavior and weight reduction methods utilized by this population. Theander's 33-year study[20] of women suffering from AN reported a crude mortality rate of 18%. This makes this disorder the deadliest of any psychiatric disorder. The majority of the physical sequelae of AN is related to the effects of starvation and is reversed by restoration of a balanced, healthy diet and weight. However, there are important differences between AN and starvation. In AN, protein intake is usually adequate, but there is limited consumption of carbohydrates, fats, and, thus, calories.[21] Vitamin deficiencies are uncommon. In starvation, the diet is lacking in protein, vitamins, and calories. Therefore, some immunological and hematological abnormalities are specific to AN, while others are also seen in starvation and malnutrition.[21] In BN, major problems relate to electrolyte imbalance and misdiagnosis and inappropriate treatment (e.g., incorrect diagnosis of pancreatitis).

Most of the major systems of the body can be affected, including cardiovascular, hematologic, gastrointestinal, renal, endocrine, and skeletal.[22] The typical AN patient looks younger than her actual age, having breast atrophy and being "petite". Lanugo (soft, downy hair), hair thinning, and carotenemia are common.

A. CARDIOVASCULAR COMPLICATIONS

Some of the most severe complications involve the cardiovascular system. Over 80% of patients suffer from cardiac abnormalities that include bradycardia, tachycardia, hypotension, ventricular arrhythmias, and cardiac failure.[21] Numerous electrocardiographic abnormalities occur including low voltage bradycardia, T-wave inversions, and ST segment depression. The most lethal findings are arrhythmias, ranging from supraventricular premature contractions to ventricular tachycardia. Prolonged QT intervals are not common, but are thought to be one etiology of sudden death.[22] The most common cardiac finding is bradycardia of less than 60 beats per minute, found in up to 87% of patients. Blood pressure less than 90/60 mmHg is seen in up to 85% of patients. One probable cause is related to chronic volume depletion which can cause dizziness/syncope.[21]

These patients are at risk for electrolyte abnormalities which may result in arrhythmias. If the patient engages in purging behavior, she may develop elevated serum bicarbonate and metabolic alkalosis.[23] Other abnormalities include hypochloremia and hypokalemia which may be further exacerbated by laxative abuse. Less frequently found are low serum bicarbonate, hypomagnesemia, and hyponatremia. Severe hypophosphatemia can occur and must be carefully monitored during the refeeding process.[24] Severe electrolyte and acid-base imbalances are the most frequent cause of death.[25]

Congestive heart failure can occur during the refeeding process, comparable to that reported in concentration camp and prisoner-of-war camp survivors in World War II. Rapid rehydration and administration of glucose-rich hyperalimentation may aggravate starvation-induced hypophosphatemia as well as place extra demands on compromised cardiac reserves.

Ipecac abuse to induce vomiting can cause irreversible myocardial damage.[22]

B. GASTROINTESTINAL COMPLICATIONS

Gastroenterologic complications are common and varied. They often involve the entire digestive tract from the mouth to the rectum, frequently interfering with nutritional rehabilitation.[23] Esophageal motility disorders have been reported, with up to half of patients with AN and one third of patients with bulimia having dysmotilities.[26,27] Indeed, Stacher et al. reported that in a total of 30 patients with AN, 7 had achalasia and 8 had other important motility disorders including diffuse spasm.[26] It has been suggested that primary esophageal motility disorders may regularly be observed in eating disorders, and/or esophageal dysmotility may contribute to the pathogenesis of the disease process. This has not been our experience, and we feel that these differences exist because our patients are all evaluated by gastroenterologists and nutritionists as well as psychiatrists in a "team approach" before the diagnosis of an eating disorder is made.[23]

Abnormal gastric emptying of solid food affects up to 80% of AN patients. In most patients, gastric emptying is delayed.[23] This delayed emptying usually responds to prokinetic agents such as cisapride or metaclopramide. A prolonged gastric emptying must be considered when refeeding the severely malnourished patient, since there have been rare reports of dilatation of the stomach with subsequent rupture.[28] More commonly, the delayed gastric emptying results in complaints of abdominal bloating and early satiety.

Small intestine functioning has not been thoroughly studied in these patients. However, several studies have reported delayed transit time.[29,30] Possible mechanisms for this include abnormalities in hypothalamic-pituitary function and/or thyroid function due to the emaciated state, disturbed sensitivity of cholinergic receptor, or impaired autonomic function.

Laxative abuse can cause episodes of diarrhea alternating with constipation. Rectal impaction has been reported in patients who have very little oral intake.[23]

Pancreatic abnormalities are associated with eating disorders.[31-33] Acute pancreatitis has been reported, sometimes in relation to the refeeding process.[32,33] Possible etiologies for the pancreatic abnormalities include severe protein calorie malnutrition, reflux into the pancreatic ducts from the duodenum due to vomiting, and inspissated secretions, if dehydration is present. In refeeding these patients, pancreatitis may develop if there is a rapid increase in caloric intake associated with a dehydrated, malnourished state.

Patients with eating disorders frequently have elevated serum amylase concentrations which may or may not be due to pancreatitis.[34-36] We measured serum amylase, lipase and isoamylase activity in 17 consecutive patients admitted to our Eating Disorder Unit.[34] Six patients had elevated amylase activity, and five of these six had isolated increases in salivary isoamylase activity. Six other patients had normal serum total amylase activity, but modest elevations in the salivary isoamylase fraction. No patient had clinical evidence of pancreatitis. Mitchell and colleagues reported that 30 of 108 consecutive outpatients seen in their eating disorder clinics had elevated serum amylase activity, which correlated with vomiting and binge eating.[35] Gwirtsman et al. reported that serum amylase helped distinguish between restrictor anorectics and bulimic anorectics.[36] More importantly, bulimics had a two- to four-fold increase in serum amylase activity after control binge eating and vomiting, whereas normal volunteers had no change in serum amylase after ingesting a large meal.[36] Most investigators have reported that the elevated serum amylase activity observed in some AN/BN patients normalizes while in the hospital in a controlled setting, which prevents binging and purging. Some physicians report that modest increases in serum amylase or isoamylase activity may be helpful in monitoring patient compliance in the outpatient setting.[36]

Associated with this hyperamylasemia may be the important physical finding of hypertrophy of the parotid glands, which may alert the physician to the possibility of an eating disorder.[23,34] This hypertrophy is usually bilateral, painless, and is often quite prominent. The etiology is poorly defined, but is thought to be related to high carbohydrate intake, alkylosis, malnutrition, and binging and purging. This usually resolves with resumption of normal eating, and is frequently associated with elevations in the serum isoamylase concentration.

In protein-calorie malnutrition, liver abnormalities are frequent, such as the fatty changes and enlarged liver seen in people suffering from kwashiorkor.[21] Clinically important liver disease directly relating to AN is quite rare. However, "nutritional hepatitis" with hypoproteinemia and hyperlipidemia, and mildly elevated serum lactate dehydrogenase and alkaline phosphatase were reported in an in-patient study in one-third of the anorexic patients.[37] Refeeding is the sole treatment recommended. The severe hypoglycemia that can occur in AN patients is thought to be related to depletion of liver glycogen stores in conjunction with fat stores not being available for gluconeogenesis.

Last, patients with eating disorders frequently have more nonspecific GI complaints such as belching, abdominal discomfort, flatulence, etc. compared to healthy age- and sex-matched controls.[23,38] These nonspecific symptoms usually improve with nutrition rehabilitation. Data are conflicting concerning whether eating disorder patients have increased problems with esophagitis and/or ulcer disease.[23] *Helicobacter pylori* is a Gram-negative spiral-shaped bacterium that resides in the antrum of the stomach and is thought to play an etiologic role in peptic ulcer disease.[39] This bacterium, when administered to normal volunteers, may induce vague abdominal discomfort similar to that seen in eating disorders.[40] However, recent unpublished data from our group show no difference in the incidence of *H. pylori* infection as determined by serology in eating disorder patients compared to age- and sex-matched controls.

C. RENAL COMPLICATIONS

Renal complications seen in AN patients include a decreased glomerular filtration rate and concentrating ability, increased blood urea nitrogen, electrolyte abnormalities, pitting edema, and hypokalemic nephropathy.[21,22,41] Different from other starvation syndromes, AN is not associated with inadequate protein intake and normal or elevated blood urea nitrogen levels are usually observed. In cases with chronic dehydration, renal calculi may develop.[42]

Electrolyte abnormalities occur more frequently in patients who abuse laxatives and/or diuretics and who engage in self-induced vomiting. Indeed, hypokalemia in an outpatient with an eating disorder suggests persistent purging and noncompliance with therapy.[43] With volume depletion that frequently occurs in these patients, a disproportionate increase in the blood urea nitrogen to creatinine ratio may be observed.[44]

Hypomagnesemia associated with refractory hypocalcemia and hypokalemia can occur. The low calcium and potassium may not improve unless magnesium is given simultaneously. Hypomagnesemia may lead to renal calculi production, as there may be increased urinary concentration of calcium.[45] Kidney stones have also been reported to occur in this population secondary to a relatively high oxalate intake (e.g., tea, spinach), chronic dehydration, low urine output, and purging.[41,42]

When there is long-standing abuse of laxatives and diuretics, hypokalemic nephropathy can occur and can lead to chronic renal failure with polyuria, polydipsia, and elevated serum creatinine.[45]

Two types of peripheral edema may occur, often when the patient is being refed.[46] A benign form, with normal plasma protein and albumin levels, is of unclear etiology and usually presents no adverse clinical sequelae. A more ominous form can follow chronic laxative abuse and vigorous purging. This may lead to hypoproteinemia with subsequent hypovolemia with fluid shifts. These patients may rarely develop shock, renal failure, and cardiovascular collapse.[45]

D. ENDOCRINE ABNORMALITIES

The individual with AN will have numerous endocrine changes that are probably related to low body fat, as well as psychological factors. By definition, the AN patient is amenorrheic. This is related to loss of more than 15% of ideal body weight. Some studies have reported that 90% of such women will begin menstruating when their body fat increases to 22% of total body weight.

In 16% of individuals with this disorder, amenorrhea develops before any weight loss. Amenorrhea may continue after weight restoration in some patients, supporting the hypothesis that the disturbance of hypothalamic function may be secondary to psychological stress.[21] Therefore, some patients must have restoration of weight as well as improvement in psychological functioning to regain normal menses.

The AN patient can also suffer from hypothalamic hypogonadism, with low basal levels of plasma luteinizing hormone (LH) and follicle stimulating hormone (FSH). The episodic release of these hormones can also be altered. The pattern of LH release is similar to that seen in puberty. These changes usually normalize with weight restoration.[21] The ovaries and uterus may be small and again normalize with weight gain (ovarian growth being related to gonadotropin functioning and uterine size to estrogen levels).[21] In the male AN patient, serum testosterone levels are decreased.[21] This is also seen in other starvation states.

Cortisol levels are elevated in eating disorder patients. This is generally due to decreased clearance and prolonged half-life. The secretion rate usually is not significantly altered.[21] This also may be seen in simple starvation.

Abnormal dexamethasone suppression is observed in 70 to 100% of eating disorder patients.[47]

Growth hormone levels may be normal or elevated with a reduced response to insulin-induced hypoglycemia.[21] Patients with AN generally have depressed levels of insulin-like growth factor-I (IGF-I), which mediates much of the anabolic aspects of growth hormone.[48] Patients with AN generally improve their IGF-I status as they regain weight.[48] It has been our experience that those with the least weight gain also have the poorest IGF-I response.[48] IGF-I is a sensitive marker of nutritional status. It is unclear in this situation whether poor weight gain in these patients is due to a poor IGF-I response or whether IGF-I is merely serving as a marker of the persisting malnutrition. Recent studies suggest that AN can be viewed as a condition of growth hormone resistance.[49,50] Body mass index was shown by Hochberg et al. to positively correlate with growth hormone responsiveness.[50] Both growth hormone and IGF-I have been used to increase nitrogen retention and weight gain in critically ill patients, and both agents have been shown to cause nitrogen retention in normal volunteers placed on a starvation diet in a clinical research setting.[51-55] Indeed, Kupfer et al. showed that a combination of both hormones was more effective at causing nitrogen retention than either one alone in food restricted normal volunteers.[52] The potential role of these two hormones alone or in combination in the nutritional therapy of severely malnourished patients remains to be determined.

Vasopressin release may be abnormal and, therefore, many patients (40%) may develop a partial neurogenic diabetes insipidus and increased urine output.[21] This is also seen in other starvation states.

There may be disturbed thyroid function. Thyroxine levels (T4) may be mildly depressed (but this generally is not clinically important). Free triiodothyronine (T3) levels may be 50% of those found in nonanorexic populations, secondary to diminished peripheral conversion of T4 to T3. Thyroxine stimulating hormone (TSH) levels are usually in the normal range. However, there may be abnormal responses to stimulation tests.[21]

Last, a recent report by Pomeroy et al. revealed increased plasma concentrations of the cytokines interleukin-6 (IL-6) and transforming growth factor-b (TGF-b) in AN patients that normalized by the end of therapy.[56] IL-6 plays an important role in the acute phase response and is thought to play a role in the anorexia seen in a variety of acute and chronic disease states. IL-6 is also thought to play a role in postmenopausal osteoporosis. Other investigators have reported increased spontaneous production of TNF from monocytes from AN patients which improved with weight gain.[57] If these observations are confirmed, this could be a potential point of therapeutic intervention for this disease process.

E. HEMATOLOGICAL COMPLICATIONS

Hematologic complications include a mild anemia and thrombocytopenia in one third of patients and leukopenia in two thirds of patients. Usually these changes are not clinically important. In severe cases, there may be a severe pancytopenia. The reduced serum complement levels that occur in other protein-calorie malnutrition states are generally not seen in AN patients. Refeeding usually normalizes any existing hematologic abnormalities.[21]

F. SKELETAL COMPLICATIONS

These patients are at increased risk to develop inadequate bone density with resulting pathological fractures and osteoporosis. Demonstrable osteoporosis is significantly correlated to the duration of illness and BMI.[58] It is hypothesized that this results from estrogen deficiency, malnutrition, increased cortisol levels, and possibly abnormal cytokine metabolism.[21] Long-term studies need to be conducted to determine how quickly the recovered anorexic individual's bone density returns to normal and whether these patients as adult women will be prone to osteoporosis and fractures of their vertebrae and long bones years after their recovery.

G. DERMATOLOGICAL AND DENTAL COMPLICATIONS

The skin is affected several ways in AN patients. Nutritional factors are linked to the development of lanugo on the extremities, back, and face seen in one third of these patients. In one fourth of cases, the skin can become dry, thin, and scaly. Carotenodermia/Carotenemia is seen in up to 80% of patients. Self-induced vomiting may lead to purpura (because of increased intrathoracic pressure associated with vomiting), and bruising.[21]

An important diagnostic sign of bulimia is skin changes over the dorsum of the hand. This is caused by trauma when the hand is used to induce vomiting. Lesions vary from elongated, superficial ulcerations to hyperpigmented calluses or scarring.[22]

Dental erosions also are a helpful diagnostic marker of bulimia. This involves the decalcification of the lingual, palatal, and posterior occlusal surfaces of the teeth. This pattern is consistent with frequent vomiting, with the acid bathing the back of the mouth.[22] Often, BN is first identified in the dental clinic, with subsequent psychiatric referral.

VI. SELECTED NUTRITIONAL DEFICIENCIES

A. VITAMINS

1. Water Soluble Vitamins

A large number of patients with eating disorders take vitamin supplements, and this practice may be one of the reasons that reports of vitamin deficiency in AN and BN are relatively infrequent.[59]

Sporadic case reports of deficiencies of water-soluble vitamins have appeared in the eating disorders literature since the early 1970s. In 1975, a South African physician reported a case of scurvy in a 25-year-old woman with AN. During her therapy, in an attempt to gain weight without ingesting large meals, she began to eat only calorie-dense carbohydrate-containing foods with the exclusion of all fruits and vegetables. This regimen resulted in the development of scurvy and iron deficiency anemia.[60]

There have been single reports of pellagra in a patient with AN and severe folate deficiency in a bulimic patient.[61,62] Numerous neurological complications of AN have been reported in the literature, some of which were the result of nutritional deficiency. A patient with Wernicke's encephalopathy was described by Handler and Perkins.[63] In a review of the records of 100 AN patients by Patchell et al., neurological complications were found in almost half. Neurological symptoms attributable to nutritional deficiency occurred in only one subject, a patient with B_{12} deficiency and paresthesias.[64]

2. Fat Soluble Vitamins

a. Vitamin A and Carotenoids

The hypercarotenemia seen in AN and BN patients has been perplexing to clinicians, since depressed serum carotene levels may be seen in other types of malnutrition. One potential explanation is that eating disorder patients emphasize foods with high carotene and vitamin A content, or supplement their diets with vitamins. However, surveys of diet composition of eating disorder patients suggests that their intake of vitamin A and carotene is actually quite low.[65,66] One study of the dietary intake of AN patients documented a mean intake of 446 ± 232 mg/day of vitamin A, much less than the RDA.

Serum retinol and retinol binding protein levels have been found to be normal in eating disorder patients despite this poor dietary intake.[67,68] To date, no manifestations of either vitamin A deficiency or excess have been described in eating disorder patients.

b. Vitamin E

Normal plasma vitamin E levels have been reported in both AN and BN patients.[66] Interpretation of vitamin E levels can be complicated by the hyperlipidemia occasionally seen in AN patients. Vitamin E is carried exclusively on lipoproteins and levels are highly correlated with total lipid level. The ratio of vitamin E level to total lipid is therefore considered to be a better reflection of body stores than a plasma level alone. The previously mentioned studies did not report the number of patients with elevated serum lipid levels. The concurrent measurement of lipids may be particularly important in these patients because the hyperlipidemia occasionally seen in eating disorders may cause plasma vitamin E levels to be normal even in the presence of inadequate body stores.

c. Vitamin K

Vitamin K deficiency has only rarely been reported in eating disorder patients. In 1983, a BN patient with coagulopathy resulting from deficiency of vitamin K-dependent clotting factors was reported.[69] In one additional study of the vitamin status of 24 AN and 8 BN patients, prolonged prothrombin time was reported in five, but vitamin K levels were not determined in these patients.[66]

In a study of vitamins and trace mineral status of women with disordered eating, Mira et al. actually found that eating disorder patients who were not taking vitamins had higher vitamin A and E levels than nonvitamin-using controls. For this reason, they suggest that supplementation with fat soluble vitamins may be contraindicated in women using self-induced vomiting as a means of weight control.[59]

B. TRACE METALS
1. Zinc

The trace mineral, zinc, plays an integral role in regulation of food intake. There are individual reports of eating disorder patients having depressed serum zinc levels and some patients who had signs and symptoms of zinc deficiency that responded to zinc supplementation.[70-72] Many individuals with AN and BN have the same symptoms and signs as persons who are zinc deficient, such as a cyclic pattern of food intake, weight loss, amenorrhea, gastric distension, alterations in mood (including depression), and skin lesions.[73]

A high frequency of biochemical zinc deficiency has been reported in a series of eating disorder patients.[74] We evaluated zinc status before and after nutritional rehabilitation (with and without zinc supplementation) in a randomized double-blind placebo-controlled study in bulimics, anorexics, and controls.[73] Pretreatment 24-h urinary zinc excretion was low in the bulimic study group and significantly depressed in the anorexic study group compared to a healthy control group. During hospitalization, serum zinc concentrations increased in all patients who received zinc supplements (vs. placebo). Urinary zinc excretion increased in both zinc supplemented and placebo-treated bulimics. Urinary zinc concentrations dramatically increased in zinc supplemented anorexics, but decreased or remained unacceptably low in the placebo group. By dietary history, controls (noneating disordered) consumed the recommended daily allowance (RDA) for zinc (11.95 ± 1.25 mg/d); anorexics 6.46 ± 1.14 mg/d; and bulimics 8.93 ± 1.29 mg/d. Thus, neither eating disorder group was consuming the RDA for zinc as an outpatient. Both the bulimic and anorexic patients who received zinc supplementation had significant improvement in biochemical zinc status when refed as inpatients. This was not seen in the AN patients who were receiving placebo. In fact, this group had a prominent worsening of zinc status during hospitalization and refeeding, in spite of consuming the RDA for zinc (probably due to increased anabolic needs for zinc during aggressive refeeding). Because aggressive nutritional rehabilitation is a mainstay of therapy for AN patients, this study strongly suggested that AN patients receive oral zinc supplementation in addition to an otherwise well-balanced diet during vigorous refeeding.

This study suggests that zinc deficiency may act as a sustaining factor for abnormal eating behavior in certain eating disorder patients and therefore could contribute to the chronicity and severity of the eating disorder symptoms.

Supporting this concept is the study by Katz et al., in which adolescents with AN were randomized to zinc supplementation or placebo. Those receiving zinc had a significant lowering of anxiety and depression.[75]

2. Copper

Casper et al. reported depressed plasma copper levels in a group of 30 patients hospitalized for therapy of AN.[76] Although they did not detect depressed ceruloplasmin levels, studies from our group demonstrated depressed copper levels in AN patients, intermediate levels in bulimia patients, and depressed ceruloplasmin levels that corresponded to copper values in both groups. Since copper deficiency has been previously shown to be associated with an increase in serum cholesterol, copper metabolism may well play a role in the hypercholesterolemia sometimes observed in these patients.[23]

VII. NUTRITIONAL AND STABILIZATION THERAPY

A. OVERVIEW

AN and BN are difficult to treat, because they are chronic processes associated with frequent relapses, and they carry a disturbingly high mortality rate. For these reasons, treatment demands a comprehensive and multidisciplinary approach including medical management, individual, group, and family psychotherapies, cognitive and behavioral strategies, nutritional counseling, and psychopharmacologic therapy.

Psychotherapy historically has been and remains the major focus of treatment, but restoring nutritional status and regular eating patterns is the first objective in patient care. Thus, the nutritionist is an important participant in the interdisciplinary treatment team and can provide nutritional counseling to the patient and family. While these patients often know the caloric and nutrient content of foods (e.g., fat, carbohydrates), healthy eating behavior needs to be encouraged and reinforced. Additionally, the nutritionist's expertise is vital in restoring a healthy diet.

B. BULIMIA NERVOSA

Most patients with BN can be treated as an outpatient unless there is severe dehydration and/or metabolic alterations requiring hospitalization. In order to structure a comprehensive nutritional therapy program for BN patients, an understanding of their eating pattern and its overall effect on attitude, mood, body perception, and energy expenditure is required. In one of the initial descriptions of BN, Russell pointed out that these patients could consume huge amounts of calories (up to 20,000 kcal) in less than a day.[77] Since then, multiple reports have documented highly chaotic eating patterns with excess caloric consumption in bulimic patients, with great individual variability. In a recent report from the NIH, Hetherington et al. observed voluntary eating patterns of bulimics and normal controls who were allowed *ad libitum* food intake in an observed setting on an inpatient eating disorder unit.[78] Bulimic subjects consumed approximately 10,000 cal/d compared to 1900 cal for normal control subjects. These investigators noted a marked variability in food intake from day to day and from individual to individual in the bulimic subjects. On average, the bulimics binged 1.6 times, purged three times, and ate one snack or one meal daily without purging. Macronutrient analysis demonstrated less energy intake from protein and more energy intake from fat in bulimics compared to controls. However, it should be noted that the RDA for protein still was exceeded in the bulimic patients. On average, patients drank 3.2 l of fluid per day (usually low-energy carbonated drinks such as diet sodas). This large amount of liquid could then facilitate a purge. An important feature observed by these investigators and others is the fact that bulimics appear to lose control of their eating. For example, a bulimic may start eating a meal or snack and subsequently lose control, binge, and then feel compelled to purge. In the study by Hetherington et al.,[78] body satisfaction increased and a feeling of being fat decreased 1 h after eating when foods had been purged compared to 1 h after a nonpurged meal. It also was noted that meals were less likely to be purged if they were preceded by a lower hunger rating and desire to eat. This and other studies have raised the possibility that bulimics have better control over their eating when they are only moderately hungry, and they are at high risk for binging and purging when they have fasted for some period of time and are hungry. Thus, one form of nutritional therapy used by many groups is to reinforce structured meals and regular eating habits.[78,79] This includes preventing long periods of fasting with the development of hunger, and the subsequent urge to binge and purge.

Several groups have suggested that purging can reduce feelings of "fatness" and nausea, and can provide relief from negative mood states. Thus, unfortunately, this altered eating pattern can provide positive reinforcement to the patient and it must be interrupted at psychotherapy and nutritional levels.[80-82]

Data relating to energy expenditure also suggest a sustaining or reinforcing role for abnormal eating patterns in BN patients. Recent research from the Rockefeller University General Clinical Research Center (GCRC) suggests that subjects may have a "set point" for maintenance of usual weight.[83] If obese patients attempted to lose weight, their energy expenditure decreased. Similar observations were seen in subjects who had never been obese. Thus, reducing and subsequently maintaining weight at 10% or below initial weight was associated with an overall reduction in energy expenditure, which would inherently make it difficult to maintain this reduced weight. On the other hand, increasing body weight to a level of 10% above usual weight was associated with increased energy expenditure. Thus, the body appears to oppose either increases or decreases in body weight that are substantially different from what the body has determined as a normal "set point". There is evidence that bulimic patients initially may have low energy expenditure, or their energy expenditure may be reduced in periods of normal eating compared to periods of binging and purging.[84] Thus, binging and purging appeared to reduce energy expenditure, and this would be a factor that reinforced abnormal eating behavior. Studies from the University of Kentucky's Eating Disorder Center showed that bulimic patients had a mean baseline resting energy expenditure that was significantly lower than controls on admission to a GCRC (1342 vs. 1549 kcal) and this overall energy expenditure decreased in bulimics to 1289 kcal after one month of in-hospital therapy.[85] When energy expenditure was expressed related to lean body mass or related to BMI, similar reductions were seen in energy expenditure in bulimics over their hospital course. Thus, it appears that bulimic patients have normal/low-normal energy expenditure in the free living setting where they are actively binging and purging, and that this energy expenditure decreases to below normal when these altered eating behaviors are interrupted.

In summary, there are many factors that reinforce the binge-purge cycle. Thus, the role of the eating disorder team and the nutritionist is to lay a firm foundation of nutritional education for the patient, to reinforce structured eating behavior, to prevent periods of starvation/hunger with subsequent over-eating, to prevent chaotic eating behavior, and to address the fears of weight gain and distorted body image.

C. ANOREXIA NERVOSA

The best outcome in AN patients is related to weight restoration and resumption of normal eating behavior. This usually needs to be accompanied by individual and family psychotherapies when the patient is medically stable.[2] Weight gain in the AN patient has been shown to improve overall body image.[86] It has been the clinical impression of many investigators including us that AN patients respond better to treatment if nutritional therapy results in early weight gain. The ultimate weight goal should be a return to an individually determined weight at which normal reproductive function resumes and bone demineralization is stopped.

Similar to BN, it is important to understand the underlying metabolic status and energy requirements in the AN patient in order to define appropriate nutritional therapy. It is well accepted that in states of malnutrition the resting energy expenditure (REE) is reduced. At the end of World War II, extensive research was conducted on starvation by Keys and colleagues in the Minnesota Experiment.[87] They demonstrated that the basal metabolic rate (BMR) of adult men decreased following six months of restricted food intake with a simultaneous loss of 25% of body weight, but energy expenditure increased again with refeeding. Their work served as the foundation for many other studies documenting adaptative hypometabolism during states of starvation. Indeed, many initial studies in patients with AN reported low energy expenditures.[88-90] Most of these studies suggested that the decreased energy expenditure was a metabolic adaptation to starvation. Some investigators such as Dempsey et al. also reported that this decreased energy expenditure improved during the course of nutritional rehabilitation.[90] However, more recent studies have suggested that energy expenditure in AN patients may not be reduced, especially if corrected for lean body mass. Indeed, studies from our laboratory suggested that AN patients may even be slightly hypermetabolic on admission to a clinical research center when the energy expenditure was corrected for lean body mass.[85] Energy expenditure normalized after 1 month of therapy in these AN patients. Studies by Obarzanek et al. from the NIMH showed somewhat similar results.[91] They related resting metabolic rate to kilogram lean body mass. They showed that resting metabolic rate was not significantly different in AN patients on admission, during early refeeding, or at target weight compared to healthy volunteers. However, during late refeeding, resting metabolic rate was significantly higher in AN patients. Thus, investigators recently questioned whether AN patients really are hypometabolic. The amount of calories consumed that are required to gain weight in AN patients is highly variable. The assumption that these patients are all hypometabolic and should easily gain weight is not necessarily correct, and this must be taken into consideration by the psychiatrist, nutritionist, and other health care workers caring for the AN patient. Thus, just because an AN patient is not gaining weight as predicted does not necessarily mean that the patient is purging or secretly exercising (although these factors must be considered).

The AN patient who is not less than 20% below average weight for height frequently can be successfully treated on an outpatient basis. Indeed, in this area of managed care, there is an even greater emphasis on outpatient therapy in these subjects. Nutritional care includes helping the AN patient change her/his ideas about food. Close monitoring is essential, and this treatment usually requires a cooperative, motivated patient with psychosocial support. Since vitamin deficiency is infrequent in these patients, even in the absence of vitamin supplementation, routine provision of therapeutic doses of vitamins is not indicated. Zinc supplementation is recommended in AN patients. Calcium supplementation and/or estrogen supplements in women with bone density below 0.8 g/cm should be considered.

Those patients who do not meet these requirements or who are medically unstable require nutritional rehabilitation in an inpatient setting.[2] A variety of inpatient treatment settings exist which use multiple methods to help these treatment-resistant patients restore weight and normal eating patterns. These include behavioral modification programs that use both positive (praise) and negative (bed rest) reinforcers to enable patients to reestablish oral caloric intake and stop pathological binging and purging.

Nasogastric tube feedings, or even total parenteral nutrition, may be required in life-threatening situations or for patients who are refractory to therapy.[2] There can be serious sequelae from rapid refeeding, including severe fluid retention, cardiac failure, and hypophosphatemia. Therefore, this must be done very cautiously with monitoring of electrolyte and cardiac status. Some patients more readily accept nasogastric feedings than eating since this is less frightening, particularly in the early phases of refeeding. We regularly attempt to place our feeding tubes in a postpyloric position so the patient will not be bothered with gastric distention. Frequently, tubes are placed endoscopically. This allows us to also rule out GI pathology as a cause of GI complaints in these patients. The potential role of anabolic hormones such as growth hormone or IGF-I in malnourished and/or treatment-resistant patients must also be determined and is a topic of current investigative attention.

Patients in the advanced stages of AN can present a difficult clinical dilemma for the treatment team, i.e., consideration of forced feeding. When this is being considered, the specific clinical circumstances, family opinion, and relevant legal and ethical issues need to be cautiously assessed.[2] Guidelines for withholding of forced nutrition in the terminally ill have been published.[92] These have been largely applied to the terminally ill and, more recently, to patients exhibiting severe incompetence, such as seen in dementia.[93] Patients with severe, treatment-resistant AN are more difficult to categorize.

The usual approach to the question of forced feeding requires an ethical analysis, considering patient autonomy (requires patient to be competent), medical benefit, and justice or fairness (considering the interests of all involved).[93] There is a weighing of benefit vs. harm that simplistically can appear objective and balanced. However, one must also consider the strong negative feelings that caregivers can subconsciously develop toward such resistant patients. The patient suffering from chronic AN is the prototype of the provoking, difficult patient. They have been described as "irascible, manipulating patients who plague concerned physicians."[93] Intractable cases can leave treatment teams feeling frustrated and paralyzed in their efforts to treat the patient. Such feelings can impair how these patients are treated, and caregivers must maintain objectivity in making difficult clinical decisions.

VIII. CONCLUSION

This chapter summarizes relevant clinical issues for the nutritionist and other health care providers working with eating disorder patients. These patients present with an intricate interaction of psychopathology, interpersonal difficulties, and complex medical issues that require a sophisticated treatment approach that demands several disciplines working together as a united force. Several unresolved issues regarding the treatment process are reviewed. It is evident that much is still unknown. However, it is clear that no meaningful psychotherapy can be accomplished until the patient is nutritionally stable and unencumbered by medical complications and nutritionally based cognitive defects.

ACKNOWLEDGMENT

This research was partially funded by the NIH #M01-RR-2602, Veterans Administration, and the McKnight Foundation.

REFERENCES

1. Mitchell, J. E. and Eckert, E. E., Scope and significance of eating disorders, *J. Consult. Clin. Psychol.*, 55, 628, 1987.
2. Yager, J., Andersen, A., Devlin, M., Mitchell, J., Powers, P., and Yates, A., Practice guideline for eating disorders, *Am. J. Psychiatry*, 150, 207, 1993.
3. *Diagnostic and Statistical Manual of Mental Disorders*, Vol. 4, American Psychiatric Association, Washington, D.C., 1994, 539.
4. Lucas, A. R., Beard, C. M., O'Fallon, W. M., and Kurlan, L. T., 50-year trends in the incidence of anorexia nervosa in Rochester, Minn.: a population-based study, *Am. J. Psychiatry*, 148, 917, 1991.
5. Kendler, K. S., MacLean, C., Neale, M., Kessler, R., Heath, A., and Eaves, L., The genetic epidemiology of bulimia nervosa, *Am. J. Psychiatry*, 148, 1627, 1991.
6. Nagel, K. L. and Jones, K. H., Sociological factors in the development of eating disorders, *Adolescence*, 27, 107, 1992.
7. Herzog, D. B., Newman, K. L., and Warshaw, M., Body image dissatisfaction in homosexual and heterosexual males, *J. Nerv. Ment. Dis.*, 179, 356, 1991.
8. Whitaker, A., Johnson, J., Shaffer, D., Rapoport, J. L., Kalikow, K., Walsh, B. T., Davies, M., Braiman, S., and Dolinsky, A., Uncommon troubles in young people: prevalence estimates of selected psychiatric disorders in a non-referred adolescent population, *Arch. Gen. Psychiatry*, 47, 487, 1990.
9. Aronson, J. K., Ed., *Insights in the Dynamic Psychotherapy of Anorexia and Bulimia*, 1993, 10.
10. Halmi, K. A., Eckert, E., Marchi, P., Sampugnaro, V., Apple, R., and Cohen, J., Co-morbidity of psychiatric diagnoses in anorexia nervosa, *Arch. Gen. Psychiatry*, 48, 712, 1991.
11. Hudson, J. I., Pope, H. G., Jr., Yurgelun-Todd, D., Jonas, J. M., and Frankenburg, F. R., A controlled study of lifetime prevalence of affective and other psychiatric disorders in bulimic outpatients, *Am. J. Psychiatry*, 144, 1283, 1987.
12. Shisslak, C. M., Perse, T., and Crago, M., Coexistence of bulimia nervosa and mania: a literature review and case report, *Compr. Psychiatry*, 32, 181, 1991.
13. Gartner, A. F., Marcus, R. N., Halmi, K., and Loranger, A. W., DSM-III-R personality disorders in patients with eating disorders, *Am. J. Psychiatry*, 146, 1585, 1989.
14. Yager, J., Landsverk, J., Edelstein, C. K., and Hyler, S. E., Screening for axis II personality disorders in women with bulimic eating disorders, *Psychosomatics*, 30, 255, 1989.
15. Zararini, M. C., Frankenburg, F. R., Pope H. G., Jr., Hudson, J. I., Yurgolon-Todd, D., and Cicchetti, C. J., Axis II co-morbidity of normal weight bulimia, *Compr. Psychiatry*, 31, 20, 1990.
16. Wilson, C. P., Hogan, C. C., and Mintz, I. L., Eds., *Fear of Being Fat: The Treatment of Anorexia Nervosa and Bulimia Nervosa*, 2nd Ed., Jason Aronson, Northvale, N.J., 1985.
17. Wilson, C. P., Hogan, C. C., and Mintz, I. L., Eds., *Psychodynamic Technique in the Treatment of Eating Disorders*, Jason Aronson, Northvale, N.J., 1992.
18. Schwartz, H. J., *Bulimia: Psychodynamic Treatment and Theory*, 2nd Ed., International Universities Press, Madison, CT, 1990.
19. Favazza A. R., DeRosear, L., and Conterio, K., Self-mutilation and eating disorders, *Suicide Life Threat. Behav.*, 19, 352, 1989.
20. Theander, S., Outcome and prognosis in anorexia nervosa and bulimia: some results of previous investigations, compared with those of a Swedish long-term study, *J. Psychiatr. Res.*, 19, 493, 1985.
21. Sharp, C. W. and Freeman, C. P. L., The medical complications of anorexia nervosa, *Br. J. Psychiatry*, 162, 452, 1993.

22. Herzog, D. and Bradburn, I., The nature of anorexia nervosa and bulimia nervosa in adolescents, in *Feeding Problems and Eating Disorders in Children and Adolescents*, Cooper, P. J. and Stein, A., Eds., Harwood Academic Publishers, Switzerland, 1992, 126.

23. McClain, C. J., Humphries, L., Hill, K., and Nickl, N., Gastrointestinal aspects of eating disorders, *J. Am. Coll. Nutr.*, 12, 466, 1993.

24. Kaysar, N., Kronenberg, J., Polliack, M., and Gaoni, B., Severe hypophosphatemia during binge eating in anorexia nervosa, *Arch. Dis. Child.*, 66, 138, 1991.

25. Winston, D., Treatment of severe malnutrition in anorexia nervosa with enteral tube feedings, *Nutr. Supp. Serv.*, 7, 24, 1987.

26. Stacher, G., Kiss, A., Weisnagrotzki, S., Bergmann, H., Hobart, J., and Schneider, C., Oesophageal and gastric motility disorders in patients categorized as having primary anorexia nervosa, *Gut*, 27, 1120, 1986.

27. Kiss, A., Bergmann, H., Abatzi, T. A., Schneider, C., Wiesnagrotzki, S., Hobart, J., Steiner-Mittelbach, G., Gaupmann, G., Kugi, A., Stacher-Janotta, G., Steinringa, H., and Stacher, G., Oesophageal and gastric motor activity in patients with bulimia nervosa, *Gut*, 31, 259, 1990.

28. Russell, G. F. M., Acute dilatation of the stomach in a patient with anorexia nervosa, *Br. J. Psychiatry*, 112, 203, 1966.

29. Haller, J. O., Slovis, T. L., Baker, C. H., Berdon, W. E., and Silverman, J. A., Anorexia nervosa: the paucity of radiologic findings in more than fifty patients, *Pediatr. Radiol.*, 5, 145, 1977.

30. Hirakawa, M., Okada, T., Iida, M., Tamai, H., Kobayoshi, N., Nakagawa, T., and Fujishima, M., Small bowel transit time measured by hydrogen breath test in patients with anorexia nervosa, *Dig. Dis. Sci.*, 35, 733, 1990.

31. Gilinsky, N. H., Humphries, L. L., Fried, M. F., and McClain, C. J., Computed tomographic abnormalities of the pancreas in eating disorders: a report of two cases with normal laparotomy, *Int. J. Eating Disorders*, 7, 567, 1988.

32. Keane, F. B., Fennell, J. S., and Tomkin, G. H., Acute pancreatitis, acute gastric dilatation and duodenal ileus following refeeding in anorexia nervosa, *Int. J. Med. Sci.*, 147, 191, 1978.

33. McDermott, W. V., Bartlett, M. K., and Culver, P. A., Acute pancreatitis after prolonged fast and subsequent surfeit. *N. Engl. J. Med.*, 279, 1956.

34. Humphries, L. L., Adams, L. J., Eckfeldt, J. H., Levitt, M., and McClain, C. J., Hyper-amylasemia in patients with eating disorders, *Ann. Intern. Med.*, 106, 50, 1987.

35. Mitchell, J. E., Pyle, R. L., Eckert, E. D., Hatsukami, D., and Lentz, R., Electrolyte and other physiologic abnormalities in patients with bulimia, *Psychol. Med.*, 13, 273, 1983.

36. Gwirtsman, H. E., Kaye, W. H., George, D. T., Carosella, N. W., Greene, R. C., and Jimerson, D. C., Hyperamylasemia and its relationship to binge-purge episodes: development of a clinically relevant laboratory test, *J. Clin. Psychiatry*, 50, 196, 1989.

37. Hall, R. C. W., Hoffman, R. S., Beresford, T. P., Wooley, B., Hall, A. K., and Kubasak, L., Physical illness encountered in patients with eating disorders, *Psychosomatics*, 30, 174, 1989.

38. Waldholtz, B. D. and Andersen, A. E., Gastrointestinal symptoms in anorexia nervosa, *Gastroenterology*, 98, 1415, 1990.

39. Nomura, A., Stemmermann, G., Chyou, P.-H., Perez-Perez, G., and Blaser, M., Helico-bacter pylori infection and the risk for duodenal and gastric ulceration, *Ann. Intern. Med.*, 120, 977, 1994.

40. Marshall, B., Armstrong, J., McGechie, D., and Glancy, R., Attempt to fulfill Koch's postulates for pyloric campylobacter, *Med. J. Aust.*, 142, 436, 1985.

41. Brotman, A. W., Stern, T. A., and Brotman, D. L., Renal disease and dysfunction in two patients with anorexia nervosa, *J. Clin. Psychiatry*, 47, 433, 1986.

42. Silber, T. J. and Kass, E. J., Anorexia nervosa and nephrolithiasis, *J. Adolesc. Health Care*, 5, 50, 1984.

43. Greenfeld, D., Mickley, D., Quinlan, D. M., and Roloff, P., Hypokalemia in outpatients with eating disorders, *Am. J. Psychiatry*, 152, 60, 1995.

44. Sheinin, J. C., Medical aspects of eating disorders, *Adolesc. Psychiatry*, 13, 405, 1986.

45. Hall, R. C. and Beresford, T. P., Medical complications of anorexia and bulimia, *Psychiatr. Med.*, 7, 165, 1989.

46. Silverman, J. A., Clinical and medical aspects of anorexia nervosa, *Int. J. Eating Disorders*, 2, 159, 1983.

47. Gerner, G. C. W. and Gwirtsman, H. E., Abnormalities of dexamethasone suppression test and urinary MHPG in anorexia nervosa, *Am. J. Psychiatry*, 138, 650, 1981.

48. Hill, K. K., Hill, D. B., McClain, M. P., Humphries, L., and McClain, C. J., Serum insulin-like growth factor-I concentrations in the recovery of patients with anorexia nervosa, *J. Am. Coll. Nutr.*, 12, 475, 1993.

49. Counts, D. R., Gwirtsman, H., Carlsson, L. M. S., Lesem, M., and Cutler, G. B., The effect of anorexia nervosa and refeeding on growth hormone-binding protein, the insulin-like growth factors (IGFs), and the IGF-binding proteins, *J. Clin. Endocrinol. Metab.*, 75, 762, 1992.

50. Hochberg, Z., Hertz, P., Colin, V., Ish-Shalom, S., Yeshurun, D., Youdim, M. B. H., and Amit, T., The distal axis of growth hormone (GH) in nutritional disorders: GH-binding protein, insulin-like growth factor-I (IGF-I), and IGF-I receptors in obesity and anorexia nervosa, *Metabolism*, 41, 106, 1992.

51. Wilmore, D. W., Catabolic illness: strategies for enhancing recovery, *Semin. Med. Beth Israel Hosp., (Boston)*, 325, 695, 1991.

52. Kupfer, S. R., Underwood, L. E., Baxter, R. C., and Clemmons, D. R., Enhancement of the anabolic effects of growth hormone and insulin-like growth factor I by use of both agents simultaneously, *J. Clin. Invest.*, 91, 391, 1993.

53. Horber, F. F. and Haymond, M. W., Human growth hormone prevents protein catabolic side effects of prednisone in humans, *J. Clin. Invest.*, 86, 265, 1990.

54. Clemmons, D. R., Smith-Banks, A., and Underwood, L. E., Reversal of diet-induced catabolism by infusion of recombinant insulin-like growth factor (IGF-I) in humans, *J. Clin. Endocrinol. Metab.*, 75, 234, 1992.

55. Manson, J. and Wilmore, D. W., Positive nitrogen balance with human growth hormone and hypocaloric intravenous feeding, *Surgery*, 100, 188, 1986.

56. Pomeroy, C., Eckert, E., Hu, S., Eiken, B., Mentink, M., Crosby, R. D., and Chao, C., Role of interluekin-6 and transforming growth factor-b in anorexia nervosa, *Biol. Psychiatry*, 36, 836, 1994.

57. Vaisman, N. and Hahn, T., Tumor necrosis factor-a and anorexia — cause or effect?, *Metabolism*, 40, 720, 1991.

58. Bachrach, L. K., Guido, D., Katzman, D., Lift, I. F., and Marcus, R., Decreased bone density in adolescent girls with anorexia nervosa, *Pediatrics*, 86, 440, 1990.

59. Mira, M., Stewart, P., and Abraham, S., Vitamin and trace element status of women with disordered eating, *Am. J. Clin. Nutr.*, 50, 940, 1989.

60. George, G., Zabow, T., and Beumont, P., Scurvy in anorexia nervosa, *S. Afr. Med. J.*, 49, 1420, 1975.

61. Rapaport, M., Pellagra in a patients with anorexia nervosa, *Arch. Dermatol.*, 121, 255, 1985.

62. Eedy, D., Cevoran, J., and Andrews, W., A patient with bulimia nervosa and profound folate deficiency, *Postgrad. Med. J.*, 62, 853, 1986.

63. James, W. and Trayhurn, P., An integrated view of the metabolic and genetic basis for obesity, *Lancet*, 2, 771, 1982.

64. Patchell, R., Fellows, H., and Humphries, L., Neurologic complications of anorexia nervosa, *Acta Neurol. Scand.*, 89, 111, 1994.

65. Beumont, P., Chambers, T., Rouse, L., and Abraham, S., The diet composition and nutritional knowledge of patients with anorexia nervosa, *J. Hum. Nutr.*, 35, 265, 1981.

66. Philip, E., Pirke, K-M., Seidl, M., Tuschl, R., Fichter, M., Eckert, M., and Wolfram, G., Vitamin status in patients with anorexia nervosa and bulimia nervosa, *Int. J. Eating Disorders*, 8(2), 209, 1988.

67. Langan, S. and Farrell, P., Vitamin E, vitamin A and essential fatty acid status of patients hospitalized for anorexia nervosa., *Am. J. Clin. Nutr.*, 41, 1054, 1985.

68. Curran-Celentano, J., Erdman, J., Nelson, R., and Grater, S., Alterations in vitamin A and thyroid hormone status in anorexia nervosa and associated disorders, *Am. J. Clin. Nutr.*, 42, 1183, 1985.

69. Niiya, K., Kitagawa, T., Fujishita, M., Yoshimoto, S., Kobayashi, M., Kubonishi, I., Taguchi, H., and Miyoshi, I., Bulimia nervosa complicated by deficiency of vitamin K-dependent coagulation factors, *J.A.M.A.*, 250, 792, 1983.

70. Esca, S. A., Brenner, W., Mach, K., and Gschnait, F., Kwashiorkor-like zinc deficiency syndrome in anorexia nervosa, *Acta Derm. Venereol. (Stockholm)*, 59, 283, 1978.

71. Safai-Kutti, S. and Kutti, J., Zinc and anorexia nervosa, *Ann. Intern. Med.*, 100, 317, 1984.

72. Safai-Kutti, S. and Kutti, J., Zinc supplementation in anorexia nervosa, *Am. J. Clin. Nutr.*, 44, 581, 1986.

73. McClain, C. J., Stuart, M. A., Vivian, B., McClain, M., Talwalker, R., Snelling, L., and Humphries, L., Zinc status before and after zinc supplementation of eating disorder patients, *J. Am. Coll. Nutr.*, 11, 694, 1992.

74. Humphries, L., Vivian, B., Stuart, M., and McMclain, C. J., Zinc deficiency and eating disorders, *J. Clin. Psychiatry*, 50, 456, 1989.

75. Katz, R., Keen, C., Litt, I., Hurley, L., Kellams-Harrison, K., and Glader, L., Zinc deficiency in anorexia nervosa, *J. Adoles. Health Care*, 8, 400, 1987.

76. Casper, R., Kirschner, B., Sandstead, H., Jacob, R., and Davis, J., An evaluation of trace metals, vitamins, and taste function in anorexia nervosa, *Am. J. Clin. Nutr.*, 33, 18011, 1980.

77. Russell, G. F., Bulimia nervosa: an ominous variant of anorexia nervosa, *Psychol. Med.*, 9, 429, 1979.

78. Hetherington, M. M., Altemus, M., Nelson, M. L., Bernat, A. S., and Gold, P. W., Eating behavior in bulimia nervosa: multiple meal analyses, *Am. J. Clin. Nutr.*, 60, 864, 1994.

79. Laessle, R. G., Beumont, P., Butow, P., et al., A comparison of nutritional management with stress management in the treatment of bulimia nervosa, *Br. J. Psychiatry*, 159, 250, 1991.

80. Kaye, W. H., Gwirtsman, H. E., George, D. T., Weiss, S. R., and Jimerson, D. C., Relationship of mood alterations to bingeing behaviour in bulimia, *Br. J. Psychiatry*, 149, 479, 1986.

81. Lingswiler, V. M., Crowther, J. H., and Parris Stephens, M. A., Emotional and somatic consequences of binge episodes, *Addict. Behav.*, 14, 503, 1989.

82. Johnson, C. and Larson, R., Bulimia: an analysis of moods and behavior, *Psychosom. Med.*, 44, 333, 1982.

83. Liebel, R., Rosenbaum, M., and Hirsch, J., Changes in energy expenditure resulting from altered body weight, *N. Engl. J. Med.*, 332, 621, 1995.

84. Altemus, M., Hetherington, M. M., Flood, M., et al., Decrease in resting metabolic rate during abstinence from bulimic behavior, *Am. J. Psychiatry*, 148, 1071, 1991.

85. Phillips, R., Humphries, L., Vivian, B., and McClain, C., The effects of treatment for anorexia and bulimia on energy expenditure and thermic response, *J. Am. Diet. Assoc.*, 89(9) (September Suppl), A82, 1989.

86. Garfinkel, P. and Garner, D., *Anorexia Nervosa: a Multidimensional Perspective*, Brunner-Mazel, New York, 1982, 217.

87. Keys, A., Brozek, J., Henschel, A., Mickelsen, O., and Taylor, H. L., Basal metabolic rate, in *The Biology of Human Starvation*, Vol. 1, University of Minnesota Press, St. Paul, 1950,

88. Walker, J., Roberts, S., Halmi, K., and Goldberg, S., Caloric requirements for weight gain in anorexia nervosa, *Am. J. Clin. Nutr.*, 32, 1396, 1979.

89. Stordy, J., Marks, V., Kalug, R., and Crisp, A., Weight gain, thermic effect of glucose and resting metabolic rate during recovery from anorexia nervosa, *Am. J. Clin. Nutr.*, 3, 138, 1977.

90. Dempsey, D., Crosby, L., Pertschub, M., Feurer, I., Busly, G., and Mullen, Weight gain and nutritional efficacy in anorexia nervosa, *Am. J. Clin. Nutr.*, 39, 236, 1984.

91. Obarzanek, E., Lesem, M. D., and Jimerson, D. C., Resting metabolic rate of anorexia nervosa patients during weight gain, *Am. J. Clin. Nutr.*, 60, 666, 1994.

92. Hastings Center, *Guidelines on the Termination of Life-sustaining Treatment and the Care of the Dying*, Indiana University Press, Bloomington, IN, 1987.

93. Herbert, P. and Weingarten, M., The ethics of forced feeding in anorexia nervosa, *Can. Med. Assoc. J.*, 2, 144, 1991.

Chapter 8

NUTRITION, CARDIOVASCULAR DISEASE, AND WOMEN

Dorothy J. Klimis-Tavantzis and Ira Wolinsky

CONTENTS

I. INTRODUCTION

Recently, there has been recognition of the need for a national agenda focusing on women's health issues. Studies to date of prevention, diagnosis, and intervention for cardiovascular disease (CVD) have either been conducted in men, or data have not been analyzed to study gender differences. Reasons given for excluding women from clinical studies are (1) that results would be confounded by women's cyclical hormonal changes; (2) study populations would be less homogenous; (3) sex-specific hypotheses or analyses require larger and more costly studies; (4) legal and ethical issues surmount potential risks to a fetus; and (5) recruitment of women is more difficult.[1] The establishment of the Office of Research on Women's Health by the National Institutes of Health (NIH) promises to place high priority on clinical and research needs for the prevention of CVD in women.

II. EPIDEMIOLOGY

Heart disease and stroke are the most common causes of death from CVD for U.S. women.[2] In the vital health statistics data collected in 1991 by the National Center for Health Statistics, 474,653 women died from CVD, which represents 45.3% of all deaths among women. Unfortunately, the focus of CVD research on males has given the impression that CVD is basically a male affliction; yet it is the leading cause of death among American women.[2-9] Although overall mortality from CVD has decreased, the decline has been greater for men than for women.[3] Additionally, coronary heart disease (CHD) and stroke still rank first and third as the causes of death for older and middle-aged women. With each decade of life the death rate from CHD increases three- to fivefold.[4] Although women develop risk for heart disease about 10 years later than men, the average 55-year-old woman can have the same risk of a heart attack as the average 55-year-old man.[4] By the year 2000, 38% of all women in the U.S. will be 45 years old or older.[5] Compared to men, women generally have a lower referral rate, more advanced disease at the time of diagnosis, poorer prognosis,[9] and are more likely to receive less aggressive treatment.[3-5]

The occurrence of clinical manifestations of CVD increases suddenly when examining the geographic patterns of heart disease mortality. Rates in the southern U.S. states are highest when men and women are considered together. There are geographic differences in the levels and rate of CHD mortality in the U.S. in all age-sex-race groups, with clusters of high death rate occurring in both men and women in the Mid-Atlantic states (New York, New Jersey, Pennsylvania, Kentucky, and West Virginia). The western mountain states rank in the lowest quartile for both men and women.[10] Different statistics between men and women by geographic area are essential for designing intervention programs.

Racial differences are also important. The age-adjusted death rates for CVD are highest for African American women as compared to white women. Mortality for CHD was 22% higher and the death rate for stroke was 78% higher in white than in African American women during 1987.[11,12] However, equitable treatment for African American women is lacking, i.e., even if they are admitted to the hospital more often than white women after a myocardial infarction, their referral for angiography is 19% lower and for coronary bypass operations, 52% lower.[12]

III. RISK FACTORS

A variety of risk factors for CVD have been identified in women. Many are similar to the ones in men.[13] In the Framingham Heart Study,[14,15] risk factors for definite coronary disease for women included glucose intolerance, elevated systolic or diastolic blood pressure, cigarette smoking, increased total serum cholesterol (TSC), low-density lipoprotein levels (LDL-C), decreased high-density lipoprotein cholesterol levels (HDL-C), and deprivation of estrogen after natural or surgical menopause.

The above studies reported that certain risk factors may affect women differently than they do men. Low levels of HDL-C, hypertriglyceridemia, and diabetes appear to be stronger risk factors for women than for men.[16-19] Obesity and sedentary life-style are also important risk factors for CVD in women.[20-22] Truncal obesity (waist/hip ratio) has also been recently recognized as a risk factor for CVD in women.[23] Other risk factors associated with the changing role(s) of women in our society deal with several psycho-social factors[24] that include type A behavior,[25] suppressed anger,[26] tension and anxiety,[27] working in clerical jobs,[28] subordinate status,[29] social isolation and loneliness,[30] being unmarried,[31] bereaved,[32] or childless.[33,34] Higher levels of depression, fatigue and exhaustion have been associated with increased risk for CVD.[35] Recent studies[36] indicate that employment in middle-aged women resulted in significantly lower TSC and fasting plasma glucose than in unemployed women. Finally, lower levels of education are associated with higher incidence of CVD in women.[37]

A. DIET-RELATED RISK FACTORS
1. Hyperlipidemia

In North American men, TSC and both low levels of HDL-C and high levels of LDL-C have been shown to be strong and independent predictors of CVD.[38,39] Lowering the concentration of TSC and LDL-C results in decreased risk of CVD in men.[39]

There are differences in lipoprotein concentrations between men and women over the life span.[40] In childhood LDL-C and HDL-C levels are similar. Beginning at puberty HDL-C levels fall in boys, while LDL-C levels are maintained into old age. Premenopausal women have lower TSC, higher HDL-C, and lower LDL-C than men of the same age.[41] The difference in HDL-C resides principally in the HDL_2 subclass, the fraction most strongly associated with atherosclerosis.[42] Longitudinal data from the Framingham Heart Study report that TSC levels increase in women following menopause,[42] coming primarily from an increase in LDL-C levels,[43] high HDL_3 subfraction[44] and triglycerides, and decreased concentrations of HDL_2 cholesterol. HDL-C levels increase slightly with age in both sexes and are higher in both white and black women ages 45 to 65 years than in men.[45] The same observations are made for apolipoprotein A-I (ApoA-I).[46] Women as a group have lower LDL-C and apolipoprotein B (ApoB) levels than do men into midlife. After the age of 55 years, women's levels of LDL-C and ApoB exceed those of men.[47] With increasing age, triglyceride (TG) levels increase in women, and remain stable in men.[48] The ApoB/ApoA-I ratio after age adjustment is lowest in premenopausal women, intermediate in postmenopausal women and highest in men.[43] These changes after menopause are associated with increased incidence of CVD seen in postmenopausal women.[45] It has been reported that the LDL particle size distribution in premenopausal women is skewed toward larger particles as compared to men.[49] Smaller LDL particle size has been associated with increased risk of CVD.[50] Lipoprotein increases with age in both sexes and is higher in women than in men.[51]

These sex differences in lipoprotein patterns seen in North American women are in contrast to studies in communities with little CVD. Sex differences in lipoprotein levels in societies with low incidence of CVD appear to be minimal compared with societies where CVD is a public health problem. The interaction of gender with perhaps socioeconomic status may explain gender differences in lipoprotein profiles observed in societies with high CVD incidence.[42]

Lipoproteins have also been found to predict CVD risk but are different between sexes, and the magnitude of risk appears to be gender related. Total serum cholesterol concentration in women was not found to be a serious positive risk factor until it exceeded 6.08 mmol/l.[48,49] Even though HDL-C is inversely related to CVD in both men and women,[47-54] epidemiologic studies have established that HDL-C is a better and more consistent predictor of CVD in women than LDL-C in contrast to findings in men. In the Lipid Research Clinics (LRC) study[53] LDL-C has been found to be a predictor of CVD risk in men, but not in women, and has only been found to be a weak predictor in the Framingham study.[52] Thus HDL-C was determined to be one of the strongest negative predictors in women[53,54] and its protective influence on CVD risk in women is about twice as strong as the atherogenic LDL effect. Thus women have a cardio-protective lipid profile, at least before menopause, largely due to their hormones.

Given the greater predictive value for HDL-C in women compared to men and the higher average TSC and LDL-C at most ages in adult women, screening in women should be done by checking the HDL-C and TSC levels before establishing a diagnosis for hypercholesterolemia.[55]

2. Obesity

Obesity is an independent risk factor for CVD in women.[56] Obesity is associated with an atherogenic lipid and lipoprotein profile in both men and women, including increases in TSC and LDL-C and decreases in HDL-C[57] and HDL$_2$; it appears to be independent of exogenous estrogen use, alcohol consumption, or smoking. National surveys report that women with high body mass index have TSC concentration 19% higher than women with low body mass index.[57] Data from the Framingham and LRC prevalence studies[57] reported that increased relative body weight is an independent risk factor for CVD and it also contributes to hypertension, low HDL-C concentrations, decreased glucose tolerance, and elevated plasma TG and cholesterol concentrations. Obese subjects have increased hepatic very-low-density lipoprotein synthesis which is associated with hypertriglyceridemia, decreased plasma HDL-C, and increased LDL production.[58] In the CARDIA study[59] with women 18 to 30 years of age, multiple linear regression analysis showed that body mass index was significantly and positively correlated with TSC and LDL-C levels and inversely correlated with HDL-C.

It has also been reported that the distribution of body fat is an important determinant of lipoprotein concentrations[60] and CVD. Women with upper-body obesity, which is a pattern usually seen in men, are more likely to have diabetes and atherosclerosis than women with lower-body obesity.[61-63] The waist-to-hip circumference is associated with adverse lipid and lipoprotein levels, is predictive of CVD, and may be able to explain the sex differences observed in TG levels HDL-C and apolipoproteins B and A-I.[64]

Women with normal TSC levels and body weight greater than 130% of recommended weight are about three times more likely to have a myocardial infarction than lean women. This degree of risk is correlated with the degree of obesity, with risk increasing to about eight times for hypercholesterolemic women. Thus, obesity is a cause of increased TSC and possible increased LDL-C concentrations.

IV. RESPONSES OF BLOOD LIPIDS AND LIPOPROTEINS TO DIETARY FAT, CHOLESTEROL, AND FATTY ACIDS IN WOMEN

Evidence suggests that blood lipid levels in women respond to dietary intervention, but not as strongly or consistently as in men. The influence of specific dietary factors including type of fat, cholesterol, fiber, and carbohydrates on the process of CVD in women has not been completely defined. This section will focus on the response(s) of blood lipids in women with changes in dietary fat, fatty acids and cholesterol.

Data from the 1987 to 1988 Nationwide Food Consumption Survey indicated that women consumed approximately 37% of kilocalories from fat.[65] Fifteen to 18% of women aged 30 to 49 years met the recommendation for fat calories. Fourteen to 23% of women met the recommendation for saturated fatty acid calories and 70 to 72% of women met the recommendation for dietary cholesterol. It can be seen that most women don't meet the dietary recommendations set by the National Academy of Sciences and the National Cholesterol Education Program.[66]

High intakes of cholesterol have been associated with hypercholesterolemia in human and nonhuman primates. In humans, high variability in their response to dietary cholesterol has been reported to result in "hyper-responders" and "hypo-responders" and postulated a genetic basis (Apo E genotype) for that response:[67] their capacity to absorb cholesterol, hepatic responsiveness, and level of obesity.[67] Shekelle and Stamler[68] presented data that more than 12% of all CVD can be attributed to excess consumption of cholesterol. Investigators[69-73] came to the conclusion that the level of dietary cholesterol has an independent serum-cholesterol raising effect that is exaggerated when the diet is high in saturated fat.[74]

The response of serum cholesterol is in proportion to baseline serum cholesterol levels as described by Keys,[75] who reported on white men. A similar relationship has been also observed in a randomized, controlled dietary trial with premenopausal women[76] and has been confirmed by studies conducted by Katan et al. with nuns in Dutch and Belgian Trappist monasteries.[77,78] Boyd et al.[76] compared, observed, and predicted changes in TSC in women with mammographic dysplasia in a controlled trial of a low-fat, high-carbohydrate diet in which total fat intake was reduced from an average of 37% of calories to 21%, and a carbohydrate intake increase from 44 to 52% of calories. Changes observed in TSC were greater than those predicted by the formulas of Hegsted and Keys for women with initial TSC in the upper tertile of the population, were not significantly different than those predicted for subjects with baseline values in the middle tertile, and were significantly less than those predicted for women whose initial TSC was in the lower tertile. The authors concluded that TSC can be used as a useful marker of change in dietary fat in women, but it depends on the TSC distribution in the study population.

The qualitative effects of blood lipids in response to different dietary fatty acids are similar in men and women,[74] but their quantitative effects have not been adequately researched. A number of studies[79,80] have reported responses of plasma lipids in men and women fed controlled diets. Results from these studies are inconclusive since most studies have not been well controlled for factors such as sample size,[83] hormonal premenopausal status, menstrual cycle, hormone replacement therapy, oral contraceptive use vs. postmenopausal status,[79,84] hyperlipidemia,[85] weight loss during the study,[86,87] and decreasing total dietary fat[84] vs. modifying the fatty acid composition of the diet and not decreasing total dietary fat.

Epidemiological studies have shown that saturated fat raises HDL-C levels in both men and women, but more markedly in women whereas a high p/s ratio decreases the HDL-C level.[88,89] Dietary cholesterol increases HDL-C, but in women only.[88] When the Food and Agricultural Organization of the United Nations examined the relationship between fat intake and HDL-C levels using food balance sheets, the HDL-C in women significantly correlated with the intake of monounsaturated fat. Saturated and monounsaturated fat correlated highly with female to male HDL-C ratio. Only monounsaturated fat correlated significantly with HDL-C levels in women. Thus significant correlations with dietary saturated and monounsaturated fatty acids, dietary cholesterol, and the female-to-male HDL-C ratio were seen.[90] A recent study by Krummel et al.[91] reported that in premenopausal women, saturated fatty acid intake was positively related to TSC, LDL-C, and HDL-C and negatively associated between intake of refined carbohydrate and HDL-C. Other studies support the above relationships.[92,93]

Kesteloot and Sasaki[90] reported that Western women show an inborn resistance to atherosclerosis, probably attributable to their ability to increase their HDL-C on a high saturated fat diet. Both saturated and monounsaturated fat and dietary cholesterol increase the female-to-male HDL-C ratio significantly, but monounsaturated fat appears to exert the major effect. Several short-term studies[94,95] have shown that a high fat intake increases HDL_2 and ApoA-I levels more in women than in men. A high saturated fat and cholesterol diet increased HDL_2 by 0.09 mmol/l in women as compared to 0.03 mmol/l in men.[94]

A gender-diet interaction likely exists in countries where fat intake is high. Women have higher HDL-C levels (8 to 10 mg/dl higher) than those of men, whereas in countries where fat intake in low, women have HDL-C levels only 4 to 5 mg/dl higher than those of men.[80,90] Some countries with low fat diets have lower rates of CHD and diet induced HDL-C lowering may not confer an increase in CHD risk. A change in LDL/HDL ratio induced by a change in total fat intake may underestimate a true reduction in CHD risk. Thus, women differ from men in their lipid and lipoprotein responses to these life-style changes.

Denke[96] studied the effect of step I low fat diet on 41 moderately hyper-cholesterolemic, postmenopausal women, and reported significant LDL-C and TSC reductions, a non-significant reduction in HDL-C levels, and no improvement in the LDL/HDL ratio. A decrease in HDL-C has been described in women on a diet with a high p/s ratio and low in saturated fat. Their HDL-C levels were reduced to the same level as in men. This is in agreement with epidemiologic studies showing similar HDL-C levels between men and women with low saturated fat and high p/s ratio diets.[97] It seems that on a low fat diet both estradiol and HDL-C levels markedly decrease in postmenopausal Western women. On a low fat diet the estradiol levels were halved and the HDL-C levels decreased from a mean of 55 to 42 mg/dl.[98] In a small cross sectional study[99] of healthy young women and men (18 to 35 years of age) that examined the association between p/s ratio and serum lipid responses, it was found that the correlation between p/s ratio and LDL-C and VLDL-C concentrations was stronger for men than for women. However, in the LRC prevalence study[100,101] no such association was found in either men or women.

Ernst et al.[102] studied the effect of an isocaloric diet with a high p/s ratio and low dietary cholesterol levels on normal and type II hyperliproteineimic women and men. In women with type II hyperlipidemia a 9% reduction was observed in both TSC and LDL-C, while HDL-C was reduced by 10%. Hyper-lipidemic men experienced higher reductions in TSC, LDL-C, and HDL-C, of 13, 11, and 25%, respectively. The greater response of men to the modified diet was also observed in normolipidemic men.

An intervention study[103] of premenopausal normocholesterolemic women who were fed a high fat diet (40% of total kilocalories) and were then switched to a low fat diet (20% of total calories) showed that even though there was only a 7% decreases in TSC, the HDL response was influenced by the p/s ratio. In women who consumed a low p/s ratio diet (0.3) their HDL-C levels decreased by 12%, while women who consumed a high p/s ratio diet (1.0) showed no change in HDL. This is in agreement with studies conducted by Brussard et al.[104] and Weisweiler et al.[105] Thus, for healthy premenopausal women with low baseline plasma cholesterol levels, a marked decrease in total fat intake on a weight-maintaining diet is not accompanied by statistically significant changes in plasma cholesterol.

In another study[79] where two diets were fed, one rich in complex carbohydrates and the other rich in olive oil, to healthy men and women, changes in HDL-C in serum were greater in men than in women, although TSC and LDL-C responses were similar in both sexes. Masarei et al.[106] placed normolipidemic men and women on a vegetarian diet and observed significant reductions in TSC, LDL-C and HDL-C, in men only. Cole et al.[107] evaluated the long-term efficacy of the American Heart Association phase 3 diet (39% kilocalories from carbohydrates, 21% kilocalories from fat, 96 mg cholesterol, p/s = 1.8) in premenopausal women with moderately elevated serum cholesterol for 5 months. They reported reduction of TSC and LDL-C by 7 and 11%, respectively, and HDL-C reduction by 5% and ApoA increases by +15%, with HDL$_3$ increasing and TG increasing by 30%. The cholesterol-lowering response to the American Heart Association phase 3 diet was one third less than predicted by the Keys equation for premenopausal women. Obese women had a smaller cholesterol-lowering response and greater triglyceride-raising response to the above dietary modifications than did their lean counterparts, which raises the question of whether these dietary recommendations are appropriate for all subgroups.

The deleterious effect of high polyunsaturated fatty acid diets is that they reduce both HDL-C and LDL-C concentration. The ideal diet would be one that would reduce LDL-C levels and increase HDL-C levels or keep them unchanged. Mata et al.[86] studied the effects of a diet enriched in monounsaturated fatty acids and one enriched in polyunsaturated fatty acids for 12 weeks (37% of total energy came from fat calories) in men and premenopausal women. The monounsaturated fatty acid diet brought about no change in TSC in men, but a rise of 9% in women. High density lipoprotein cholesterol increased by 17% in men and by 30% in women. The atherogenic index fell significantly in both sexes. No significant changes occurred in LDL-C or TGs. Thus, a habitual diet rich in monounsaturated fatty acids with a relatively low p/s has essentially the same effects on plasma LDL-C as does a diet high in polyunsaturated fatty acids. This diet also increases HDL-C concentration which may be of a greater benefit to women than men in Western countries that tend to have relatively high fat intakes.

Mata et al.[83] also studied the effect of a saturated fat diet followed by a monounsaturated fat diet rich in olive oil, followed by a sunflower oil rich diet in pre- and postmenopausal, normolipidemic women. Again they found that a monounsaturated fatty acid diet not only lowered TSC and LDL-C but increased HDL-C and ApoAI when compared to the poly and saturated-rich periods. They also reported that these effects were independent of menopausal status. In short-term dietary studies with men and premenopausal normolipidemic women, Mensink et al.[81] reported that in men HDL-C levels fell slightly, but not significantly, with diets enriched with monounsaturated or polyunsaturated fatty acids, but similar observations were not made in women.

In summary, the data suggest that dietary intake (diets of high p/s and low cholesterol) affects serum lipid and lipoprotein concentrations in women, but the magnitude of lipid reductions appears to be less than in men, with a less detrimental decrease of HDL-C in women. It may be that endogenous hormone secretion in women modifies or overrides the modifying effect of diet.

Thus, since gender[108] differences exist in HDL-C response, well-controlled studies are needed to determine gender differences in dietary responsiveness and their public applications to the general population of U.S. women.

V. RECOMMENDATIONS FOR DIETARY CHANGE

The general population-based recommendation for both men and women is the adoption of American Heart Association step I diet to lower LDL-C (i.e., 30% kilocalories from fat, 10% saturated fat and <300 mg cholesterol with a high p/s ratio). Will these guidelines reduce risk for CVD equally in both men and women? The above dietary alteration lowers LDL-C but tends to also reduce the HDL-C. Data from studies with women who followed a step I diet reduced both LDL-C and HDL-C levels.[70,73,109] Similar studies in men[69,71,72] showed smaller decreases in LDL-C and no change or very small decreases in HDL-C. High density lipoprotein cholesterol is usually reduced by an increased dietary p/s ratio.[110] Thus, for low risk women the benefits of a low fat diet are far from clear. Since low fat diets have the disadvantage of lowering HDL-C cholesterol, enriching the diet with monounsaturated fatty acid is now being studied. Monounsaturated fatty acids do not decrease HDL-C, a change observed in increased polyunsaturated fatty acid or restricted total fat kilocalorie diets.

Furthermore, even though a step I diet would reduce LDL-C levels in most women, there is little evidence that this will reduce their CVD risk. LDL-C is not as strong a predictor of CVD risk in women as it is in men, though some investigators have reported that the step I diet has minimal effects on lowering HDL-C. Since in low-risk women HDL-C is a stronger predictor of CVD risk, the present dietary advice for women needs to be reexamined. Meanwhile, women should follow the time-tested recommendation of reducing dietary fat to 30% of calories and they should maintain low intakes of saturated fat and dietary cholesterol.

REFERENCES

1. Kumanyika, S. K., Women and health research: rewriting the rules, *Perspect. Appl. Nutr.*, 2, 10, 1994.
2. Heart Memo, The Cardiovascular Health of Women, Special Edition, National Heart, Lung and Blood Institute, National Institutes of Health, Bethesda, MD, 1994.

3. National Cholesterol Education Program (NCEP), *Report of the Expert Panel on Population Strategies for Blood Cholesterol Reduction,* NIH Publ., U.S. Department of Health and Human Services, Public Health Service, NIH, National Heart, Lung and Blood Institute, Bethesda, MD, 1990, 3046.

4. Sempos, C. T., Cleeman, J. I., Carroll, M. D., Johnson, C. L., Bachorik, P. S., Gordon, D. J., Burt, V. L., Briefel, R. R., Brown, C. D., Lippel, K., and Rifkind, B. M., Prevalence of high blood cholesterol among U.S. adults: an update based on guidelines from the Second Report of the National Cholesterol Education Program Adult Treatment Panel, *J. Am. Med. Assoc.,* 269, 3009, 1993.

5. U.S. Senate Special Committee on Aging, Aging America: Trends and Projections, U.S. Department of Health and Human Services, Washington, D.C., 1988.

6. Langer, R. D. and Barrett-Connor, E., Coronary heart disease prevention in women, *Pract. Cardiol.,* 17, 45, 1991.

7. Keil, J. E., Gazes, P. C., Loadholt, C. B., Tyrolen, H. A., Sutherland, S., Gross, A. J., Knowles, M., and Rust, P. F., Coronary heart disease mortality and its predictors among women in Charleston, South Carolina, in *Coronary Heart Disease in Women,* Eaker, E.D., Packard, B., Wenger, N. K., Clarkson, T. B., and Tyroler, H. A., Eds., Haymarket Doyma Inc., New York, 1987, 90.

8. Steingart, R. M., Packer, M., Hamm, P., Goglianese, M. E., Gersh, B., Geltman, E. M., Sollano, J., Katz, S., Moye, L., Basta, L. L., Lewis, S. J., Gottlier, S. S., Bernstein, V., McEwan, P., Jacobson, K., Brown, E. J., Kukin, M. L., Kantrowitz, N. E., and Pfefeer, M. A., Sex differences in the management of coronary artery disease, *N. Engl. J. Med.,* 325, 226, 1991.

9. Eaker, E. D., Packard, B., and Thom, T. J., Epidemiology and risk factors for coronary heart disease in women, *Cardiovasc. Clin.,* 19, 129, 1989.

10. Coronary Heart Disease in Women, a summary of proceedings, National Health, Lung and Blood Institute, NIH, Bethesda, MD, 1986.

11. Wenger, N. K., Coronary disease in women, *Annu. Rev. Med.,* 36, 285, 1985.

12. Holm, K., Penckofer, S., Keresztes, P., Biordi, D., and Chandler, P., Coronary artery disease in women: assessment, diagnosis, intervention and strategies for life style change, *A WHONN'S Clin.,* 4, 272, 1993.

13. Eaker, E. D. and Castelli, W. P., Coronary heart disease and its risk factors among women in the Framingham study, in *Coronary Heart Disease in Women,* Eaker, E.D., Packard, B., Wenger, N.K., Clarkson, T.B., and Tyroler, H.A., Eds., Haymarket Doyma Inc., New York, 1987, 122.

14. Kahn, H. S., Williamson, D. F., and Stevens, F. A., Race and weight change in U.S. women: the roles of socioeconomic and marital status, *Am. J. Public Health,* 81, 319, 1991.

15. Barrett-Connor, E. and Bush, T. L., Estrogen and coronary heart disease in women, *J. Am. Diet. Assoc.,* 265, 1861, 1991.

16. Higgins, M., Keller, J. B., and Ostrander, L. D., Risk factors for coronary heart disease in women: Tecumseh community health study, 1959 to 1980, in *Coronary Heart Disease in Women,* Eaker, E. D., Packard, B., Wenger, N. K., Clarkson, T.B., and Tyroler, H. A., Eds., Haymarket Doyma Inc., New York, 1987, 83.

17. Bush, T. L., Criqui, M. H., Cowan, L. D., Barrett-Conner, E., Wallace, R. B., Tyroler, H. A., Suchindran, C. M., Cohn, R., and Rifkind, B. M., Cardiovascular disease mortality in women: results from the Lipid Research Clinics follow-up study, in *Coronary Heart Disease in Women,* Eaker, E. D., Packard, B., Wenger, N. K., Clarkson, T. B., and Tyroler, H. A., Eds., National Heart, Lung, and Blood Institute, NIH, Bethesda, MD, 1987, 106.

18. Wingard, D. L. and Cohn, B. A., Coronary heart disease mortality among women in Alameda County, 1965 to 1973, In *Coronary Heart Disease in Women,* Eaker, E. D., Packard, B., Wenger, N. K., Clarkson, T. B., Tyroler, H. A., Eds., Haymarket Doyma Inc., New York, 1987, 99.

19. Stampfer, M. J., Colditz, G. A., Willett, W. C., Rosner, B., Speizer, F. E., and Hennekers, C.H., Coronary heart disease risk factors in women: the Nurses' Health Study experience, in *Coronary Heart Disease in Women*, Eaker, E. D., Packard, B., Wenger, N. K., Clarkson, T. B., and Tyroler, H. A., Eds., Haymarket Doyma Inc., New York, 1987, 112.

20. Barrett-Connor, E. L., Obesity, atherosclerosis, and coronary artery disease, *Ann. Intern. Med.,* 103, 1010, 1985.

21. Hubert, H. B., Feinleib, M., McNamara, P. M., and Castelli, W. P., Obesity as an independent risk factor for cardiovascular disease: a 26-year follow-up of participants in the Framingham heart study, *Circulation,* 678, 968, 1983.

22. Manson, J. E., Stampfer, M. J., Hennekens, C. H., and Willett, W. C., Body weight and longevity: a reassessment, *J. Am. Med. Assoc.,* 257, 353, 1987.

23. Kissebah, A. H., Vydelingum, N., Murray, R., Evans, D., Hartz, A., Kalkhoff, R., and Adams, P., Relation of body fat distribution to metabolic complications of obesity, *J. Clin. Endocrinol. Metab.*, 54, 254, 1982.

24. Powell, L. H., Shaker, L. A., Jones, B. A., Vaccarino, L. V., Thoresen, C. E., and Pattillo, J. R., Psychosocial predictors of mortality in 83 women with premature acute myocardial infarction, *Psychosom. Med.*, 55, 420, 1993.

25. Haynes, S. G., Feinleib, M., and Kannel, W. B., The relationship of psychosocial factors to coronary heart disease in the Framingham study. III. Eight-year incidence of coronary heart disease, *Am. J. Epidemiol.*, 111, 37, 1980.

26. Haynes, S. G. and Feinleib, M., Women, work and coronary heart disease: prospective findings from the Framingham heart study, *Am. J. Public Health*, 70, 133, 1980.

27. Hallstrom, T., Lapidum, L., Bengtsson, C., and Edstrom, K., Psychosocial factors and risk of ischemic heart disease and death in women: a 12-year follow-up of participants in the population study of women in Gothenburg, Sweden, *J. Psychosom. Res.*, 30, 451, 1986.

28. Eaker, E. D., Pinsky, J., and Castelli, W. P., Myocardial infarction and coronary death among women: psychosocial predictors from a 20-year follow-up of women in the Framingham study, *Am. J. Epidemiol.*, 135, 854, 1992.

29. Clarkson, T. B., Adams, M. R., Kaplan, J. R., and Shively, C. A., Pathophysiology of coronary artery atherosclerosis: animal studies of gender differences, in *Heart Disease in Women*, Douglas, P. S., Ed., F.A. Davis, Philadelphia, 1989.

30. Berkman, L. F. and Breslow, L., Health and Ways of Living. The Alameda County Study, Oxford University Press, New York, 1983.

31. Cottington, E. M., Matthews, K. A., Talbott, E., and Kuller, L. H., Environmental events preceding sudden death in women, *Psychosom. Med.*, 42, 567, 1980.

32. Talbott, E., Kuller, L. H., Perper, J., and Murphy, P. A., Sudden unexpected death in women. Biologic and psychosocial origins, *Am. J. Epidemiol.*, 114, 671, 1981.

33. Matthews, K. A., Kelsey, S. F., Meilahn, E. N., Kuller, L. H., and Wing, R. P., Educational attainment and behavioral and biologic risk factors for coronary heart disease in middle-aged women, *Am. J. Epidemiol.*, 129, 1132, 1989.

34. Conference on Women, Behavior, and Cardiovascular Disease: Task Force on Psychosocial Factors in Cardiovascular Disease Treatment, Recovery, and Rehabilitation in Women, National Heart, Lung and Blood Institute, Chevy Chase, MD, September 1991.

35. Chesney, M. A., Social isolation, depression and heart disease: research on women broadens the agenda, *Psychosom. Med.*, 55, 429, 1993.

36. Kirtz-Silverstein, D., Wingard, D. L., and Barrett-Connor, E., Employment status and heart disease risk factors in middle-aged women: the Rancho Bernardo study, *Am. J. Public Health*, 82, 315, 1992.

37. Winkleby, M. A., Jatulis, D. E., Frank, E., and Pertmann, S. P., Socioeconomic status and health: how education, income, and occupation contribute to risk factors for cardiovascular disease, *Am. J. Public Health*, 82, 816, 1992.

38. Lipid research clinics program. The lipid research clinics coronary primary prevention trial results. I. Reduction in incidence of coronary heart disease, *J. Am. Med. Assoc.*, 251, 351, 1984.

39. Lipid research clinics program. The lipid research clinics coronary primary prevention trial results. II. The relationship of reduction in incidence of coronary heart disease to cholesterol lowering, *J. Am. Med. Assoc.*, 251, 365, 1984.

40. LaRosa, J.C., Lipids and cardiovascular disease do the finding and therapy apply equally to men and women?, *WHI*, 20, 102, 1992.

41. Gordon, D. J., Probstfield, J. L., Garrison, R. J., Neaton, J. D., Castelli, W. P., Knoke, J. D., Jacobs, D. R., Jr., Bangdiwala, S., and Tyroler, H.A., High-density lipoprotein cholesterol and cardiovascular disease: Four prospective studies, *Circulation*, 79, 8, 1989.

42. Eaker, E. D. and Castelli, W. P., Coronary heart disease and its risk factors among women in the Framingham study, in *Coronary Heart Disease in Women*, Eaker, E. D., Packard, B., Wenger, N., Clarkson, T. B., and Tyroler, H. A., Eds., Haymarket Doyma Inc., New York, 1987, 122.

43. Brunner, E. J., Marmot, M. G., White, I. R., O'Brien, J. R., Etherington, M. D., Slavin, B. M., Kearney, E. M., and Davey Smith, G., Gender and employment grade differences in blood cholesterol, apolipoproteins and haemostatic factors in the Whitehall II study, *Atherosclerosis*, 102, 195, 1993.

44. Stevenson, J. C., Crook, D., and Godsland, I. F., Influence of age and menopause on serum lipids and lipoproteins in healthy women, *Atherosclerosis*, 98, 3, 1993.

45. Seed, M., Sex hormones, lipoprotein and cardiovascular risk, *Atherosclerosis*, 90, 1, 1991.

46. Higgins, M. and Keller, J., Cholesterol, coronary heart disease, and total mortality in middle-aged and elderly men and women in Tecumseh, *AEP*, 2, 69, 1992.

47. Kannel, W. B., Castelli, W. P., and Gordon, T., Cholesterol in the prediction of atherosclerotic disease, *Ann. Intern. Med.*, 90, 85, 1979.

48. Bush, T. L., Barrett-Connor, E., Cowan, L. D., Criqui, M. H., Wallace, R. B., Suchindran, C. M., Tyroler, H. A., and Rifkind, B. M., Cardiovascular mortality and noncontraceptive use of estrogen in women: results from the Lipid Research Clinics' program follow-up study, *Circulation,* 75, 1102, 1987.

49. Kannel, W. B., Castelli, W. P., Gordon, T., and McNamara, P. M., Serum cholesterol, lipoproteins, and the risk of coronary heart disease, *Ann. Intern. Med.*, 74, 1, 1971.

50. Gordon, T., Kannel, W. B., Castelli, W. P., and Dawber, T. R., Lipoproteins, cardiovascular disease, and death, *Arch. Intern. Med.*, 141, 1128, 1981.

51. Utermann, G., Menzel, H. J., Kraft, H. G., Duba, N. C., Kemmler, H. G., and Seitz, C., Lp(a)-lipoprotein concentrations in plasma, *Hum. Genet.*, 78, 47, 1988.

52. Lemer, D. J. and Kannel, W. B., Patterns of coronary heart disease morbidity and mortality in the sexes: a 26-year follow-up of the Framingham population, *Am. Heart J.,* 111, 383, 1986.

53. Jacobs, D., Jr., Shrikant, I., Bangdiwala, I., Criqui, M., and Tyroler, M., High density lipoprotein cholesterol as a predictor of cardiovascular disease mortality in men and women, *Am. J. Epidemiol.*, 131, 32, 1990.

54. Gordon, T., Kannel, W. P., Hortland, M. C., Kannel, W. B., and Dawber, T. R., High density lipoprotein as a protective factor against coronary heart disease, *Am. J. Med.*, 62, 707, 1977.

55. National Center for Health Statistics, Dietary intake and cardiovascular risk factors. II. Serum urate, serum cholesterol, and correlates: U.S., 1971–75, Vital and Health Statistics, Series 11, No. 227, Department of Health and Human Services Publ. No. (PHS) 83-1677, Public Health Service, U.S. Government Printing Office, Washington, D.C., March 1983.

56. Kissebath, A. H., Freedman, D. S., and Peiris, A. N., Risks of obesity, *Med. Clin. North Am.,* 73, 111, 1989.

57. Glueck, C. J., Taylor, H. L., Jacobs, D., Morrison, J. A., Beaglehole, R., and Williams, O. D., Plasma high-density lipoprotein cholesterol: association with measurements of body mass. The Lipid Research Clinics Program Prevalence Study, *Circulation*, 62, 62, 1980.

58. Kesaniemi, Y. A. and Grundy, S. M., Increased low density lipoprotein production associated with obesity, *Arteriosclerosis,* 3, 170, 1983.

59. Katan, M. B., Diet and HDL, in *Clinical and Metabolic Aspects of High-density Lipoprotein,* Miller, N. E. and Miller, G. J., Eds., Elsevier, Amsterdam, 1984, 103.

60. Larsson, B., Svärdsudd, K., Welin, L., Wilhelmsen, L., Björntorp, P., and Tibblin, G., Abdominal adipose tissue distribution, obesity, and risk of cardiovascular disease and death: 13 year follow up of participants in the study of men born in 1913, *Br. Med. J.,* 288, 1401, 1984.

61. Anderson, A. L., Sobocinski, K. A., Freedman, D. S., Barborial, J. J., Rimm, A. A., and Gruchow, H. W., Body fat distribution, plasma lipids, and lipoproteins, *Arteriosclerosis,* 8, 88, 1988.

62. Stern, M. P. and Haffner, S. M., Body fat distribution and hyperinsulinemia as risk factors for diabetes and cardiovascular disease, *Arteriosclerosis,* 6, 123, 1986.

63. Hartz, A. J., Rupley, D. C., Kalkhoff, R. D., and Rimm, A. A., Relationship of obesity to diabetes: influence of obesity level and body fat distribution, *Prev. Med.,* 12, 351, 1983.

64. Freedman, F., Jacobsen, J., Brboriak, J., Sobocinski, K., Anderson, A., Kissebah, A., Sasse, E., and Gruchow, H., Body fat distribution and male/female differences in lipids and lipoproteins, *Circulation,* 81, 1498, 1980.

65. Murphy, S. P., Rose, D., Hudes, M., and Viteri, F. E., Demographic and economic factors associated with dietary quality for adults in the 1987–88 Nationwide Food Consumption Survey, *J. Am. Diet. Assoc.,* 92, 1352, 1992.

66. Kris-Etherton, K. and Krummel, D., Role of nutrition in the prevention and treatment of coronary heart disease in women, *J. Am. Diet. Assoc.,* 93, 987, 1993.

67. Cobb, M. M., Teitlebaum, H., Risch, N., Jekel, J., and Ostfield, A., Influence of dietary fat, apolipoprotein E phenotype, and sex on plasma lipoprotein levels, *Circulation,* 86, 849, 1992.

68. Shekelle, R. B. and Stamler, J., Dietary cholesterol and ischaemic heart disease, *Lancet,* 1, 1177, 1989.

69. Grundy, S. M., Nix, D., Whelen, M. F., and Franklin, L., Comparison of three cholesterol lowering diets in normolipidemic men, *J. Am. Med. Assoc.,* 256, 2351, 1986.

70. Jones, D. Y., Judd, J. T., Taylor, P. R., Campbell, W. S., and Nair, P. P., Influence of caloric contribution and saturation of dietary fat of plasma lipids in premenopausal women, *Am. J. Clin. Nutr.,* 45, 1451, 1987.

71. Brussard, J. H., Dallinga-Thie, G., Groot, P. H. E., and Katan, M. B., Effects of amount and type of dietary fat on serum lipids, lipoproteins, and apolipoproteins in man, *Atherosclerosis,* 36, 515, 1980.

72. Coulston, A. M., Liu, G. C., and Reaven, G. M., Plasma glucose, insulin, and lipid responses to high-carbohydrate low-fat diets in normal humans, *Metabolism,* 32, 52, 1983.

73. Kohlmeier, M., Strickler, G., and Schlierf, G., Influences of "normal" and "prudent" diets on biliary and serum lipids in healthy women, *Am. J. Clin. Nutr.,* 42, 1201, 1985.

74. Report of the expert panel of detection, evaluation and treatment of high blood cholesterol in adults, in National Institutes of Health Publication, National Heart, Lung and Blood Institute, Bethesda, MD, 1988, 2925.

75. Keys, A., Anderson, J. T., and Grande, F., Serum cholesterol response to changes in the diet. IV. Particular saturated fatty acids in the diet, *Metabolism,* 14, 776, 1965.

76. Boyd, N.F., Cousins, N., Beaton, M., Kriukov, V., Lockwood, G., and Tritchler, D., Quantitative changes in dietary fat intake and serum cholesterol in women: results from a randomized, controlled trial, *Am. J. Clin. Nutr.,* 52, 470, 1990.

77. Katan, M. B., van Gastel, A. C., de Rover, C. M., van Montfort, M. A. J., and Knuiman, J. T., Differences in individual responsiveness of serum cholesterol to fat-modified diets in man, *Eur. J. Clin. Invest.,* 18, 644, 1988b.

78. Clifton, P., Kestin, M., Abbey, M., Drysdale, M., and Nestel, P., Relationship between sensitivity to dietary fat and dietary cholesterol, *Arteriosclerosis,* 10, 394, 1990.

79. Mensink, R. P. and Katan, M. B., Effect of monounsaturated fatty acids vs. complex carbohydrates on high-density lipoprotein in healthy men and women, *Lancet*, 1, 122, 1987.

80. Barnard, R. J., Effects of life-style modification on serum lipids, *Arch. Intern. Med.*, 151, 1389, 1991.

81. Mensink, R. P. and Katan, M. B., Effect of a diet enriched with monounsaturated or polyunsaturated fatty acids on levels of low-density and high-density lipoprotein cholesterol in healthy women and men, *N. Engl. J. Med.*, 321, 436, 1989.

82. Mensink, R. P. and Katan, M. B., Effect of dietary trans fatty acids on high-density and low-density lipoprotein cholesterol levels in healthy subjects, *N. Engl. J. Med.*, 323, 439, 1990.

83. Mata, P., Garrido, J. A., Ordovas, J. M., Blazquez, E., Alvarez-Sala, L. A., Rubio, M. J., Alonso, R., and de Oya, M., Effect of dietary monounsaturated fatty acids on plasma lipoproteins and apolipoproteins in women, *Am. J. Clin. Nutr.*, 56, 77, 1992.

84. Ng, T. K. W., Hayes, K. C., DeWitt, G. F., Jegathesan, M., Satgunasigam, N., Ong, A. S. H., and Tan, D., Dietary palmitic and oleic acids exert similar effects on serum cholesterol and lipoprotein profiles on normocholesterolemic men and women, *J. Am. Coll. Nutr.*, 11, 383, 1992.

85. Jenkins, D. J. A., Wolever, T. M. S., Rao, A. V., Hegele, R. A., Mitchell, S. J., Ransom, T. P. P., Boctor, D. L., Spadofora, P. J., Jenkins, A. L., Mehline, C., Relle, L., Connelly, P. W., Story, J. A., Furumoto, E. J., Corey, P., and Wursch, P., Effect on blood lipids of very high intakes of fiber in diets low in saturated fat and cholesterol, *N. Engl. J. Med.*, 329, 21, 1993.

86. Mata, P., Alvarez-Sala, L. A., Rubio, M. J., Nuño, J., and De Oya, M., Effects of long-term monounsaturated- vs polyunsaturated-enriched diets on lipoproteins in healthy men and women, *Am. J. Clin. Nutr.*, 55, 846, 1992.

87. Wood, P. D., Stefanik, M. L., Williams, P. T., and Haskell, W. l., The effects on plasma lipoproteins of a prudent weight-reducing diet, with or without exercise, in overweight men and women, *N. Engl. J. Med.*, 325, 461, 1991.

88. Kesteloot, H., Geboers, J., and Joossens, J. V., On the within-population relationship between nutrition and serum lipids: the B.I.R.N.H. study, *Eur. Heart J.*, 10, 196, 1989a.

89. Kesteloot, H., Oviasu, V. O., Obashohan, A. O., Cobbaert, C., and Lissens, W., Serum lipid and apolipoprotein levels in a Nigerian population sample, *Atherosclerosis*, 78, 33, 1989b.

90. Kesteloot, H. and Sasaki, S., On the relationship betweeen nutrition, sex hormones and high-density lipoproteins in women, *Acta Cardiol.*, 4, 355, 1993.

91. Krummel, D., Mashaly, M., and Kris-Etherton, P., Prediction of plasma lipids in a cross-sectional sample of young women, *J. Am. Diet. Assoc.*, 92, 942, 1992.

92. Van Horn, L., Ballew, C., Liu, K., Ruth, K., McDonald, A., Hilner, J., Burke, G., Savage, P., Bragg, C., Caan, B., Jacobs, D., Slattery, M., and Sidney, S., Diet, body size, and plasma lipids-lipoproteins in young adults: differences by race and sex. The coronary artery risk development in young adults (CARDIA) study, *Am. J. Epidemiol.*, 133, 9, 1991.

93. Knuiman, J. J., West, C. E., Katan, M. B., and Hautvast, J. G. A. J., Total cholesterol and high density lipoprotein cholesterol levels in populations differing in fat and carbohydrate intake, *Arteriosclerosis*, 7, 612, 1987.

94. Baggio, G., Fellin, T., Baiocchi, M. R., Martini, S., Baldo, G., Manzato, E., and Crepaldi, G., Relationship between triglyceride-rich lipoprotein (chylomicrons and VLDL) and HDL_2 and HDL_3 in the postprandial phase in humans, *Atherosclerosis*, 37, 271, 1980.

95. Clifton, P. M. and Nestel, P. J., Influence of gender, body mass index, and age on response of plasma lipids to dietary fat plus cholesterol, *Arterioscler. Thromb.*, 12, 955, 1992.

96. Denke, M., Individual responsiveness to a cholesterol-lowering diet in postmenopausal women with moderate hypercholesterolemia, *Arch. Intern. Med.*, 154, 1977, 1994.

97. Kesteloot, H., Changing trends in mortality, in *New Horizons in Preventing Cardiovascular Diseases*, Yamori, Y. and Strasser, T., Eds., Elsevier, New York, 1989, 101.

98. Heber, D., Ashley, J. M., Leaf, D. A., and Barnard, R. J., Reduction of serum estradiol in postmenopausal women given free access to low-fat high-carbohydrate diet, *Nutrition,* 7, 137, 1991.

99. Pometta, D., James, R., and Suenram, A., HDL and coronary heart disease: a familial trend, in *Lipoprotein and Atherosclerosis,* Malmendier, C. L. and Alaupovic, P., Eds., Plenum Press, New York, 1986, 219.

100. Ernst, N., Fisher, M., Smith, W., Gordon, T., Rifkind, B. M., Little, J. A., Mischkel, M. A., and Williams, O. D., The association of plasma high-density lipoprotein cholesterol with dietary intake and alcohol consumption. The Lipid Research Clinics program prevalence study, *Circulation,* 62, 41, 1980.

101. Gordon, T., Fisher, M., Ernst, N., and Rifkind, B. M., Relation of diet to LDL cholesterol, VLDL cholesterol, and plasma total cholesterol and triglycerides in white adults. The Lipid Research Clinic prevalence study, *Arteriosclerosis,* 2, 502, 1982.

102. Ernst, N., Fisher, M., Bowen, P., Schaefer, E. J., and Levy, R. I., Changes in plasma lipids and lipoproteins after a modified fat diet, *Lancet,* 2, 111, 1980.

103. Jones, D. Y., Judd, J. T., Taylor, P. R., Campbell, W. S., and Nair, P. P., Influence of caloric contribution and saturation of dietary fat on plasma lipids in premenopausal women, *Am. J. Nutr.,* 45, 1451, 1987.

104. Brussard, J. H., Katan, M. B., Groot, P. H. E., Havekes, L. M., and Hautvast, J. G. A. J., Serum lipoproteins of healthy persons fed a low-fat diet or a polyunsaturated fat diet for three months, *Atherosclerosis,* 42, 205, 1982.

105. Weisweiler, P., Janetschek, P., and Schwandt, P., Influence of polyunsaturated fats and fat restriction on serum lipoproteins in humans, *Metabolism,* 34, 83, 1985.

106. Masarei, J. R. L., Rouse, I. L., Lynch, W. J., Robertson, K., Vandongen, R., and Beilin, L. J., Effects of a lacto-ovo vegetarian diet on serum concentrations of cholesterol, triglyceride, HDL-C, HDL_2-C, HDL_3-C, apolipoprotein-B, and $Lp(a)^{1-3}$, *Am. J. Clin. Nutr.,* 40, 468, 1984.

107. Cole, T., Bowen, P., Schmeisser, D., Prewitt, E., Aye, P., Langenberg, P., Dolecek, T., Brace, L., and Kamath, S., Differential reduction of plasma cholesterol by the American Heart Association phase 3 diet in moderately hypercholesterolemic, premenopausal women with different body mass indexes, *Am. J. Clin. Nutr.,* 55, 385, 1992.

108. Brownell, K. D. and Stunkard, A. J., Differential changes in plasma high-density lipoprotein-cholesterol levels in obese men and women during weight reduction, *Arch. Intern. Med.,* 141, 1142, 1981.

109. Zanni, E. E., Annis, V. I., Blum, C. B., Herbert, P. N., and Breslow, J. L., Effect of egg cholesterol and dietary fats on plasma lipids, lipoproteins, and apoproteins of normal women consuming natural diets, *J. Lipid Res.,* 28, 518, 1987.

110. Shepard, J., Packard, C. J., Patsch, J. R., Botto, A. M., and Taunton, O. D., Effects of dietary polyunsaturated and saturated fat on the properties of high density lipoproteins and the metabolism and apolipoprotein A-I, *J. Clin. Invest.,* 61, 1582, 1978.

Chapter 9

PREMENSTRUAL SYNDROME — NUTRITIONAL IMPLICATIONS

Jaime S. Ruud

CONTENTS

I. INTRODUCTION

Premenstrual syndrome (PMS) is a phenomenon that has existed throughout history. Literary accounts of PMS date back 2600 years.[1] Accounts of rituals and beliefs surrounding premenstrual distress can be found.

0-8493-8502-4/96/$0.00+$.50

In recent years, a proliferation of interest and research on PMS has increased our knowledge of the diagnosis and management of this phenomenon. Many factors contribute to PMS and several nutritional, hormonal, and psychosocial theories, exist. Yet, PMS has not been clearly defined and the cause is still unknown.[2] In the meantime, PMS sufferers are searching for ways to cope with monthly physical and psychological symptoms.

II. DEFINITION

The symptom of what was originally known as "premenstrual tension" was first described by Frank in 1931.[3] He theorized that premenstrual tension was caused by high levels of female sex hormones in the blood. He used calcium lactate, either alone or in combination with caffeine preparations, to relieve symptoms.

In 1953, Greene and Dalton[4] changed the term to "premenstrual syndrome" because "tension is only one of the many components of the syndrome." They attributed symptoms of PMS to water retention caused by abnormal estrogen/progesterone ratios and treated it with progesterone.

Since that time, the definition and classification of PMS has been controversial. According to Reid,[5] PMS is "the cyclic recurrence in the late luteal phase of the menstrual cycle, of a combination of distressing physical, psychologic, and/or behavioral changes of sufficient severity to result in deterioration of interpersonal relationships and/or interference with normal activities."

In 1987, the American Psychiatric Association (APA) concluded that severe PMS is actually a psychiatric disorder. They introduced a new definition entitled "late luteal phase dysphoric disorder" (LLPDD) to the appendix of the Diagnostic and Statistical Manual of Mental Disorders.[6] The major symptoms of LLPDD are listed in Table 1. According to the APA's definition, the essential feature of LLPDD is a "pattern of clinically significant emotional and behavioral symptoms that occur during the last week of the luteal phase and remit within a few days after the onset of the follicular phase." Diagnosis of LLPDD is based on retrospective reports (past events and experiences). Two symptomatic cycles are needed to confirm the diagnosis. Preliminary data by Hurt et al.[7] indicated that between 14 and 45% of women with PMS in their study met the criteria for LLPDD.

III. SYMPTOMS

PMS symptoms vary, ranging from mild to incapacitating. More than 150 symptoms have been attributed to PMS.[8-10] Smith and Schiff[11] categorized PMS symptoms into three groups: psychologic, physical, and behavioral (Table 2). The most common symptoms are abdominal bloating and/or pain, backache, headache, constipation, breast tenderness, food cravings (carbohydrates,

TABLE 1
Diagnostic Criteria for Late Luteal Phase Dysphoric Disorder

In most menstrual cycles during the past year, symptoms in B occurred during the last week of the luteal phase and remitted within a few days after onset of the follicular phase; in menstruating females, these phases correspond to the week before, and a few days after, the onset of menses (in nonmenstruating females who have had a hysterectomy, the timing of luteal and follicular phases may require measurement of circulating reproductive hormones)

At least five of the following symptoms have been present for most of the time during each symptomatic later luteal phase, at least one of the symptoms being one of the first four below

    Marked affective lability e.g., feeling suddenly sad, tearful, irritable, or angry

    Persistent and marked anger or irritability

    Marked anxiety, tension, feelings of being "keyed up", or "on edge"

    Markedly depressed mood, feelings of hopelessness, or self-deprecating thoughts

    Decreased interest in usual activities, e.g., work, hobbies

    Easy fatigability or marked lack of energy

    Subjective sense of difficulty in concentrating

    Marked change in appetite, overeating, or specific food cravings

    Hypersomnia or insomnia

    Other physical symptoms, such as breast tenderness or swelling, headaches, joint or muscle pain, a sensation of "bloating", weight gain

The disturbance seriously interferes with work or with usual social activities or relationships with others

The disturbance is not merely an exacerbation of the symptoms of another disorder, such as major depression, panic disorder, dysthymia, or a personality disorder (although it may be superimposed on any of these disorders)

Criteria above are confirmed by prospective daily self-ratings during at least two symptomatic cycles (the diagnosis may be made provisionally prior to this confirmation)

Note: For coding purposes, record: 300.90 Unspecified Mental Disorder (late luteal phase dysphoric disorder).

sweets, chocolate, salt), fatigue, irritability, and symptoms related to depression.

Bancroft and co-workers[12] studied four groups of women in terms of their premenstrual complaints, menorrhagia (excessive bleeding), and dysmenorrhea (menstrual cramping) and found considerable overlap in a number of symptoms. However, the premenstrual group was significantly more depressed than the other two groups during the premenstrual phase. Other symptoms that stood out for the PMS group included food cravings and clumsiness. In another study, Siegel et al.[13] evaluated symptoms in a group of women with severe PMS and reported two distinct clusters of emotional/behavioral symptoms — "withdrawn mood" and "anxious/tense mood." They also noted two clusters of physical symptoms "physical discomfort" and "water retention". Similar results were described previously in a study by Abraham.[14]

To further complicate matters, PMS complaints may also be the result of an underlying disease. Thyroid disease, hyperprolactinemia, diabetes mellitus, and hypoglycemia can cause physical and psychological symptoms similar to PMS.[15]

TABLE 2
Psychological, Physical, and Behavioral Symptoms of PMS

Psychological Symptoms

Anxiety related	Depression related	Other
Nervous tension	Anxious-depression	Insomnia
Mood swings	Crying	Forgetfulness
Irritability	Loneliness	Confusion
Restlessness	Low self-image	Reduced concentration
		Distractability

Physical Symptoms

Tension headaches	Generalized achiness	Dizziness
Migraine headaches	Weight gain	Nausea
Breast tenderness	Hot flashes	Heart pounding
Abdominal bloating	Faintness	Fatigue
Peripheral edema	Abdominal cramps	

Behavioral Symptoms

Increased appetite
Food cravings
Avoidance of social or work activities
Staying at home
Increased alcohol consumption
Increased or decreased libido

Adapted from Smith, S. and Schiff, I., *Fertil. Steril.*, 52, 527, 1989.

IV. MENSTRUAL CYCLE

For a better understanding of PMS, a review of the basic facts about menstruation is necessary. The average menstrual cycle lasts about 28 d, although cycles vary from woman to woman and even in the same woman at different times. The menstrual cycle can be divided into four phases: the menstrual phase (4 d beginning with the first day of menstruation); the follicular phase (the fifth day after menstruation to the periovulatory phase); the periovulatory phase (4 d to the approximate time of ovulation); and the luteal phase (the days between the periovulatory phase and the day before the beginning of menstruation).[16]

During the follicular phase, estrogen and progesterone levels are low. The pituitary gland secretes follicle-stimulating hormone (FSH), which stimulates growth in one of the follicles in a woman's ovary. Toward the end of the follicular phase, estrogen levels increase, signaling the lining of the uterus to prepare for a fertilized egg. Rising estrogen levels stimulate the pituitary gland to secrete luteinizing hormone (LH), which causes the follicle to release the mature egg.

In the luteal phase, the follicle continues to secrete estrogen and the level of LH increases. This produces progesterone, the hormone responsible for changes in the uterine endometrium in the luteal phase of the menstrual cycle. If conception does not occur, hormone levels decrease and the lining of the uterus is shed by menstruation.

To be diagnosed with PMS, a woman's symptoms must correspond with the luteal phase and be absent during the follicular phase of the menstrual cycle. It is the timing of the appearance and disappearance of symptoms, rather than a specific symptom, that leads to the diagnosis of PMS. Two symptomatic cycles are needed, and symptoms must be severe enough to disrupt normal daily activities.

V. PREVALENCE

The prevalence of PMS varies depending on the diagnostic tool used to measure symptoms. The Moos' Menstrual Distress Questionnaire (MDQ) is one of the most widely used self-rating instruments for diagnosis of PMS.[17] It requires women to rate 47 symptoms on a scale of one to six, with six being "acute or partially disabling". Woods et al.[18] administered the MDQ to a group of women and found 30% or more reported common PMS symptoms such as weight gain, cramps, anxiety, fatigue, painful breasts, mood swings, or tension, although only 2 to 8% of women found these symptoms severe or disabling.

Fisher and colleagues[19] administered the Premenstrual Assessment Form (PAF) to 207 adolescent females. The PAF, developed by Halbreich et al.,[20] consists of 95 items describing premenstrual changes in mood, behavior, and physical condition. Items are rated on a six-point scale, from "no change" to "extreme change".

Mortola et al.[21] developed a simple prospective inventory, the Calendar of Premenstrual Experiences, which includes the 10 most common physical and 12 most common behavioral (affective) symptoms of PMS. Each symptom is rated daily on a four-point Likert scale where symptom severity is based on interference with ability to perform daily activities. The calendar is a reliable and practical tool, applicable to some clinical and research settings.

Plouffe et al.[22] used the Calendar of Prospective Records of the impact and severity of menstrual symptoms to determine the number of women who met the criteria for PMS. A total of 43 women had previously been diagnosed as having PMS by other physicians. However, results showed that only 19 of those 43 women were confirmed as having PMS. This study demonstrates the importance of appropriate prospective documentation.

In summary, there are several types of questionnaires used to rate PMS symptoms. Questionnaires can be retrospective, based on past events and experiences, or prospective, based on actual events as they occur. Although prospective measures are thought to underestimate symptom prevalences, retrospective measures may overestimate actual prevalence rates because of recall bias.[23]

VI. ETIOLOGY

The etiology of PMS is unknown, but the fact that PMS is a female disorder makes hormones a major suspect. Levels of estrogen and progesterone change dramatically the week before menstruation and thus can affect many psychological and physiological functions. This may explain why progesterone therapy is widely prescribed for PMS even though there are few well-controlled studies demonstrating its efficacy. Freeman and co-workers[24] conducted a randomized, placebo-controlled, double-blind crossover study of 168 women receiving progesterone suppositories in doses of 400 and 800 mg/d, or a placebo. PMS symptoms were not significantly improved in any measure used in the study.

Among American women, researchers have even speculated that symptoms of PMS are the result of learned attitudes and expectations. In a classic study by Ruble[25] in 1977, 44 women at Princeton University were told they were participating in a new technique for predicting the expected date of menstruation. Unknown to the subjects, the scheduled day of testing corresponded with the sixth or seventh day before her next period. Subjects were told they were either premenstrual (due in 1 or 2 d) or intermenstrual (due in 7 or 10 d). Women who were led to believe they were premenstrual reported a significantly higher degree of water retention, menstrual pain, and changes in eating habits than did women who were led to believe they were intermenstrual. The results of this study are important to researchers, clinicians and physicians who treat PMS because it shows that psychosocial factors can influence self-reports of menstrual-related symptoms in some women.

Several other theories have been advanced in PMS including endogenous opiate withdrawal, prostaglandin deficiency, fluid retention and hypoglycemia. For a more comprehensive review of the etiology of PMS, the reader is referred to Smith and Schiff.[11] The following section will focus on recent nutritional factors implicated in the cause and/or treatment of PMS.

VII. NUTRITIONAL IMPLICATIONS

A. VITAMIN B_6

Perhaps one of the most widely held nutritional theories regarding PMS is that it results from a deficiency of vitamin B_6. As such, supplementation with vitamin B_6 has been a popular approach to treating PMS. Arguments for the use of vitamin B_6 are based on its role as a cofactor for several enzymes, and its association with low levels of the neurotransmitter serotonin and depression.[26] Williams et al.[27] reported a significant improvement in women receiving 100 to 200 mg of vitamin B_6 per day compared to those receiving a placebo. Another study observed favorable trends in symptom improvements with dietary modification and 250 mg/d of vitamin B_6 in an experimental group compared to a control group.[28] However, differences in these two groups were not significant. Although the RDA for vitamin B_6 is 1.6 mg/d for women ages 19 to 50,[29] some women have been known to take 50 to 300 mg/d supplemented by a number of multivitamin preparations.[30] Because excessive amounts of vitamin B_6 are known to produce neurological disorders,[31] caution is indicated and indiscriminate use is not advised.

B. MAGNESIUM

Abraham and Lubran[32] theorized that a magnesium (Mg) deficiency may cause PMS. They reported significantly lower mean levels of serum magnesium in a group of PMS patients compared to a control group. Magnesium is involved in the synthesis of dopamine and thus a deficiency may produce changes in behavior.

Magnesium supplementation has reportedly been successful in relieving premenstrual mood fluctuations in PMS sufferers. Facchinetti et al.[33] conducted a double-blind randomized study involving 28 women with confirmed PMS. For 2 months, magnesium carboxylic acid (360 mg) or a placebo was administered three times a day from the 15th day of the menstrual cycle to the onset of menstrual flow. Magnesium supplementation was shown to be more effective than the placebo in improvement of PMS mood, providing preliminary evidence that this nutrient may have pharmacologic benefits in instances of magnesium deficiency.

Dietary intake of Mg in the U.S. is generally lower than the RDA of 280 mg/d for women of reproductive age. Alcohol abuse, vomiting, diarrhea, or endocrine disorders may contribute to a deficiency of Mg. Legumes, seeds, nuts and green vegetables are good sources of Mg. A balanced diet generally contains an adequate supply.

C. VITAMIN E

Vitamin E (alpha-tocopherol) has also been implicated in PMS because of its effects on PMS symptoms through regulation of aberrant prostaglandin synthesis.[34] Research has shown improvement in breast tenderness and other PMS symptoms in women receiving vitamin E supplements.[34] In a more recent study, however, Chuong et al.[35] examined whether changes in vitamin E levels in the blood were associated with PMS symptoms and found no association.

Mira et al.[36] measured plasma levels of magnesium, zinc, vitamin A, and vitamin E during the luteal phase and midfollicular phase in 38 women with PMS. They found no evidence of nutritional deficiencies including vitamin E. The authors concluded that vitamin E supplementation can only be considered an empirical theory for PMS until further studies are conducted.

D. CAFFEINE

Most dietary guidelines for PMS recommend avoiding caffeine even though it has not been shown to cause PMS. In most cases, this recommendation is based on personal experiences of some women with PMS who have reported improvements in symptoms with caffeine reduction. Rossignol et al.[37] found that consumption of caffeine-containing beverages affected the prevalence and severity of PMS. In women with more severe symptoms, the effect was higher, per amount of exposure, for consumers of tea and coffee than for soft drink consumers over the range of consumption studied (0 to 8 cups of soft drink, and 0 to 3 cups of tea or coffee). The authors suggested that women with PMS consider eliminating caffeine from their diets and then evaluate any changes in the severity of symptoms after several months.

More recently, Cann et al.[38] examined the association between alcohol and caffeine consumption and PMS and found no significant difference in total caffeine intake or in the individual caffeine-containing beverages consumed during the premenstrual period. PMS subjects were more likely to be heavy consumers of decaffeinated coffee or herbal tea than control subjects.

E. FOOD CRAVINGS

Increased hunger and food cravings are symptoms frequently reported by women who suffer from PMS. Cravings for sweets and chocolate are particularly strong. It has been suggested that these food cravings are related to abnormal serotonin activity in the brain which, in turn, may affect mood and appetite. The treatment approach has been to reduce intake of refined carbohydrates especially during the late luteal phase of the menstrual cycle. However, research now suggests that eating carbohydrates may actually relieve PMS symptoms and improve mood.

Wurtman et al.[39] examined the effect of nutrient intake on premenstrual depression in 19 PMS patients and nine control subjects. Compared to the control group, women with PMS significantly increased their consumption of calories, carbohydrates, and fat during the late luteal phase of the cycle. Caloric intake from meals increased from 1455 to 1729 kcal and from snacks from 437 to 666 kcal. Carbohydrate intake increased by 24% from meals and by 43% from snacks. The types of carbohydrates eaten included both sweets and starches such as cookies, potatoes, pasta, bread, and rolls.*

F. SEROTONIN THEORY

According to recent theories, serotonin, the neotransmitter synthesized from the amino acid tryptophan, plays an important role in PMS. Rapkin et al.[40] found that compared to a control group serotonin levels of women with PMS were significantly ($p \leq 0.05$) lower during the midluteal, late luteal, and premenstrual phases which may account for some of the psychological symptoms of PMS such as depression, anxiety, sleeplessness, headaches, and mental confusion. Low serotonin levels may also trigger early ovulation and a shift in estrogen and progesterone patterns, which could account for some of the

---

* Results of this study suggest that increasing carbohydrate intake during the luteal phase of the menstrual cycle may alleviate PMS symptoms.

physical symptoms of PMS such as breast tenderness, abdominal bloating, water retention, acne, and food cravings.

Although it is not known exactly how a deficiency of serotonin relates to PMS symptoms, the amino acid tryptophan may play an important role. According to Fernstrom,[41] tryptophan and other large neutral amino acids such as valine, leucine, and phenylalanine compete for the same saturable carrier protein for transport across the blood-brain barrier. Data suggest that the ratio of plasma tryptophan to the sum of those competing amino acids predicts the level of tryptophan and thus serotonin levels in the brain.[41] In 1991, Rapkin and co-workers[42] tested the hypothesis that diminution of central nervous system L-tryptophan uptake in women with PMS could account for the symptoms seen in the luteal phase of the menstrual cycle. Results showed no significant differences between PMS and control subjects in L-tryptophan-to-competing amino acid ratios.

Tryptophan was a popular nutritional supplement for PMS, insomnia, depression, and weight loss until it was linked to a blood disorder in 1989. At that time the Food and Drug Administration ordered a recall of all dietary supplements containing L-tryptophan because the rare blood disorder eosinophilia-myalgia syndrome was associated with the use of this amino acid. One study indicated that the cause was due to a contaminant in a product manufacturered by a single company under specific operating conditions.[43] Nevertheless, tryptophan is no longer available to the public.

VIII. TREATMENT

PMS symptoms can be physical, psychological, and/or behavioral. Therefore, treatment must address all three areas. Women with mild symptoms may respond well to a combination of diet, exercise, and life-style changes. However, for women with severe PMS symptoms, drug therapy and psychiatric counseling are probably necessary. Treatment depends on the individual and the severity of her symptoms. Practical experience shows that most women prefer not to use medication.

Health professionals who care for women with PMS need to provide support and encourage their patients. Many PMS clinics report that symptoms improve as a result of a caring relationship between the patient and health professional. A sense of hopefulness about a woman's situation may be one of the most important factors in the treatment of PMS.[22]

A. DIETARY RECOMMENDATIONS

Most dietary recommendations include simple modifications such as limiting caffeine, salt, and sugar. These recommendations, however, are empirically based and may or may not work for everyone.

A diet high in complex carbohydrates, such as whole grains, vegetables, breads, pasta, and cereals is encouraged. These foods contain important vitamins and minerals, such as vitamin B_6, and magnesium, and fiber, which helps prevent constipation. Eating carbohydrates may also reduce PMS symptoms by increasing serotonin levels in the brain.

B. EXERCISE

Regular exercise plays a therapeutic role in treating PMS. Studies show that women who are physically active tend to suffer less from PMS. Prior and colleagues[44] conducted a 3-month controlled study involving six sedentary women and eight women who began an exercise training program. The exercising women reported significant decreases in breast tenderness and fluid retention after 3 months of gradual training. In another study, Steege and Blumenthal[45] found that women who participated in aerobic exercise for 60 min three times a week showed significant improvements in PMS symptoms, especially premenstrual depression.

The most persuasive evidence linking exercise to PMS involves beta-endorphin, a chemical in the brain associated with emotion and behavior. One study showed that PMS subjects had lower levels of plasma beta-endorphin during the luteal phase of the menstrual cycle.[46] Because exercise stimulates endorphin production[47] exercise may provide some relief from PMS symptoms. However, further research is needed to confirm this observation.

IX. CONCLUSIONS

PMS is a cyclic disorder that occurs during the luteal phase of the menstrual cycle, producing a number of physical and emotional changes. Commonly reported symptoms include abdominal bloating, backache, breast tenderness, food cravings, fatigue, irritability, and symptoms related to depression. Research shows that it is the timing of the appearance and disappearance of symptoms, rather than a specific symptom, that leads to the diagnosis of PMS.

The direct cause of PMS is unknown. Numerous theories have been proposed and investigated, but none can be proven. The nutritional factors that have been studied include Vitamin B_6, magnesium, vitamin E, caffeine, tryptophan, and food cravings.

Some research suggests that low levels of the neurotransmitter serotonin may account for some of the physical as well as psychological symptoms of PMS. Increasing complex carbohydrates in the diet may relieve PMS symptoms by increasing serotonin levels in the brain.

At present, guidelines for PMS include a combination of diet, exercise, and life-style changes. Most women prefer not to use medication. In addition, support and encouragement are important considerations in the treatment of PMS.

REFERENCES

1. Speroff, L., Historical and social perspectives, in *The Premenstrual Syndrome*, Keye, W. R., Ed., W. B. Saunders, Philadelphia, 1988, 3.
2. Rubinow, D. R., The premenstrual syndrome, *J.A.M.A*, 268, 1908, 1992.
3. Frank, R. T., The hormonal causes of premenstrual tension, *Arch. Neurol. Psychiatr.*, 26, 1053, 1931.
4. Greene, R. and Dalton, K., The premenstrual syndrome, *Br. Med. J.*, 1, 1007, 1953.
5. Reid, R. L., Premenstrual syndrome, *N. Engl. J. Med.*, 324, 1208, 1991.
6. American Psychiatric Association, *Diagnostic and Statistical Manual of Mental Disorders — DSM-III-R*, 3rd Ed., American Psychiatric Association, Washington, D.C., 1987, 367.
7. Hurt, S. W., Schnurr, P. P., Severino, S. K., Freeman, E. W., Gise, L. H., Rivera-Tovar, A., and Steege, J. F., Late luteal phase dysphoric disorder in 670 women evaluated for premenstrual complaints, *Am. J. Psychiatry*, 149, 525, 1992.
8. Reid, R. L., Premenstrual syndrome, *Curr. Probl. Obstet. Gynecol. Fertil.*, 8, 1, 1985.
9. Moos, R. H., Typology of menstural cycle symptoms, *Am. J. Obstet. Gynecol.*, 103, 390, 1969.
10. Abraham, G. E., Nutritional factors in the etiology of the premenstrual tension syndromes, *J. Reprod. Med.*, 28, 446, 1983.
11. Smith, S. and Schiff, I., The premenstrual syndrome — diagnosis and management, *Fertil. Steril.*, 52, 527, 1989.
12. Bancroft, J., Williamson, L., Warner, P., Rennie, D., and Smith, S. K., Perimenstrual complaints in women complaining of PMS, menorrhagia, and dysmenorrhea: toward a dismantling of the premenstrual syndrome, *Psychosom. Med.*, 55, 133, 1993.
13. Siegel, J. P., Myers, B. J., and Dineen, M. K., Premenstrual tension syndrome symptom clusters, *J. Reprod. Med.*, 32, 395, 1987.
14. Abraham, G. E., Premenstrual tension, *Curr. Prob. Obstet. Gynecol.*, 3, 5, 1980.
15. Chuong, C. J., Pearsall-Otey, L. R., and Rosenfeld, B. L., Revising treatments for premenstrual syndrome, *Contemp. Obstet. Gynecol.*, 66, 1994.
16. Gong, E. J., Garrel, D., and Calloway, D. H., Menstrual cycle and voluntary food intake, *Am. J. Clin. Nutr.*, 49, 252, 1989.
17. Moos, R. H., The development of menstrual distress questionnaire, *Psychosom. Med.*, 30, 853, 1968.
18. Woods, N. F., Most, A., and Dery, G. K., Prevalence of perimenstrual symptoms, *Am. J. Public Health*, 72, 1257, 1982.
19. Fisher, M., Trieller, K., and Napolitano, B., Premenstrual symptoms in adolescents, *J. Adolesc. Health Care*, 10, 369, 1989.
20. Halbreich, V., Endicott, J., Schacht, S., and Nee, J., The diversity of premenstrual changes as reflected in the premenstrual assessment form, *Acta Psychiatr. Scand.*, 65, 177, 1980.
21. Mortola, J. F., Girton, L., Beck, L., and Yen, S. S. C., Diagnosis of premenstrual syndrome by a simple, prospective, and reliable instrument: the calendar of premenstrual experiences, *Obstet. Gynecol.*, 76, 302, 1990.
22. Plouffe, L., Stewart, K., Craft, K. S., Maddox, M. S., and Rausch, J. L., Diagnostic and treatment results from a southeastern academic center-based premenstrual syndrome clinic: the first year, *Am. J. Obstet. Gynecol.*, 169, 295, 1993.
23. Rubinow, D. R., Roy-Byrne, P., and Hobban, M. C., Premenstrual mood changes: characteristic patterns in women with and without premenstrual syndrome, *J. Affect. Dis.*, 10, 85, 1986.
24. Freeman, E., Rickels, K., Sondheimer, S. J., and Polansky, M., Ineffectiveness of progesterone suppository treatment for premenstrual syndrome, *J.A.M.A.*, 264, 349, 1990.
25. Ruble, D. N., Premenstrual symptoms: a reinterpretation, *Science*, 197, 291, 1977.

26. Rose, D. P., The interactions between vitamin B_6 and hormones, *Vitam. Horm.*, 36, 53, 1978.

27. Williams, M. J., Taylor, M. L., and Dean, B. C., Controlled trial of pyridoxine in the premenstrual syndrome, *J. Int. Med. Res.*, 13, 174, 1985.

28. Berman, M. K., Taylor, M. L., and Freeman, E., Vitamin B_6 in premenstrual syndrome, *J. Am. Diet. Assoc.*, 90, 859, 1990.

29. Food and Nutrition Board, *Recommended Dietary Allowances*, 10th Ed., National Academy of Sciences, Washington, D.C., 1989.

30. Dalton, K., Pyridoxine overdose in premenstrual syndrome, *Lancet*, 1, 1168, 1985.

31. Schaumburg, H., Kaplan, J., Windebank, A., Nicholas, V., Rasmus, S., Pleasure, D., and Brown, M. J., Sensory neuropathy from pyridoxine abuse, *N.Engl. J. Med.*, 309, 445, 1983.

32. Abraham, G. E. and Lubran, M. M., Serum and red cell magnesium levels in patients with premenstrual tension, *Am. J. Clin. Nutr.*, 34, 2364, 1981.

33. Facchinetti, F., Borella, P., Sances, G., Fioroni, L., Nappi, R. E., and Genazzani, A. R., Oral magnesium successfully relieves premenstrual mood changes, *Obstet. Gynecol.*, 78, 177, 1991.

34. London, R. S., Murphy, L., Kitlowski, K. E., and Reynolds, M. A., Efficacy of alpha-tocopherol in the treatment of the premenstrual syndrome, *J. Reprod. Med.*, 32, 400, 1987.

35. Chuong, C. J., Dawson, E. B., and Smith, E. R., Vitamin E levels in premenstrual syndrome, *Am. J. Obstet. Gynecol.*, 163, 1591, 1990.

36. Mira, M., Stewart, P. M., and Abraham, S. F., Vitamin and trace element status in premenstrual syndrome, *Am. J. Clin. Nutr.*, 47, 636, 1988.

37. Rossignol, A. M. and Bonnlander, H., Caffeine-containing beverages, total fluid consumption, and premenstrual syndrome, *Am. J. Public Health*, 80, 1106, 1990.

38. Cann, B., Duncan, D., Hiatt, R., Lewis, J., Chapman, J., and Armstrong, M. A., Association between alcoholic and caffeinated beverages and premenstrual syndrome, *J. Reprod. Med.*, 38, 630, 1993.

39. Wurtman, J. J., Brzezinski, A., Wurtman, R. J., and Laferrere, B., Effect of nutrient intake on premenstrual depression, *Am. J. Obstet. Gynecol.*, 161, 1228, 1989.

40. Rapkin, A. J., Edelmuth, E., Chang, L. C., Reading, A. E., McGuire, M. T., and Tung-Ping, S., Whole-blood serotonin in premenstrual syndrome, *Obstet. Gynecol.*, 70, 533, 1987.

41. Fernstrom, J. D., Role of precursor availability in control of monoamine biosynthesis in brain, *Physiol. Rev.*, 63, 484, 1983.

42. Rapkin, A. J., Reading, A. E., Woo, S., and Goldman, L. M., Tryptophan and neutral amino acids in premenstrual syndrome, *Am. J. Obstet. Gynecol.*, 165, 1830, 1991.

43. Belongia, E. A., Hedberg, C. W., Gleich, G. J., White, K. E., Mayeno, A. N., Loegering, D. A., Dunnette, S. L., Pirie, P. L., MacDonald, K. L., and Osterholm, M. T., An investigation of the cause of the eosinophilia-myalgia syndrome associated with tryptophan use, *N. Engl. J. Med.*, 323, 357, 1990.

44. Prior, J. C., Vigna, Y., and Alojada, N., Conditioning exercise decreases premenstrual symptoms, *Eur. J. Appl. Physiol.*, 55, 349, 1986.

45. Steege, J. F. and Blumenthal, J. A., The effects of aerobic exercise on premenstrual symptoms in middle-aged women: a preliminary study, *J. Psychosom. Res.*, 37, 127, 1993.

46. Chuong, C. J., Coulam, C. B., and Kao, P. C., Neuropeptide levels in premenstrual syndrome, *Fertil. Steril.*, 44, 760, 1985.

47. Thoren, P., Floras, J. S., Hoffmann, P., and Seals, D. R., Endorphins and exercise: physiological mechanisms and clinical implications, *Med. Sci. Sports Exerc.*, 22, 417, 1990.

Chapter 10

ORAL CONTRACEPTION AND NUTRITION

Priscille G. Massé

CONTENTS

I. INTRODUCTION

Oral contraceptives (OCs) are among the most thoroughly studied drugs. In our modern society, women are becoming sexually active earlier, delaying the birth of their first child and limiting their total number of children. As a consequence, approximately 14 million women in the U.S. and 150 million worldwide, averaging 85% of reproductive age women, choose oral contraceptives for birth control because of their convenience and efficiency. The new generation of OCs includes both the low-dose combined estrogen-progestogen pill (containing less than 50 μg estrogen and less than 1.5 mg progestogen) as well as the progestogen-only pill. In the first category, more than two dozen preparations are currently marketed. The majority are modifications of the "first generation" higher dose combined estrogen-progestogen.

During the past decade, the major development in hormone contraceptive technology has been the introduction of triphasic preparations (e.g., Triphasil®, Wyeth Ltd.). These new combinations of low-dose hormones are specifically tailored to minimize estrogen- and progestogen-related side effects, to mimic the woman's physiologic hormonal cycle, and to provide effective contraception.[1] These objectives are achieved by gradually increasing the progestogen (levonorgestrel) dose from 50 μg for the first 6 d of the cycle to 75 μg for the next 5 d, and then to 125 μg for the remaining 10 d. Estrogen (ethinyl estradiol) doses are 30, 40, and 30 μg for the same periods. As a result, total monthly progestogen content is 39% less, and the estrogen dose 8% more than that of the lowest fixed-dose OCs now available.

II. PHARMACOKINETICS OF CONTRACEPTIVE STEROIDS

All of the combined preparations contain one of two estrogens (namely, ethinyl estradiol and mestranol) and one of four progestogens (namely, ethynodiol diacetate, norethindrone acetate, norethynodrel, and norgestrel). The bioavailability of both synthetic estrogens is equal, any differences observed being due to the metabolic conversion time.[2] The degradation of mestranol and estradiol appears identical, with the major urinary metabolite being estradiol glucuronide. Other products include estradiol sulfate and various hydroxylated compounds. The progestative steroid is a 19-nortestosterone compound that exhibits a progesterone-like activity and is used because progesterone itself is inactive when administered orally. The fate of progestogens is more complex than the synthetic estrogens due to extensive metabolism. Over 30 metabolites have been identified for the various progestogens.[2] Ethynodiol diacetate and norethindrone acetate undergo metabolism to norethindrone as a principal metabolic pathway. This steroid is then hydroxylated and undergoes rapid bond reduction and conjugation before excretion. For *d*-norgestrel, considerably more active than the ℓ-isomer, the metabolism is similar to that of norethindrone, but the rate of metabolism and conjugation is slower.

III. ESTABLISHMENT OF METABOLIC CHANGES

The assessment of any drug-induced metabolic effects implies the evaluation of the nutritional status which requires laboratory tests on easily available body fluids such as blood and urine. They should be specific, simple, inexpensive, and reveal tissue depletion at an early stage. The choice of the blood component is guided by the concentration of the vitamin in it and its sensitivity to deficiency states. Vitamin B_{12} measurements are generally made in the serum or plasma, whereas for most other water-soluble vitamins, plasma as well as blood cells are used. For the fat-soluble vitamins, only plasma is used because the concentrations of these vitamins or their metabolites in blood cells are very low.[3] Under some circumstances the distribution of vitamins between tissues is known to be altered. One such example which has been studied recently is oral contraceptive use.

In the case of vitamins, nutritional status can be evaluated basically by *two types of biochemical tests*:

- Those based on the measurement of either the vitamin or its metabolites in blood or urine
- Those based on the measurement of one or more of their enzymatic and metabolic functions (functional tests)

It has been possible to develop functional tests, in the case of the B complex vitamins, since most of their biochemical functions are well established. In the interpretation of their results, it is advisable to take into account the basal enzyme activity as well as its activation with coenzyme, known as the *in vitro* stimulation test which is expressed as activation coefficient (AC). Examples of functional enzymatic tests are transketolase for thiamin, glutathione reductase for riboflavin, and alanine and aspartate aminotransferases for pyridoxine (vitamin B_6). In metabolic tests, a rise in the concentration of a metabolite in blood or urine as a result of a vitamin deficiency-mediated enzymatic lesion is measured, preferably after administering a load of an appropriate precursor. Examples of such tests are the tryptophan load test inherent to the evaluation of pyridoxine status (e.g., urinary level of xanthurenic acid), histidine and valine load tests to assess folic acid, and vitamin B_{12} status by the formiminoglutamic acid (abbreviated as FIGLU) and methylmalonic acid excretions in urine, respectively. Sauberlich et al.[4] have described tentative guidelines for the interpretation of laboratory tests currently available for assessing vitamin nutrition status. Tables 1 and 2 indicate the test pertinent to our discussion. These will be referred to throughout this chapter.

A. OC-INDUCED METABOLIC CHANGES

The enthusiastic acceptance and widespread usage of OCs have withdrawn attention from their potential side effects. This subject has been documented previously on several occasions. Either estrogens or progestogens, or their combination, modulate a number of physiological processes that are metabolic and nutritional in nature. In general, their ingestion has been shown to affect a number of metabolic processes in either an insignificant or advantageous manner. Examples will be given to highlight both cases.

TABLE 1

Tentative Guidelines for the Interpretation of Blood Vitamin Levels and Enzyme Tests

	Deficient (high risk)	Low (medium risk)
Erythrocyte aspartate aminotransferase — AC[a]	≥1.5–2.0	
Erythrocyte alanine aminotransferase — AC	≥1.25	
Serum folate (ng/mℓ)	<3.0	3.0–5.9
Erythrocyte folate (ng/mℓ)	<140	140–159
Serum vitamin B_{12} (pg/mℓ)	<150	150–200

[a] AC: activation coefficient.

Adapted from Sauberlich, H.E., Scala, J. H., and Dowdy, R. P., *Laboratory Tests for the Assessment of Nutritional Status,* CRC Press, Boca Raton, FL, 1974.

TABLE 2

Tentative Guidelines for Acceptable Urinary Excretion of Vitamins or Metabolites in Adults

	Per Day	Per Gram Creatinine
Pyridoxine (µg)	—	>20
4-Pyridoxic acid (mg)	≥0.8	—
Xanthurenic acid (mg)	<25	—
FIGLU mg/8 h	<30	—
Methylmalonic acid (mg)	<24	—

Adapted from Sauberlich, H.E., Scala, J. H., and Dowdy, R. P., *Laboratory Tests for the Assessment of Nutritional Status*, CRC Press, Boca Raton, FL, 1974..

The significance of the alterations in nutrient metabolism becomes a matter of concern when OCs are used on a long-term basis. Table 3 summarizes the recognized metabolic modifications that occur in women upon exposure to the "pill". In brief, serum concentrations tend to rise for iron, copper, and vitamin A, while reductions are reported in circulating levels of selected B vitamins, ascorbic acid, and zinc.[5-9] The most significant decreases are found in water-soluble vitamins: thiamin, riboflavin, pyridoxine, cobalamin, and folic acid. Clinical effects of severe vitamin deficiencies are rare (Table 4). However, a marginal (or subclinical), vitamin deficiency can occur. It describes a condition in which vitamin status is poor (depleted reserves) but no overt symptoms of a deficiency are present. The increases of vitamin A, iron, and copper are not large enough to cause clinical effects and may be beneficial in some instances.

TABLE 3
Oral Contraceptives and Nutritional Status

Nutrient	Observed Modifications in Nutritional Status
Vitamins	↑ circulating levels of vitamin A
	↓ circulating levels of carotene, vitamin E, folacin, vitamin B_{12}, vitamin B_6, vitamin C
	↑ in vitro stimulation of erythrocyte B_1-dependent transketolase, B_2-dependent glutathione reductase, and B_6-dependent aminotransferases with thiamine, riboflavin and pyridoxine, respectively
	Biochemical signs of vitamin B_6 deficiency in some women (low urinary pyridoxic acid, plasma pyridoxal phosphate, and erythrocyte aminotransferases); occasionally accompanied by depression
	↓ circulating levels of calcium, phosphorus, magnesium, and zinc
Minerals	↑ circulating levels of iron and copper

TABLE 4
Some Vitamin Deficiency Diseases and Symptoms

Vitamin	Deficiency Disease/Major Symptoms
A (retinol)	Xerophtalmia, night blindness, blindness
Thiamin (B_1)	Beriberi, numbness, muscle weakness, cardiac disturbance; Wernicke's encephalopathy, polyneuropathy
Riboflavin (B_2)	Glossitis, dermatitis, cheilosis
Niacin	Pellagra, dermatitis, diarrhea, mental disturbance
B_6 (pyridoxine)	Sideroblastic anemia, dermatitis, depression, convulsions
B_{12} (cobalamin)	Pernicious anemia, peripheral neuritis, spinal cord degeneration
C (ascorbic acid)	Scurvy, sore gums, capillary bleeding
Folic acid (folate, folacin)	Megaloblastic anemia, macrocytic anemia

IV. EFFECTS OF OCs ON VITAMIN NUTRITION

Studies have been conducted on the effects of OCs on several vitamins, namely, retinol (vitamin A), thiamin (vitamin B_1), riboflavin (vitamin B_2), pyridoxine (vitamin B_6), folic acid, cobalamin (vitamin B_{12}), ascorbic acid (vitamin C), α-tocopherol (vitamin E), and vitamin K.[6,10,11] This chapter will emphasize vitamins B_6, B_{12}, and folic acid due to the significance of their metabolic alterations in terms of psychological side effects.

A. IMPAIRMENT OF VITAMIN B_6 STATUS
1. Indirect Evidence: Abnormalities in Tryptophan Metabolism

As previously mentioned in section III of this chapter, one biochemical indirect method to evaluate the vitamin B_6 status consists of measuring the amount of xanthurenic acid (XA) excreted in urine after administration of a tryptophan load test. One of the main roles of vitamin B_6 after it is converted to the coenzyme (active) form, pyridoxal phosphate (PLP), is to act as a catalyst in the formation of niacin from tryptophan, an essential amino acid. This metabolic pathway is illustrated in Figure 1. The first enzyme of this pathway, tryptophan pyrrolase (TPase), appears to be particularly susceptible to the direct effect of OCs or to their secondary stimulating action on glucocorticoid secretion by adrenal glands. Whatever the mechanism, this induction of hepatic TPase directs more tryptophan into the niacin pathway than usual, with the result of a higher metabolic demand for vitamin B_6 since a number of the steps are B_6 dependent. The results are the accumulation of tryptophan intermediates and a consequent relative deficiency of the vitamin.

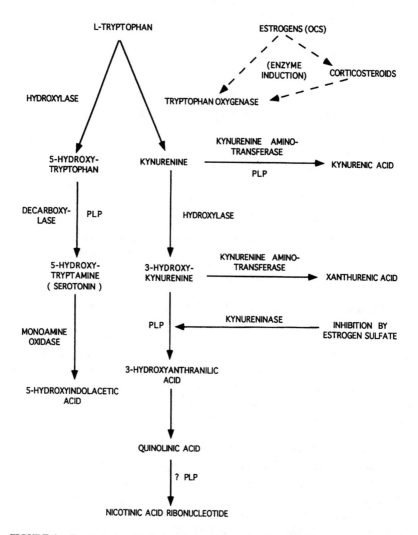

FIGURE 1. Tryptophan metabolism in liver and in brain. (From Bamji, M. S., in *Vitamins in Human Biology and Medicine*, Briggs, M. H., Ed., CRC Press, Boca Raton, FL, 1981. With permission.)

The suspicion that OCs might affect vitamin B_6 status arose in part from the analogy drawn with the state of pregnancy. In fact, the same abnormality in the tryptophan pathway has been demonstrated in women taking a variety of combined estrogen-progestogen contraceptive preparations.[12] This disturbance has been demonstrated after a tryptophan load and also without loading.[13] Several investigators have consistently shown that urinary excretion of XA in women taking OCs is higher as compared to nonusers.[14-16] This increase in the excretion of XA was interpreted for years as evidence for pyridoxine deficiency, although at that time the mode of action by which estrogen modified tryptophan metabolism was not clear. Various investigators have proposed that the activation of liver tryptophan catabolism by estrogen was the result of increased TPase activity.[17-20] Consequently, a tryptophan oral loading will cause a relative shortage of PLP coenzyme due to the stimulation of aminotransferases (refer to Figure 1) to transaminate the extra amount of kynurenine and hydroxykynurenine deriving from the accelerated degradation of tryptophan.

A relative vitamin B_6 deficiency at the level of B_6-dependent kynureninase might well be responsible for the accumulation of tryptophan metabolites.[21] More recently, Bender et al.[22] concluded that abnormalities of tryptophan metabolism in women receiving estrogens can be accounted for by the inhibition of this enzyme by estrogen metabolites and not to a stimulation of TPase activity. It is still not clear whether inhibited kynureninase activity or stimulated TPase activity is the cause of changes in tryptophan metabolism. Despite this uncertainty, there seems to be general agreement that consumption of OCs can contribute to vitamin B_6 deficiency as a result of the perturbation in tryptophan metabolism.

However, the validity of the tryptophan load test as an index of vitamin B_6 deficiency has often been questioned. One study showed that the urinary excretion of XA was poorly correlated with plasma PLP.[23] Leklem[24] reported a significant difference between users of OCs and nonusers in the tryptophan load test, but no significant difference in other indices of B_6 status, such as urinary cystathionine, urinary pyridoxic acid, plasma PLP, and erythrocyte alanine and aspartate aminotransferases. The use of the tryptophan load as an index of B_6-status was also criticized on the grounds that inhibition of kynureninase by estrogens or their metabolites would give results indistinguishable from vitamin B_6 deficiency. In effect, being a PLP-dependent enzyme, the activity of kynureninase is also impaired in this deficiency, leading to increased excretion of kynurenic and XA acids. As previously mentioned, the inhibition of this enzyme has been demonstrated in rats when given estrogens (estrone sulfate), but the dose used was approximately three times the dose that is used clinically.[22]

Another relevant question persists in regard to the clinical significance of the tryptophan metabolic abnormality. It has been suggested that the increased TPase activity could be the cause of the depression observed among women taking OCs.[25] In effect, the induction of this enzyme by OCs might decrease the amount of brain tryptophan available for the synthesis of serotonin (5-hydroxytryptamine, 5-HT), known to play a role in mood control. This aspect will be discussed in more detail in the following section.

a. Psychoaffective Disturbances

There exists a link between depressive mood changes and abnormalities in tryptophan metabolism. First, a direct inhibition of cerebral uptake of tryptophan by the synthetic steroids could reduce the amount available for 5-HT synthesis. Second, 5-hydroxytryptophan decarboxylase (another B_6-dependent enzyme), involved in this synthesis, may be susceptible to competition for pyridoxal phosphate by estrogen conjugates. Third, a disturbance in liver tryptophan metabolism during oral contraception may cause, indirectly, depression through changes in the level of brain serotonin, as already mentioned in the previous section. Our discussion will focus on this metabolic cerebral alteration which has been the most explored.

The synthetic estrogens (and the 50-fold increased endogenous estrogen secretion during pregnancy), by stimulating TPase, contribute to the diversion of tryptophan metabolism from its minor cerebral serotonin pathway to its major kynurenine-niacin pathway in the liver.[26] This shift of tryptophan metabolism toward the kynurenine-niacin pathway, evidenced by increased urinary xanthurenic acid excretion, is at the expense of serotonin synthesis (Figure 1). The reduced 24-h urinary output of 5-hydroxyindolacetic acid (5-HIAA, end product of 5-HT) has been demonstrated by Shaaraway et al.[27]

Studies carried out on the psychological side effects of hormonal contraception have focused on the depressive syndrome, although other various emotional states do occur. In fact, psychological side effects related to OCs use are multidimensional in nature.[28] The recent literature suggests that depression associated with OCs may differ significantly from non-organic major depressive episodes.[29] Depression has been recognized as a complication of estrogen-progestogen contraceptives, although only a small number of women develop this syndrome. Its incidence is still disputed, but it probably occurs in about 5 to 6% of women.[2,30,31] In agreement with Kutner and Brown's study,[32] Massé and Roberge[33] have been unable to support a relationship between oral contraception and depression. The depression scale of OC users, when administered by MMPI (Minnesota Multiphasic Personality Inventory) after a long-term use (4 years on average) of a relatively low-dose (30 μg ethinyl estradiol) combined preparation (Figure 2), was identical to that of control nonusers. None of the OC users suffered depression. Our recent specific study on Triphasil® also revealed no psychoaffective changes at an early stage of utilization, e.g., at the sixth menstrual cycle (unpublished data).[120] The strength of the last three aforementioned studies lies in the use of an objective and comprehensive rating instrument such as MMPI.

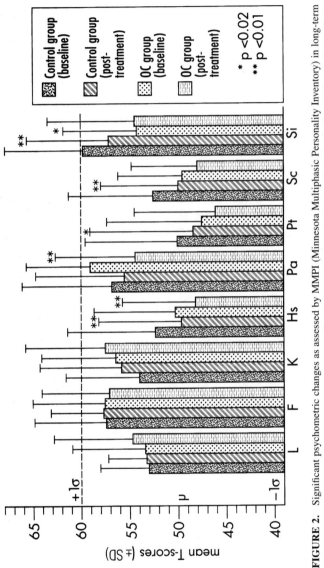
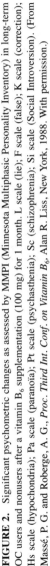

FIGURE 2. Significant psychometric changes as assessed by MMPI (Minnesota Multiphasic Personality Inventory) in long-term OC users and nonusers after a vitamin B_6 supplementation (100 mg) for 1 month. L scale (lie); F scale (false); K scale (correction); Hs scale (hypochondria); Pa scale (paranoïa); Pt scale (psychasthenia); Sc (schizophrenia); Si scale (Social Introversion). (From Massé, P. G. and Roberge, A. G., *Proc. Third Int. Conf. on Vitamin B_6*, Alan R. Liss, New York, 1988. With permission.)

2. Direct Evidence: Abnormalities in Vitamin B_6 Metabolism

Some controversy also exists when the B_6-dependent alanine and aspartate aminotranferase enzymes, commonly known as transaminases, are used to assess vitamin B_6 status. When a significant change in basal or activated enzymatic activity is reported, both enzymes are generally affected. An early review of the extensive literature pertaining to the activity of these enzymes in serum showed disparate results. Our laboratory did not show any changes in regard to both serum aminotransferases (transaminases).[33] This biochemical parameter which reflects liver functions is known to be a poor indicator of B_6 nutritional status. As judged by the basal activity of specific alanine (ALT) aminotransferase in erythrocytes, the B_6 status of OC users is either similar to nonusers[34,35] or different enough to be considered significant.[14,36] The basal activity of specific aspartate (AST) aminotransferase in erythrocytes indicated a deficiency in OC users consuming a nonsupplemented diet.[15,37,38] Recently, van der Vange et al.[39] reported no significant change in the activation coefficient (a more reliable parameter than the basal activity) of this enzyme in erythrocyte after 6 months of low-dose OCs. Our recent longitudinal study on young college students taking a triphasic preparation (Triphasil®) confirmed this negative finding (unpublished data). In the former study, subjects (n = 70) were taking seven different varieties of monophasic, biphasic, and triphasic OC preparations.[39] Table 5 summarizes our data relative to vitamin B_6 and other nutrients.

TABLE 5
Effect of a 6-Month Treatment with Triphasil® on Nutritional Status Relative to Iron, Folic Acid, Vitamins B_6 and B_{12}

	Serum iron (μmol/l)	Serum ferritin (μg/l)	Serum folic acid (ηmol/l)	Serum vitamin B_{12} (pmol/l)	Erythrocyte PLP (ηmol/l)	Plasma B_6-aldehydes (ηmol/l)
Before	15.2 ± 8.3[a]	19.5 ± 15.8	15.5 ± 9.7	370 ± 126	52.4 ± 10.2	70.8 ± 12.7
After	15.8 ± 10.2	28.3 ± 18.5	12.6 ± 4.1	273 ± 120	51.6 ± 11.7	70.1 ± 17.4
	ns	ns	ns	ns	ns	ns
Normal range	5–28[b]	10–200[b]	6–39[b]	148–840[b]	37–144[c]	78.1[d]

[a] Mean ± SD; ns = nonsignificant. B_6-aldehydes = pyridoxal phosphate (PLP) + pyridoxal (PL).
[b] Reference values used in our laboratory according to standardized methods.
[c] Reference values used in TNO Nutrition and Food Research Laboratory, Zeist, The Netherlands.
[d] Average value published by Barnard, H. C., Vermaak, W. J. H., and Potgieter, G. M., *Int. J. Vitamin Nutr. Res.*, 56, 351, 1986.

Alternative approaches to the assessment of vitamin B_6 status are direct measurements of the vitamin and its metabolites. Attempts to define the nutritional status of vitamin B_6 during oral contraception by direct measurement, particularly in blood, but also in urine, have also led to a range of conclusions.

Both enzymatic and microbiological assays have been used. The latter method often lacks specificity, which may account for some conflicting results. Chemical and enzymatic methods have been proven to be more reliable and reproducible.

According to Bender et al.,[22] the administration of estrone sulfate to rats caused a slight reduction in the concentration of PLP in plasma. In several past human studies, this biochemical indicator of B_6 status was found to be significantly lower in OC users as compared with nonusers,[38,40,41] even when compared with pretreatment levels within the first 3 months of use.[23] It is noteworthy to mention that most of these women returned to their normal PLP values by the sixth month of utilization. A similar observation has been made recently by van der Vange et al.[39] According to most recent human studies, there exists no real difference between OC users and nonusers in regard to plasma PLP level.[33,39] Our current longitudinal and specific study on Triphasil®, based on specific biochemical parameters such as PLP level and *in vitro*-stimulated activity of AST aminotransferase in erythrocytes, also showed no significant changes after six consecutive menstrual cycles. Only 1 subject of 14 exhibited a decline in erythrocyte PLP level at the third menstrual cycle. There was no return to normal value at the sixth month of use. This finding was consistent with a continuous elevation of AST activation coefficient throughout the study. In addition to using other criteria, several investigators also studied the urinary excretion of 4-pyridoxic acid. Generally, OCs do not change the level of this metabolite, despite the excretion of abnormal amounts of tryptophan metabolites.[28,40,42,43] Although a high percentage (evaluated to be approximately 80% by Luhby et al.[44]) of women who take OCs exhibit abnormal tryptophan metabolism, only a minority show biochemical evidence of vitamin B_6 deficiency, the number depending on the criterion employed. It seems that the causes of altered vitamin B_6 metabolism are diverse.

B. IMPAIRMENT OF FOLIC ACID STATUS

There is evidence that OCs interfere with and impair the body's metabolism of folic acid, or folate, and vitamin B_{12}. However, the following two sections will show that several investigators have reported results that negate these findings. This discrepancy, independent of biochemical indicators used, has created some confusion and controversy.

Clinical and biochemical indicators frequently examined to assess the folate nutritional status have been the following: (1) the incidence of megaloblastic anemia and cervical dysplasia, (2) serum and erythrocyte folate concentrations, (3) the urinary formiminoglutamic acid (FIGLU) excretion, and (4) the intestinal absorption of polyglutamates. Numerous cases of megaloblastic anemia attributed to OCs have been reported.[45] In some of these cases there were associated contributory factors, such as a mild malabsorption syndrome or dietary folate deficiency, and it is not clear whether megaloblastic anemia would have occurred in the absence of these factors. The literature pertinent to the association between OC use and folic acid status is divergent. Some reports that have demonstrated that women using OCs have a lower serum level of folate than nonusers[46,47] have been contradicted by others showing no statistical difference.[48-50] The subject is also considered controversial when the erythrocyte level (a better biochemical marker than serum level and more representative of tissue metabolism) is used to assess nutritional status. A number of investigators have reported that the mean red cell level of folate in groups of women taking OCs, as assessed by microbiological techniques, was significantly lower than that of control groups.[47,51-53] Other studies have failed to show any statistical differences.[50,54,55]

Although conflicting data still exist as to the effects of OCs on folic acid status, the majority of reports tend to support the observation that there is a parallel lowering of the folic acid concentration in erythrocytes and an increase in urinary FIGLU excretion simultaneously with the reduction in serum folate levels. FIGLU is an intermediary product of the metabolism of histidine that requires the reduced form of folic acid to be further metabolized. Shojania[51] found that women using OCs excreted significantly more FIGLU in the urine after a histidine load than controls and that the levels decreased to normal within 2 to 4 months after their use was stopped. It is not clear whether this increase is due to folate deficiency induced by OCs or to a physiologic effect that mimics early pregnancy. A higher level of FIGLU is also excreted during pregnancy.[56]

The mechanism of the impairment of folic acid metabolism by OCs, both in experimental animals and in humans, remains unclear. The difference in the intestinal absorption between the usual dietary folate and folic acid in therapeutic vitamin preparations, in OC users, has been underlined in several medical reports.[51-56] Polyglutamates, the major dietary source of folic acid, must be enzymatically deconjugated in the small intestine before absorption takes place. Streiff[57] has described cases of women on OCs showing a defect in utilization or absorption between polyglutamates and monoglutamate.

Initially, the inhibition of the activity of folate conjugase by OCs and the consequent malabsorption of folate polyglutamates seemed to have provided a satisfying explanation for the impairment of folic acid metabolism. However, a subsequent report failed to show any malabsorption of folate polyglutamates in OC users or any inhibitory effect of these compounds on folate conjugase.[58] The hormonal alterations found during pregnancy do not selectively change polyglutamate absorption, suggesting that oral synthetic estrogens and progestogens may act in a different manner than do the naturally occurring hormones, at least as far as intestinal absorption of folic acid is concerned. Another mechanism has been proposed for the impairment of folic acid metabolism in association with the use of OCs. The increased excretion of folates in the urine, which is also reported in pregnant women, may in part explain the lower levels of folic acid in the serum and erythrocytes of some OC users.[59]

C. IMPAIRMENT OF VITAMIN B_{12} STATUS

OC users have been reported to exhibit significantly reduced levels of serum vitamin B_{12} whether the level is determined by microbiologic[52,54,60] or radioisotope[60-62] assays. It is difficult to explain the mechanism behind this phenomenon. Serum levels of vitamin B_{12} may be lowered, to subnormal values in some cases, but this finding is not necessarily associated with evidence of tissue depletion (sign of a true deficiency). However, the clinician may suggest that the patient temporarily stop taking "the pill" to see if the serum level of vitamin B_{12} is decreased. A Schilling test (a radioactive absorption assay) is usually performed to exclude the possibility that the problem is caused by vitamin B_{12} malabsorption. Results from our current longitudinal (six menstrual cycles) study on young women taking Triphasil® in regard to vitamin B_{12} and other nutrients are summarized in Table 5. Mean serum vitamin B_{12} level was reduced by 26% but the difference was not significant (due to high variance of data), despite the fact that the blood sample was withdrawn at the same period of menstrual cycle for all subjects.

Besides malabsorption problems, proposed explanations for the serum vitamin B_{12} reduction have included an increased renal excretion and an impaired production of vitamin binders. Hjelt et al.[63] measured vitamin B_{12} absorption and excretion by means of a sensitive whole-body counting technique. Since none of the OC users suffered from dietary insufficiency, the findings of normal absorption and excretion indicated that the vitamin B_{12} stores were normal. This is in accordance with others who have found a normal Schilling test and no changes in erythrocyte levels and urinary excretion of methylmalonic acid (another biochemical marker for vitamin B_{12} status).[60,61,63]

The low serum vitamin B_{12} level is most likely associated with defective serum vitamin B_{12} binders. In fact, OCs can inhibit the production of transcobalamin I (TC-I), a glycoprotein synthesized by leukocytes. This binder, 70 to 100% saturated, is not essential for vitamin B_{12} transport to the tissues and is more concerned with its transport in plasma. Total serum level of TC-I has been found to be reduced[60] or not significantly changed[61,62] in OC users. Since about 90% of vitamin B_{12} is bound to TC-I, a low level could contribute to the low serum vitamin B_{12} level. Transcobalamin II is a beta globuline and is 90 to 95% unsaturated, but it plays the major role in vitamin B_{12} transport to the tissues. Larsson-Cohn[64] suggested that OC treatment increases the tissue avidity for vitamin B_{12} resulting in a redistribution of the vitamin within the different tissue compartments. This is unlikely to occur according to Shojania and Wylie,[60] because TC-II is unaffected by OCs.

D. METABOLIC INTERRELATIONSHIPS BETWEEN VITAMINS B_6, B_{12}, AND FOLIC ACID

Low serum vitamin B_{12} may be secondary to folate deficiency. Kornberg et al.[65] reported a case of a 34-year-old woman having developed megaloblastic anemia and peripheral polyneuropathy following the use of OCs for 4 years.

Both levels of folic acid and vitamin B_{12} were low. The poor response to vitamin B_{12} alone, and the development of anemia and polyneuropathy 4 months after cessation of vitamin B_{12} therapy, suggested that folate deficiency was the primary problem. However, according to Wertalik et al.,[61] oral administration of folic acid has no effect on serum vitamin B_{12} values, suggesting that the serum vitamin B_{12} decrease is not secondary to folate deficiency. Although OCs are widely used, the aforementioned symptoms of folate deficiency rarely develop. It is possible that a minor effect of the drug may unmask a pre-existent subclinical vitamin deficiency caused by nutritional factors, hidden malabsorption, or increased metabolism.

There may be some relation between the low serum levels of vitamin B_{12} and impaired pyridoxine (tryptophan) metabolism. Boots et al.[66] demonstrated that baboons treated with OCs had lower serum vitamin B_{12} levels than controls, but that the lowering of serum vitamin B_{12} levels could be prevented with pyridoxine. It has been reported that deficiencies of folate and vitamin B_{12} can lead to pathological homocysteinemia with levels comparable to those in heterozygotes for homocystinuria.[67-72] Based on these observations, one can hypothesize that the occurrence of vascular events reported during the use of OCs may be induced, at least partially, by pathological homocysteinemia caused by depressed levels of one of the three vitamins playing an important role in the metabolism of sulfur amino acids (Figure 3). Steegers-Theunissen et al.[55] showed that the homocysteine levels in fasting serum of long-term users of a monophasic sub-50 OC*(Marvelon®), on the third day of the menstrual cycle, were significantly higher in comparison with control women not taking OCs. However, this difference was not significant in the high hormonal phase (50 µg), i.e., on the 21st day. Serum and red blood cell folate and vitamin B_{12} levels were not reduced. However, on both days, the fasting whole-blood PLP concentrations were slightly but significantly lower in OC users. A possible explanation of the difference observed in serum homocysteine levels between the two groups is this decrease in the PLP concentration of OC users. This active form of vitamin B_6 is coenzyme in the conversion of homocysteine to cystathionine.[73]

V. EFFECTS OF OCs ON MINERAL NUTRITION

OCs use can also affect the metabolism of minerals. For instance, it can depress the physiologic level of zinc and elevate those of iron and copper (Table 3). Here we will focus on iron to underline a positive side of OCs other than its contraceptive action. Another positive effect in relation to bone mineralization has been recently discovered and could mean a reduced risk of postmenopausal bone loss for past long-term users (6 years or more). In effect, Kritz-Silverstein and Barrett-Connor[74] examined bone mineral density of 239

---

* 30 µg ethinyl estradiol/0.15 mg desogestrel.

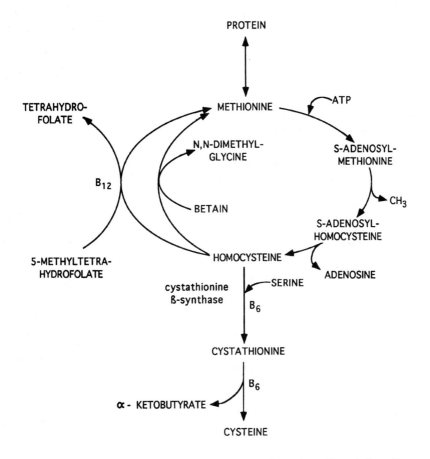

FIGURE 3. Role of vitamins B_6, B_{12} and folic acid in sulfur amino acid metabolism. (From Smolin, L.A. and Benevenga, N. J., *J. Nutr.,* 114, 103, 1984. With permission.)

postmenopausal women, 35.1% of whom reported prior oral contraceptive use. Women who had used OCs for 6 or more years had significantly higher bone densities of the lumbar spine and femoral neck than women who never used them. However, cross-sectional studies of bone density among pill users have yielded discrepant results. Data from another recent study on a cohort of 46,000 women do not support the hypothesis that pill use protects women against the occurrence of osteoporotic fractures in later life.[75]

Although the metabolic effects of OCs have been studied for a number of years, reports are scarce in regard to iron status as compared to vitamin nutriture. The most notable effect of OCs is the reduction in menstrual blood loss that occurs in about 60 to 80% of the women who use them. The mode of action of this reduction is known to be due to several different factors. Atrophy of the endometrium is considered the main reason for the reduction in menstrual blood loss induced by OCs. The contraceptive steroids are also known to influence coagulation and fibrinolysis as well as prostaglandin synthesis, which may also contribute to the observed changes in menstrual blood loss during oral contraception.[76,77]

OC users may lose one third to one half the menstrual blood iron of non-OC users.[78,79] Most studies on this subject were performed more than 20 years ago and were carried out in women using combined OCs containing quantities of estrogen and progestogen well in excess of those found in modern OCs now in use. However, a recent study has shown comparable results with a modern low-dose combined OC, containing 30 μg estradiol and 0.15 mg desogestrel.[80] The menstrual blood loss was reduced by approximately 44%. If there is such a marked reduction in menstrual iron excretion, the iron status of women of child-bearing age would be significantly improved. This will be particularly beneficial in the prevention of anemia during pregnancy and for teenagers using OCs. In fact, iron requirements of this target group are not adequately met due to notoriously bad food habits.

The use of steroid contraceptives has been associated with an improved iron status due to the reduction in menstrual loss. In regard to the effect of OCs on hemoglobin content and blood and tissue iron levels, there are conflicting data in the literature.[9,81,82] Walters and Lim[83] performed a longitudinal study which showed that hemoglobin level was reduced significantly during OC use because of a 10% increase in plasma volume. This 10% increase in plasma volume was accompanied by a mean decrease in hemoglobin of 0.3 mg/dl and in hematocrit of 1.2%, which is less than 10%. It is possible that the change in plasma volume could be responsible for masking any benefits that OCs use might entail for iron status.

Both serum iron and total iron binding capacity (TIBC) are elevated in OC users.[9] However, it has been observed that although changes in TIBC or transferrin occur very rapidly after the onset of treatment with contraceptive drugs, this increase is not followed immediately by an increase in serum iron. Thus, the possibility remains that there may be separate mechanisms affecting serum iron levels and iron-binding capacities.[85] The mechanism by which serum transferrin and TIBC levels are raised may be a function of the stimulatory effect of estrogen on the liver biosynthesis of protein.[86] Moreover, little is known about the mechanism(s) controlling fluctuations in serum iron levels, but fever, time of day, and day of the menstrual cycle, as well as iron deficiency, are well-known factors associated with variations in serum iron levels.[87-89]

Serum ferritin is the most reliable single parameter for determination of iron status. Pilon et al.[90] found that for a given individual, serum ferritin varied less from day to day than did serum iron and percent iron saturation. In Frassinelli-Gunderson's study,[91] a comparison of serum ferritin and other parameters of iron status was made between 46 women taking OCs for 2 or more years continuously and 71 women who never took OCs. The mean serum ferritin level for the OC users was significantly higher (p <0.001) than that of the control group. Their serum transferrin and serum iron values were also significantly greater than those of the control nonusers as demonstrated by other investigators.[9,84] Hemoglobin was identical in both groups. The major differences between the study groups were (1) the lesser quantity and shorter duration of menstrual blood loss for OC users, (2) the longer menstrual cycle for the controls, and (3) the higher heme iron content of the OCs users' diet. The heme iron content of the diet was about 0.5 mg/d higher for the OC users, but this alone could not account for the magnitude of the difference in serum ferritin levels, according to the investigators. In effect, since the total iron content of the diet was not significantly different (and this finding was confirmed by our dietetic study[92]), they figured out that the net amount of absorbed iron would be about 0.05 mg higher for the OC users based on the assumption that the absorption of heme iron is about 20%, and for nonheme iron is about 10%. The additional 0.05 mg of iron per day over 3 years would then result in a storage of about 55 mg of iron, which is still well below the estimated 113 mg of additional iron stored by the OC users.[91]

In a cross-sectional study on the effects of long-term (4 years on average) use of OCs, Massé and Roberge[84] found that serum ferritin level of OC users was comparable to that of non-OC users. However, their mean serum iron concentration was significantly (p <0.001) higher. The discrepancy between these two sets of biochemical data might reflect a shift of minerals from one body pool to another as a result of OCs, as postulated by Lei et al.[93] Body iron reserves as assessed by serum ferritin levels were considered to be low in both groups of women. This finding might reflect a lack of highly available iron in the diet. Most of the iron in plant sources is in the less bioavailable nonheme form. To provide a more accurate means of estimating the adequacy of diets with respect to iron metabolism, it has been proposed, in addition, to discriminate the chemical nature of iron ingested (heme and nonheme), to take into consideration the dietary ascorbic acid intake, because this vitamin can enhance the intestinal absorption of nonheme iron.[94,95]

Table 5 summarizes our most recent data on iron status of young women after a short-term use of Triphasil®. It is noteworthy to mention the 1.5-fold increase (although not significant) in the serum ferritin concentration that occurred early after the sixth month of administration. Serum ferritin levels fluctuated very much (as judged by high variance of data) despite the fact the blood sample was withdrawn during the same period of the menstrual cycle for all subjects. Serum ferritin levels were not expected to vary as much as serum iron levels. This study confirmed our previous finding that iron body reserves in women, as assessed by serum ferritin, are borderline independent of the choice of contraception. Mean serum iron level did not increase contrary to our previous study including five different OC preparations taken on a long-term basis.

Mechanisms beyond higher serum ferritin levels in some OC users have not yet been elucidated. More evidence is required, first of all, to substantiate the physiological significance of this metabolic difference between OC users and nonusers, and second, to understand why the ferritin concentration in the OC users decreases to levels which are similar to those of non-users during iron supplementation (ferrous fumarate equivalent to 16 mg).[96] In order to conclude that the higher serum ferritin level actually represents a greater amount of stored iron for OC users, further study is needed to determine whether induction of apoferritin synthesis can be produced by sex steroids independent from iron. If the stimulatory effect of estrogen on ferritin biosynthesis is similar to that for transferrin, then the relationship between serum ferritin and bone marrow stores would be weakened.

VI. IMPACT OF OCs ON NUTRITIONAL REQUIREMENTS

Although the effects of OCs on several metabolic routes have been well documented, little information exists about their impact on nutritional requirements. Since the reduction of serum vitamin B_{12} has been observed within a few months of the administration of OCs and since the possibility does exist that related folate deficiency-induced megaloblastic anemia might result from long-term use, it has been proposed that the requirement for vitamin B_{12} of women on OCs be considered to be the same as those of pregnant women.[97] As previously mentioned, the first factor thought to be the cause of higher serum iron level in women taking OCs is that progestogens cause atrophy of the endometrium and induce a scanty withdrawal bleeding which is less than in a normal cycle. This is the reason why the nutritional iron requirement of women, in other words, their dietary need for iron, might be lowered while receiving OC treatment.[6,97] This contention is supported by the observation that steroid contraceptives not only decrease the menstrual blood loss, but also increases iron absorption from the gut.[82]

More than 60 research articles have dealt with the effects of OC use on pyridoxine status. This considerable interest was triggered by reports in the 1960s that women using oral contraception exhibited abnormal tryptophan metabolism, which was corrected by a vitamin B_6 supplement. If urinary XA excretion is used as the sole criterion, one might conclude that a significant proportion of OC users require additional vitamin B_6 beyond that which they normally consume. However, nutritionists universally agree with the conclusion that this tryptophan metabolite is not a good indicator of vitamin B_6 status. A more direct and accurate biochemical indicator, plasma PLP level, suggests that a significant number of OC users do not require additional dietary pyridoxine.[23] Moreover, the results of depletion and repletion studies based on a diversity of parameters are not in favor of an increased requirement during oral contraception.[16,42,98,99] Donald and Bossé[99] concluded that the requirement for this vitamin, in the majority of cases, was close to that for women not using oral contraception. According to the American Academy of Sciences, there is no evidence to support a greater dietary allowance for OC users based on the fact that their plasma PLP levels are not deficient and therefore their vitamin B_6 status does not appear to be compromised.[100]

However, there are several observations justifying the concern for an adequate requirement for vitamin B_6 during oral contraception. One is that lower (about 10 to 20%) plasma PLP levels have consistently (although not statistically significant) been observed in some OC users. Second, the level of PLP in whole blood was found to be lowered significantly[55,101] and erythrocyte PLP concentration as well, but slightly.[98] The latter biochemical parameter is a very good indicator of tissue metabolism, but unfortunately is not usually used for assessing vitamin B_6 status. Third, a B_6-dependent enzyme such as alanine aminotransferase (commonly known as GPT transaminase), considered to have a relatively constant activity as opposed to aspartate aminotransferase which can be influenced directly by sex steroids, can be *in vitro* stimulated with PLP. This is an excellent method to confirm a metabolic lack of vitamin B_6 as already discussed in a previous section. Finally, the effect of long-term use of OCs on the vitamin B_6 status of pregnant and lactating women is a real concern to nutritionists. According to a report by Roepke and Kirksey,[102] these women may be at risk of developing vitamin B_6 deficiency after a long-term use of OCs. These investigators suggested that long-term use of OCs before conception reduces the reserves of vitamin B_6, compounding the effects of hormonal changes that affect vitamin B_6 in normal pregnancy. According to Miller,[103] vitamin B_6 status should be monitored and evaluated in women using OCs, especially those who are postponing pregnancy and intending to breast-feed their infants. Reynolds et al.[104] revealed that the vitamin B_6 intakes of upper-income-class pregnant and lactating women were only half of the recommended dietary allowances.

A. PERTINENCE OF ORAL SUPPLEMENTATION

The elevation of iron body stores by OC use entails health considerations. Supplementation with iron might impose a risk of iron overload for some OC users. Any proposal for further enrichment of food with iron needs to be reassessed in light of the recent study having shown a 3.5 times greater risk of myocardial infarction for past OC users (depending on the duration of its use).[105] Vitamin A levels can also be increased during oral contraception.[6,8,54] Caution is needed regarding daily supplementation of this vitamin, especially periconceptionally, to avoid toxic or teratogenic levels; supplementation of 1000 IU of vitamin A does not approach these levels.

Folic acid deficiency may not necessarily be the cause of megaloblastic anemia if it is present in OC users. Certain underlying disorders in absorption and metabolism may be the principal factors involved. Other factors can be also related to megaloblastic anemia, such as insufficient diet, alcoholism, and disease. Folic acid supplementation is advisable for high-risk groups, such as women who become pregnant within 6 months after the interruption of OC utilization and women with increased folate needs caused by repeated pregnancies, malnutrition, iron deficiency, malnutrition, or anticonvulsant use. It is well known that pregnancy increases the metabolic demand for this vitamin.[3] Women living in marginal economic conditions and teenagers having poor food habits and taking "the pill" need a folic acid supplement. Martinez and Roe[106] suggest a daily dose varying between 50 µg and 1 mg.

High dose (10 mg folic acid tablet) has been tested to reduce the progression of dysplasia and to help to reduce the risk of cervical cancer in women taking OCs. At present, there is no epidemiologic evidence that OCs increase the risk of this form of cancer in the population as a whole. Butterworth et al.[107] measured red blood cell folate concentration and assigned biopsy scores to 47 cervical dysplasia patients and controls. Initially, folate concentrations were lower in OC users than nonusers, and lowest in users with dysplasia. After a double-blind, 3-month placebo-controlled trial, using 10 mg folic acid, treated subjects had significantly better biopsy scores than controls. A summary of early reports concluded that approximately one fifth of OC users had megaloblastic changes in the cervicovaginal epithelium that were completely reversed by folic acid supplementation.[108] A striking finding is that these changes were found even in women with normal serum folate levels.

Lower cobalamin concentrations in OC users are seen both in populations with adequate and inadequate nutritional conditions. According to Hjelt et al.,[63] absorption and excretion of this vitamin in OC users are not different from other women. No sign of pernicious anemia has ever been associated with OCs. According to Mooij et al.,[54] multivitamin supplementation did not change the vitamin B_{12} concentration, suggesting that the lower vitamin B_{12} in OC users does not reflect a situation of higher vitamin B_{12} demand. However, such a situation can prevail during pregnancy, usually due to an underlying condition.[105] Briggs and Briggs[109] reported that the low serum vitamin B_{12} levels of pregnant women could be corrected with a supplementary multivitamin preparation that provided 5 mg of pyridoxine and 4 µg of vitamin B_{12} a day. It was not clear whether the correction was due to the pyridoxine or the vitamin B_{12} supplementation.

Significant improvements in B_6 status occur when pyridoxine hydrochloride is administered, usually at dose levels of 20 to 40 mg daily.[10] Several years ago, Rose and Adams[110] showed that the administration of supplementary (10 mg pyridoxine hydrochloride) vitamin B_6 could restore tryptophan metabolism to normal when a relatively high dose of estrogen (50 µg ethinyl estradiol or more) was used. Improvement in the metabolic response of subjects to OCs containing a relatively low dose (30 µg ethinyl estradiol) has also been reported.[7]

Winston[111] made the first attempt to treat OC-induced depression with a vitamin B_6 supplement. In 1969, he reported beneficial effect with a 50 mg dose, administered daily. Subsequently, Baumblatt and Winston[112] observed that the administration of vitamin B_6 supplement to 58 women taking OCs, complaining of premenstrual depression, relieved the symptoms in 18 and caused an improvement in a further 26. According to these studies, vitamin B_6 therapy seemed to be successful in alleviating the symptoms of depression, although they have been criticized for not being well controlled.

In our nutritional intervention study,[33] OC users (n = 34) and control nonusers (n = 33) were given a 100-mg vitamin B_6 supplement during a complete menstrual cycle. Blood samples were taken and a psychometric test (MMPI) (refer to previous Section IV.A.1.a for definition) was administered twice, prior to and after the experimental period, at the same period of the menstrual cycle for all the subjects. Significant positive changes were observed for half of the ten clinical scales as depicted in Figure 2. According to lie (L) and false (F) scales, subjects in both groups coped similarly with the psychometric test prior to and after the experimental period. At baseline, the two groups were comparable, except for the social introversion scale (Si). Incidently, women taking OCs performed better in this respect than control subjects ($p < 0.02$). Their scores on hypochondria (Hs) and psychastenia (Pt) scales were lower and the score relative to paranoia (Pa) scale was higher. None of these scores showed significant differences between the two groups prior to B_6 supplementation. However, they changed significantly at the end of the experimental period.

Few investigators reported on advantages of OCs other than their well-recognized contraceptive action. This aforementioned study presented OC users as being more social and less introspective than women using another method of contraception. This finding is confirmed by a higher T score on the correction (K) scale. Besides being used as a correction factor, this scale has its own clinical significance. A moderate elevation of the score on this scale can be observed in social, dynamic, and enthusiastic persons.[113] The baseline significant difference on Si scale between the two groups disappeared after the B_6 supplementation. The psychoaffective improvement observed in control nonusers was also detectable on their K scale as judged by the slight increase of the T score. Whereas the mean T score on the depression (D) scale was not modified by the B_6 supplement, it improved significantly in subjects having a baseline T score equal or superior to 60 whatever the groups. Plasma PLP levels in both groups were three-fold increased by the end of the supplementation period. No case of deficient or marginal values was reported in this study. In the group of depressed women studied by Adams et al.[114] only those having absolute vitamin B_6 deficiency responded to the administration of pyridoxine supplement.

Our positive psychological response to a 100-mg supplemental dose of vitamin B_6 may be attributed to the stimulating dopaminergic activity of pyridoxine in the central nervous system as has been demonstrated by pharmacological studies on humans and animals.[115-117] In effect, this vitamin is a coenzyme in the decarboxylation reaction that converts dopa to dopamine. Our results suggest a role for the vitamin B_6 supplement as a psychostimulant agent. However, replication of studies at different research centers with larger numbers of subjects is desirable.

VII. CONCLUSIONS

The nutritional status of a woman reflects her dietary habits which are influenced by several factors and life styles, including consumption of "the pill." Although a dietetic study revealed that OC users and nonusers have comparable nutrient intakes,[92] numerous biochemical studies have clearly demonstrated that the use of OCs was associated with decreased or increased plasma levels of some vitamins and minerals. OC users represent a selected group at risk of poor vitamin status in the U.S. population.[118] As an example, the percent of population having an inadequate vitamin B_6 and folate status is estimated to be 10.4. In view of the role of these vitamins in the growth and functioning of the central nervous system, adequate nutritional status of all pregnant and lactating women, in general, and those who use OCs before conception, in particular, should be of concern.

While the absence of obvious malnutrition is considered to represent good nutrition, the importance of preventing functional metabolic disturbances that can evolve into overt clinical symptoms has been recognized.[119] This is the reason it is recommended that women be encouraged to adopt good dietary habits during oral contraception. Table 6 summarizes the best dietary sources of nutrients to favor during oral contraception in order to minimize the risks of nutritional deficiencies. Recommended dietary allowances (RDAs) of the U.S. National Research Council are also indicated.[100] There is little or no need for nutritive supplements for OC users who have an adequate diet. Vitamin and mineral supplementation are indicated only if deficiency symptoms become apparent and cannot be corrected through dietary adjustments. At present, supplements are advised only for high-risk groups where other factors, such as diet, pregnancy, and disease, could increase the chances for a deficiency to develop. More research is needed to determine which groups of women may need supplements and in what amounts.

TABLE 6
Major Dietary Sources of Vitamins and Minerals
Recommended During Oral Contraception

U.S. RDA[a]

Vitamin A and carotenes	1000 μg RE[b]	Milk, butter, fortified margarine, liver, eggs, leafy green and yellow vegetables (e.g., carrots)
Thiamin	1.5 mg	Enriched bread and cereals, liver, peas and lima beans, leafy green vegetables
Riboflavin	1.7 mg	Eggs, liver, lean meats, enriched bread and cereals, leafy green vegetables, milk
Vitamin B_6 (includes pyridoxine, pyridoxamine, and pyridoxal)	2 mg	Liver, meats, fish, eggs, whole grain cereals, green leafy and yellow vegetables, bananas, grapes, pears
Vitamin B_{12}	6 μg	Liver, other meats, clams, sardines, salmon, oysters, herring, other fish, cheeses, milk, eggs
Ascorbic acid[c]	60 mg	Lemons, oranges, grapefruit, tangerines, strawberries, cantaloupe, citrus fruit juices, canned fruit beverages fortified with vitamin C, sweet peppers, broccoli, brussels sprouts, cabbage, turnip greens, collards, cauliflower, spinach, collard greens, kale, tomatoes, onions
Folate[c]	400 μg	Liver (beef, calf, lamb, pork, chicken), asparagus, spinach, lettuce, onions, brussels sprouts, cauliflower, broccoli, cabbage, peas, beans, nuts, orange juice, berries
Zinc	15 mg	Liver, other animal protein foods
Calcium	1000 mg	Milk, buttermilk, ice cream and ice milk, cheese, cottage cheese
Magnesium	400 mg	Dried beans and peas, soybeans, nuts

[a] *U.S. Recommended Daily Allowances,* National Academy of Sciences, National Academy Press, Washington, D.C., 1989.

[b] Retinol equivalents.

[c] Major losses occur due to storage or cooking.

REFERENCES

1. De Cecco, L., Capitanio, G., Venturini, P., Tuo, F., Marketti, L., and Gherardi, S., The efficiency of triphasic oral contraceptives and effects on the pituitary-ovarian axis in younger women compared with other types of oral contraceptives, in *New Considerations in Oral Contraception*, Brosens, I., Ed., Biomedical Information Corporation Publications, New York, 1982, 191.

2. De Lia, J. E. and Emery, M. G., Clinical pharmacology and common minor side effects of oral contraceptives, in *Clinical Obstetrics and Gynecology — Update on Oral Contraception*, Beck, W. W., Ed., Harper & Row, Scranton, PA, 1981, 879.

3. Bamji, M. S., Laboratory tests for the assessment of vitamin nutritional status, in *Vitamins in Human Biology and Medicine*, Briggs, M. H., Ed., CRC Press, Boca Raton, FL, 1981,

4. Sauberlich, H. E., Scala, J. H., and Dody, R. P., *Laboratory Tests for the Assessment of Nutritional Status*, CRC Press, Boca Raton, FL, 1974.

5. Worthington, B. S., Nutrition during pregnancy, lactation, and oral contraception, *Nurs. Clin. North Am.*, 14, 269, 1979.

6. Webb, J. L., Nutritional effects of oral contraceptive use. A review, *J. Reprod. Med.*, 25, 150, 1980.

7. Prema, K., Ramalakshmi, B. A., and Babu, S., Serum copper and zinc in hormonal contraceptive users, *Fertil. Steril.*, 33, 267, 1980.

8. Thorp, V. J., Effect of oral contraceptive agents on vitamin and mineral requirements, *J. Am. Diet. Assoc.*, 76, 581, 1980.

9. Prasad, A. S., Oberleas, D., Lei, K. Y., Moghissi, K. S., and Stryker, J. C., Effect of oral contraceptive agents on nutrients. I. Minerals, *Am. J. Clin. Nutr.*, 28, 377, 1975.

10. Tonkin, S. Y., Oral contraceptives and vitamin status, in *Vitamins in Human Biology and Medicine*, Briggs, M. H., Ed., CRC Press, Boca Raton, FL, 1981, 29.

11. Tyrer, L. B., Nutrition and the pill, *J. Reprod. Med.*, 29, 547, 1984.

12. Rose, D. P., Excretion of xanthurenic acid in the urine of women taking progestogen-oestrogen preparations, *Nature*, 210, 196, 1966.

13. Tonkin, S. Y., Oral contraceptives and vitamin status, in *Vitamins in Human Biology and Medicine*, Briggs, M. H., Ed., CRC Press, Boca Raton, FL, 1981, 29.

14. Faisy, A. and Mahtab, B. S., Vitamin supplements to women using oral contraceptives, *Contraception*, 14, 309, 1976.

15. Faisy, A., Bamji, M. S., and Iyengar, L., Effect of oral contraceptive agents on vitamin nutrition status, *Am. J. Clin. Nutr.*, 28, 606, 1975.

16. Leklem, J. E., Brown, R. R., Rose, D. P., Linkswiler, H. M., and Arend, R. A., Metabolism of tryptophan and niacin in oral contraceptive users receiving controlled intakes of vitamin B_6, *Am. J. Clin. Nutr.*, 28, 146, 1975.

17. Rose, D. P., The influence of oestrogens on tryptophan metabolism in man, *Clin. Sci.*, 31, 265, 1966.

18. Leonard, B. E. and Hamburger, A. D., Sex hormones, tryptophan oxygenase activity and cerebral monoamine metabolism in the rat, *Biochem. Soc. Trans.*, 2, 1351, 1974.

19. Manning, B. D. and Mason, M., Kynurenine metabolism in rats: some hormonal factors affecting enzyme activities, *Life Sci.*, 17, 225, 1975.

20. Kanke, Y., Suzuki, K., Hirakawa, S., and Goto, S., Oral contraceptive steroids: effects on iron and zinc levels and on tryptophan pyrrolase and alkaline phosphatase activities in tissues of iron-deficient anemic rats, *Am. J. Clin. Nutr.*, 33, 1244, 1980.

21. Green, A. R., Bloomfield, M. R., Woods, H. F., and Seed, M., Metabolism of oral tryptophan load by women and evidence against the induction of tryptophan pyrrolase by oral contraceptives, *Br. J. Clin. Pharmacol.*, 5, 233, 1978.

22. Bender, D. A., Tagoe, C. E., and Vale, J. A., Effects of oestrogen administration on vitamin B_6 and tryptophan metabolism in the rat, *Br. J. Nutr.*, 47, 609, 1982.

23. Lumeng, L., Cleary, R. E., and Li, T.K., Effect of oral contraceptives on the plasma concentration of pyridoxal phosphate, *Am. J. Clin. Nutr.*, 27, 326, 1974.

24. Leklem, J. E., Vitamin B_6 requirement and oral contraceptive use — a concern?, *J. Nutr.*, 116, 475, 1986.

25. Herzberg, B. N., Johnson, A. L., and Brown, S., Depressive symptoms and oral contraceptives, *Br. J. Med.*, 4, 142, 1970.

26. Rose, D. P. and Braidman, I. P., Excretion of tryptophan metabolites as affected by pregnancy, contraceptive steroids, and steroids, *Am. J. Clin. Nutr.*, 24, 673, 1971.

27. Shaaraway, M., Fayard, M., Nagui, A.R., and Azim, S. A., Serotonin metabolism and depression in oral contraceptive users, *Contraception*, 26, 193, 1982.

28. Chang, A. M. Z., Chick, P., and Milburn, S., Mood changes as reported by women taking the oral contraceptive pill, *Aust. N. Z. Obstet. Gynaecol.*, 22, 78, 1982.

29. Patten, S. B. and Lamarre, C. J., Can drug-induced depression be identified by their clinical features?, *Can. J. Psychiatry,* 37, 213, 1992.

30. Herzberg, B. and Copper, A., Changes in psychological symptoms in women taking oral contraceptives, *Br. J. Psychiatry*, 116, 161, 1970.

31. Malek-Ahmadi, P. and Behrmann, P. J., Depressive syndrome induced by oral contraceptives, *Dis. Nerv. Sys.*, 37, 406, 1976.

32. Kutner, S. J. and Brown, W. L., Types of oral contraceptives, depression and pre-menstrual symptoms, *J. Nerv. Ment. Dis.*, 155, 153, 1972.

33. Massé, P. G., and Roberge, A. G., The psychoaffective profile of women taking oral contraceptives in relation to vitamin B_6 status, in *Current Topics in Nutrition and Disease: Clinical and Physiological Applications of Vitamin B_6, — Vol. 19, Proc. Third Int. Conf. on Vitamin B_6*, Reynolds, R. D. and Leklem, J. E., Eds., Alan R. Liss, New York, 1988, 381.

34. Joshi, U. M., Lahiri, A., Kora, S., Dikshit, S. S., and Virkar, K., Short-term effect of Ovral and Norgestrel on the vitamin B_6 and B_1 status of women, *Contraception*, 12, 425, 1975.

35. Miller, L. T., Dow, M. J., and Kokkeler, S. C., Methionine metabolism and vitamin B_6 status in women using oral contraceptives, *Am. J. Clin. Nutr.*, 31, 619, 1978.

36. Driskell, J. A., Geders, J. M., and Urban, M. C., Vitamin B_6 status of young men, women, and women using oral contraceptives, *J. Lab. Clin. Med.*, 87, 813, 1976.

37. Kishi, H., Kishi, T., Williams, R. H., Watanabe, T., Folkers, K., and Stahl, M. L., Deficiency of vitamin B_6 in women taking contraceptive formulations, *Res. Commun. Chem. Pathol. Pharmacol.*, 17, 283, 1977.

38. Prasad, A. S., Lei, K. Y., Oberleas, D., Moghissi, K. S., and Stryker, J. C., Effect of oral contraceptive agents on nutrients. II. Vitamins, *Am. J. Clin. Nutr.*, 28, 385, 1975.

39. van der Vange, N., van den Berg, H., Kloosterboer, H. J., and Haspels, A. A., Effects of seven low-dose combined contraceptives on vitamin B_6 status, *Contraception*, 40, 377, 1989.

40. Miller, L. T., Benson, E. M., Edwards, M. A., and Young, J., Vitamin B_6 metabolism in women using oral contraceptives, *Am. J. Clin. Nutr.*, 27, 797, 1974.

41. Shane, B. and Contractor, S. F., Assessment of vitamin B_6 status. Studies on pregnant women and oral contraceptive users, *Am. J. Clin. Nutr.*, 28, 739, 1975.

42. Brown, R. R., Rose, D. P., Leklem, J. E., Linkswiler, H., and Anand, R., Urinary 4-pyridoxic acid and plasma pyridoxal phosphate, and erythrocyte aminotransferase levels in oral contraceptive users receiving controlled intakes of vitamin B_6, *Am. J. Clin. Nutr.*, 28, 385, 1975.

43. Leklem, J. E., Brown, R. R., Rose, D. P., and Linkswiler, H. M., Vitamin B_6 requirements of women using oral contraceptives, *Am. J. Clin. Nutr.*, 28, 535, 1975.

44. Luhby, A. L., Brin, M., Gordon, M., Davis, P., Murphy, M., and Spiegel, H., Vitamin B_6 metabolism in users of oral contraceptive agents. I. Abnormal urinary xanthurenic acid excretion and its correction by pyridoxine, *Am. J. Clin. Nutr.*, 24, 684, 1971.

45. Shojania, A. M., Oral contraceptives: effects on folate and vitamin B_{12} metabolism, *Can. Med. Assoc. J.*, 126, 244, 1982.

46. Prasad, A. S., Lei, K. Y., Moghissi, K. S., Stryker, J. C., and Oberleas, D., Effect of oral contraceptives on nutrient. III. Vitamins B_6, B_{12} and folic acid, *Am. J. Obstet. Gynecol.*, 125, 1063, 1976.

47. Pietarinen, G. J., Leichter, J., and Pratt, R. F., Dietary folate intake and concentration of folate in serum and erythrocytes in women using oral contraceptives, *Am. J. Clin. Nutr.*, 30, 375, 1977.

48. Paine, C. J., Crafton, W. D., Dickson, V. L., and Eichner, E. R., Oral contraceptives, serum folate and hematological status, *J.A.M.A.*, 231, 731, 1975.

49. Ross, C. E., Stone, M. K., Reagan, J. W., Wentz, W. B., and Kellermeyer, R. W., Lack of influence of oral contraceptives on serum folate, hematologic values, and cervical cytology, *Semin. Hematol.*, 13, 233, 1976.

50. Karlin, R., Dumont, M., and Long, B., Etude des taux sanguins d'acide folique au cours des traitements oestroprogestatifs, *J. Gynecol. Obstet. Biol. Reprod. (Paris)*, 6, 489, 1977.

51. Shojania, A. M., The effect of oral contraceptives on folate metabolism, *Am. J. Obstet. Gynecol.*, 111, 782, 1971.

52. Areekul, S., Panatampon, P., Doungbarn, J., Yamarat, P., and Vongyuthithum, M., Serum vitamin B_{12}, serum and red cell folic acid binding proteins in women taking oral contraceptives, *Southeast Asian J. Trop. Med. Public Health*, 8, 480, 1977.

53. Ahmed, F., Bamji, M. S., and Iyengar, L., Effect of oral contraceptive agents on vitamin nutrition status, *Am. J. Clin. Nutr.*, 28, 606, 1975.

54. Mooij, P. N. M., Thomas, C. M. G., Doesburg, W. H., and Eskes, T. K., Multivitamin supplementation in oral contraceptive users, *Contraception*, 44, 277, 1991.

55. Steegers-Theunissen, R. P. M., Boers, G. H. J., Steegers, E. A. P., Trijbels, F. J. M., Thomas, C. M. G., and Eskes, T. K., Effects of sub-50 oral contraceptives on homocysteine metabolism: a preliminary study, *Contraception*, 45, 129, 1992.

56. Courtney, M. G., McPartlin, J. M., McNulty, H. M., Scott, J. M., and Weir, D. G., The cause of folate deficiency in pregnancy is increased catabolism of the vitamin, *Gastroenterology*, 92, 1355, 1987.

57. Streiff, R. R., Folate deficiency and oral contraceptives, *J.A.M.A.*, 214, 105, 1970.

58. Stephens, M. E. M., Craft, I., Peters, T. J., and Hoffbrand, A. V., Oral contraceptives and folate metabolism, *Clin. Sci.*, 42, 405, 1972.

59. Fleming, A. F., Urinary excretion of folate in pregnancy, *J. Obstet. Gynecol. Br. Commonw.*, 79, 916, 1972.

60. Shojania, A. M., and Wylie, B., The effect of oral contraceptives on vitamin B_{12} metabolism, *Am. J. Obstet. Gynecol.*, 135, 129, 1979.

61. Wertalik, L. F., Metz, E. N., LoBuglio, A. F., and Balcerzak, S. P., Decreased serum B_{12} levels with oral contraceptive use, *J.A.M.A.*, 221, 1371, 1972.

62. Costanzi, J. J., Young, B. K., and Carmel, R., Serum vitamin B_{12} and B_{12}-binding protein levels associated with oral contraceptives, *Tex. Rep. Biol. Med.*, 36, 69, 1978.

63. Hjelt, K., Brynskov, J., Hippe, E., Lundström, P., and Munck, O., Oral contraceptives and the cobalamin (vitamin B_{12}) metabolism, *Acta Obstet. Gynecol. Scand.*, 64, 59, 1985.

64. Larsson-Cohn, U., Oral contraceptives and vitamins: a review, *Am. J. Obstet. Gynecol.*, 121, 84, 1975.

65. Kornberg, A., Segal, R., Theitler, J., Yona, R., and Kaufman, S., Folic acid deficiency, megaloblastic anemia and peripheral polyneuropathy due to oral contraceptives, *Isr. J. Med. Sci.*, 25, 142, 1989.

66. Boots, L., Cornwell, P. E., and Beck, L. R., Effect of ethynodiol diacetate and mestranol on serum folic acid and vitamin B_{12} levels and tryptophan metabolism in baboons, *Am. J. Clin. Nutr.*, 28, 354, 1975.

67. Stabler, S. P., Marcell, P. D., Podell, E. R., Allen, R. H., Savage, D. G., and Lindenbaum, J., Elevation of total homocysteine in the serum of patients with cobalamin or folate deficiency detected by a capillary gas chromotography mass spectrometry, *J. Clin. Invest.*, 81, 466, 1988.

68. Brattström, L. E., Israelsson, B., Lindgärde, F., and Hultberg, B., Higher total plasma homocysteine in vitamin B_{12} deficiency than in heterozygosity for homocystinuria due to cystathionine β-synthase deficiency, *Metabolism*, 37, 175, 1988.
69. Böttiger, L. E., Boman, G., Eklund, G., and Westerholm, B., Oral contraceptives and thromboembolic disease: effects of lowering estrogen content, *Lancet*, 1, 1097, 1980.
70. Maguire, M. G., Tonascia, J., Sartwell, P. E., Stolley, P. D., and Tockman, M. S., Increased risk of thrombosis due to oral contraceptives: a further report, *Am. J. Epidemiol.*, 110, 188, 1979.
71. Mishell, D. R., Contraception, *N. Engl. J. Med.*, 320, 777, 1989.
72. Vessey, M. P., Oral contraceptives and cardiovascular disease: some questions and answers, *Br. Med. J.*, 284, 615, 1982.
73. Smolin, L. A. and Benevenga, N. J., Factors affecting the accumulation of homocysteine in rats deficient in vitamin B_6, *J. Nutr.*, 114, 103, 1984.
74. Kritz-Silverstein, D. and Barrett-Connor, E., Bone mineral density in postmenopausal women as determined by prior oral contraceptive use, *Am. J. Public Health*, 83, 100, 1993.
75. Cooper, C., Hannaford, P., Croft, P., and Kay, C. R., Oral contraceptive pill use and fractures in women: a prospective study, *Bone*, 14, 41, 1993.
76. Siegban, A. and Ruusuvaara, L., Age dependence of blood fibrinolytic components and the effects of low-dose contraceptives on coagulation and fibrinolysis in teenagers, *Thromb. Haemostas.*, 60, 361, 1988.
77. Lundström, V. and Gréen, K., Endogenous levels of prostaglandin F_2 and its metabolites in plasma and endometrium of normal and dysmenorrheic women, *Am. J. Obstet. Gynecol.*, 130, 640, 1978.
78. Thein, M., Beaton, G. H., Milne, H., and Veen, M. J., Oral contraceptive drugs: some observations on their effect on menstrual loss and hematological indices, *Can. Med. Assoc. J.*, 101, 73, 1969.
79. Newton, J., Barnard, G., and Collins, W., A rapid method for measuring menstrual blood loss using automatic extraction, *Contraception*, 16, 269, 1977.
80. Larsson, G., Milsom, I., Lindstedt, G., and Rybo, G., The influence of a low-dose combined oral contraceptive on menstrual blood loss and iron status, *Contraception*, 46, 327, 1992.
81. Briggs, M. H. and Briggs, M., Effects of steroid pharmaceuticals on plasma zinc, *Nature*, 232, 480, 1971.
82. Margen, S. and King, J. C., Effect of oral contraceptive agents on the metabolism of some trace minerals, *Am. J. Clin. Nutr.*, 28, 392, 1975.
83. Walters, W. A. W. and Lim, Y. L., Haemodynamic changes in women taking oral contraceptives, *J. Obstet. Gynaecol. Br. Commonw.*, 77, 1007, 1970.
84. Massé, P. G. and Roberge, A. G., Long-term effect of low-dose combined steroid contraceptives on body iron status, *Contraception*, 46, 243, 1992.
85. Zilva, J. F., Oral contraceptives and serum proteins, *Br. Med. J.*, 3, 521, 1970.
86. Mcknight, G. S., Lee, D. C., and Palmiter, R. D., Transferrin gene expression. Regulation of mRNA transcription in chick liver by steroid hormones and iron deficiency, *J. Biol. Chem.*, 255, 148, 1980.
87. Elin, R. J., Wolff, S. M., and Finch, C. A., Effect of induced fever on serum iron and ferritin concentrations in man, *Blood*, 49, 147, 1977.
88. Mardell, M. and Zilva, J. F., Effect of oral contraceptives on the variations in serum-iron during the menstrual cycle, *Lancet*, 2, 1325, 1967.
89. Cook, J. D., Finch, C. A., and Smith, N. J., Evaluation of the iron status of a population, *Blood*, 48, 449, 1976.
90. Pilon, V. A., Howanitz, P. J., Howanitz, J. H., and Domres, N., Day-to-day variation in serum ferritin concentration in healthy subjects, *Clin. Chem.*, 27, 78, 1981.
91. Frassinelli-Gunderson, E. P., Margen, S., and Brown, J. R., Iron stores in users of oral contraceptive agents, *Am. J. Clin. Nutr.*, 41, 703, 1985.
92. Massé, P. G., Nutrient intakes of women who use oral contraceptives, *J. Am. Diet. Assoc.*, 91, 1118, 1991.

93. Lei, K. J., Prasad, A. S., Bowersox, E., and Oberleas, D., Oral contraceptives, norethindrone and mestranol: effects on tissue levels of minerals, *Am. J. Physiol.*, 231, 98, 1976.

94. Monsen, E. R., Halberg, L., Larysse, M., Hegsted, D. M., Cook, J. D., Mertz, W., and Finch, C. A., Estimation of available dietary iron, *Am. J. Clin. Nutr.*, 31, 134, 1978.

95. Henderson-Sabry, J. and Grief, H., Calculated available iron, heme iron and non-heme iron in diets of a group of men, *J. Can. Diet. Assoc.*, 43, 132, 1982.

96. Mooij, P. N. M., Thomas, C. M. G., Doesburg, W. H., and Eskes, T. K. A. B., The effects of oral contraceptives and multivitamin supplementation on serum ferritin and hematological parameters, *Int. J. Clin. Pharmacol. Ther. Toxicol.*, 30, 57, 1992.

97. Theur, R. C., Effect of oral contraceptive agents on vitamin and mineral needs: a review, *J. Reprod. Med.*, 8, 13, 1972.

98. Bossé, T. R. and Donald, E. A., The vitamin B_6 requirement in oral contraceptive users. I. Assessment by pyridoxal level and transferase activity in erythrocytes, *Am. J. Clin. Nutr.*, 32, 1015, 1979.

99. Donald, E. A. and Bossé, T. R., The vitamin B_6 requirement in oral contraceptive users, *Am. J. Clin. Nutr.*, 32, 1023, 1979.

100. Food and Nutrition Board, *Recommended Dietary Allowances*, 10th ed., National Academy of Sciences, Washington, D. C., 1989.

101. Amatayakul, K., Uttaravichai, L., Singkamani, R., and Ruckphapunt, S., Vitamin metabolism and the effects of multivitamin supplementation in oral contraceptive users, *Contraception*, 30, 179, 1984.

102. Roepke, J. L. B. and Kirksey, A., Vitamin B_6 nutriture during pregnancy and lactation. II. The effect of long-term use of oral contraceptives, *Am. J. Clin. Nutr.*, 32, 2257, 1979.

103. Miller, L. T., Do oral contraceptive agents affect nutrient requirements — vitamin B_6?, *J. Nutr.*, 116, 1344, 1986.

104. Reynolds, R. D., Polansky, M., and Moser, P. B., Analysed vitamin B_6 intakes of pregnant and postpartum lactating and nonlactating women, *J. Am. Diet. Assoc.*, 84, 1339, 1984.

105. Slone, D., Shapiro, S., Kaufman, D., Rosenberg, L., Miettinen, O. S., and Stolley, P. D., Risk of myocardial infarction in relation to current and discontinued use of oral contraceptives, *N. Engl. J. Med.*, 305, 420, 1981.

106. Martinez, O. and Roe, D. A., Effect of oral contraceptives on blood folate levels in pregnancy, *Am. J. Obstet. Gynecol.*, 128, 255, 1977.

107. Butterworth, C. E., Hatch, K. D., Gore, H., Mueller, H., and Krumdieck, C. L., Improvement in cervical dysplasia associated with folic acid therapy in users of oral contraceptives, *Am. J. Clin. Nutr.*, 35, 73, 1982.

108. Lindenbaum, J., Whitehead, N., and Reyner, F., Oral contraceptive hormones, folate metabolism, and the cervical epithelium, *Am. J. Clin. Nutr.*, 28, 346, 1975.

109. Briggs, M. and Briggs, M., Changes in biochemical indices of vitamin nutrition in women using oral contraceptives during treatment with "Surbex 500", *Curr. Med. Res. Opin.*, 2, 626, 1974–75.

110. Rose, D. P. and Adams, P. W., Oral contraceptives and tryptophan metabolism: effect of estrogen with a low progestogen and a low progestogen (megesterol acetate) given alone, *J. Clin. Pathol.*, 25, 252, 1972.

111. Winston, F., Oral contraceptives, pyridoxine and depression, *Am. J. Psychiatry*, 130, 1217, 1973.

112. Baumblatt, M. J. and Winston, F., Pyridoxine and the pill, *Lancet*, 2, 832, 1970.

113. Gilberstadt, H. and Duker, J., *Handbook for Clinical and Actuarial MMPI Interpretation*, W. B. Saunders, New York, 1982.

114. Adams, P. W., Rose, D. P., Folkard, J., Wynn, V., Seed, M., and Strong, R., Effect of pyridoxine hydrochloride (vitamin B_6) upon depression associated with oral contraception, *Lancet*, 28, 897, 1973.

115. LeChat, P. G., Streichenberger, G., Boismare, F., and Letteron, N., Modification par la pyridoxine des propriétés pharmacologiques antiparkinsoniennes de la L-Dopa, *J. Pharmacol.*, 28, 479, 1977.

116. Roberge, A. G., Differentiation in brain and liver DOPA/5-HTP decarboxylase activity after L-DOPA administration with or without pyridoxine in cats, *J. Neurochem.*, 28, 479, 1977.

117. Cassachia, M., Boni, B., and Meco, G., Pyridoxine and depression: neuroendocrine aspects, *Acta Vitaminol. Enzymol.*, 4, 55, 1982.

118. Gaby, S. K., Bendich, A., Singh, V. N., and Machlin, L. J., *Vitamin Intake and Health: A Scientific Review*, Marcel Dekker, New York, 1991, 7.

119. Pietrzik, K., Concept of borderline vitamin deficiencies, *Int. J. Vitam. Nutr. Res. Suppl.*, 27, 61, 1985.

Chapter 11

NUTRITIONAL FACTORS IN WOMEN'S CANCERS: BREAST, CERVICAL, ENDOMETRIAL, AND OVARIAN

Barbara C. Pence

CONTENTS

0-8493-8502-4/96/$0.00+$.50
© 1996 by CRC Press, Inc.

I. INTRODUCTION

Many investigators have examined the impact of diet and nutrition on both total cancer incidence and mortality. These results are based on evaluating the relationship between dietary factors and the observed cancer risk, migrant studies in which there are definite shifts in site-specific cancer rates among those peoples migrating to the U.S., supportive evidence from animal studies, as well as the biological relevance of diet to a particular type of cancer.[1] In 1981 Doll and Peto[2] estimated that 35% of all cancer mortality in the United States was related to diet, and previously, Wynder and Gori[3] estimated that nearly 40% of cancers among women are related to diet. Although it is not possible to quantify the contribution of diet to cancer risk for a particular site, it is sufficient to say that, excluding colon cancer which is not specific to women, there appears to be a significant role for diet and nutrition in the etiology of women's cancers. In this chapter the role of nutrition in the potential causation of those cancers specific to women will be discussed, by site (breast, cervical, endometrial, and ovarian) and by nutrient class.

II. BREAST CANCER

Breast cancer is the second most common cause of cancer mortality in U.S. women. It is second only to lung cancer, which obviously is not a nutritionally related cancer. Cancer at this site is associated with hormonal activity, but diet has long been suspected as a major cause.[4] Many descriptive epidemiologic studies of migrants have demonstrated an association between life-style factors and risk for breast cancer. Diet has been implicated extensively in the etiology of this disease, especially dietary fat, but results are inconclusive to date and have been the subject of much controversy in recent years.

Several types of studies will be discussed providing evidence supporting the importance of dietary factors in breast cancer: descriptive epidemiological studies, correlation studies, evaluation of nutritionally mediated risk factors, case control, and cohort studies. This review will focus solely on human studies, with animal data mentioned only where it might add pertinent support.

A. DESCRIPTIVE EPIDEMIOLOGICAL STUDIES

The evidence from descriptive epidemiological studies suggests that cultural factors or life-style, especially diet, are important etiological factors in the development of breast cancer. Kolonel[5] reported that Japanese migrant women living in Hawaii have a higher incidence of this disease than those Japanese women living in Japan. Migrant studies have shown that the incidence of breast cancer among premenopausal Japanese-American women living in California is now almost as high as that for Caucasian women, whereas the incidence of cancer among them was similar to the low rate in Japan when they first migrated.[6] Other descriptive studies[7] have shown that changes in cancer incidence for certain populations can be related to changes in life-style of successive birth cohorts.

B. CORRELATION STUDIES

A second type of evidence for dietary factors in breast cancer has been provided by studies correlating breast cancer incidence and mortality with per capita intake of total fat and other nutrients in different countries[8] and the U.S. Early correlation studies[9] with various dietary constituents have shown a correlation between dietary fat and mortality from breast cancer in a number of countries. Gaskill et al.[10] found a direct correlation between cancer mortality and intake of milk, table fats, beef, calories, protein, and fat, and an inverse correlation with intake of eggs.

C. NUTRITIONALLY MEDIATED FACTORS

Factors that are considered nutritionally related, but are not nutrients themselves, have been analyzed with respect to breast cancer risk. These include weight, height, body mass (which is dependent on weight and height), and age at menarche. Women who experience menarche at an early age, especially before age 12, are at higher risk.[4,11] Evidence that body weight and food intake are related to early onset of estrus in rats[12] supports the hypothesis that the rat's body must contain a minimum amount of fat for estrus to occur. This also appears to be essential for menarche in women,[13] although not all studies have confirmed these findings.[14] To confuse the results further, an evaluation of the effects of per capita intake of total fat and animal protein on the international incidence and mortality rates for breast cancer found a significant effect of these variables, even after controlling for height, weight, and age at menarche.[15] Most studies examining height and breast cancer risk support an association of height with increased breast cancer risk.[16] Recently, in the Nurses' Health Study, a significant positive association was seen between height and breast cancer risk in postmenopausal women.[17] As an additional variable, the body mass index (weight/height^2) has been studied, suggesting an interaction between body mass index, breast cancer, and menopausal status.[18] Eleven out of 13 case-control studies of body mass index and breast cancer risk show a greater relative risk for postmenopausal women in the highest body mass index category,[16] but this is an inverse association in premenopausal women. In the Nurses' Health Study, a similar inverse association was seen between weight at age 18 and risk of breast cancer in premenopausal women.[17]

D. CASE-CONTROL OR COHORT STUDIES

Case-control or cohort studies should provide the most conclusive evidence we have on dietary factors and breast cancer risk. An early case-control study reported in 1975 five categories of foods which were associated with breast cancer: fried foods, fried potatoes, hard fat used for frying, dairy products except milk, and white bread, with the relative risks ranging from 1.6 to 2.6.[19]

In another early case-control study[20] the strongest association for dietary factors and breast cancer risk was seen for total fat consumption, in both premenopausal and postmenopausal women, although the relative risks were low and there was no dose-response. Yet another study[21] reported that the relative risk of breast cancer increased significantly with more frequent consumption of beef and other red meat, pork, and sweet desserts. More recent studies have not supported the connection between dietary fat and breast cancer. Graham et al.[22] compared the fat intake of 2024 breast cancer cases with 1463 controls and found that both animal fat and total fat intake were nearly identical in the two groups. A number of smaller case-control studies have been summarized in a meta-analysis by Howe et al.[23] Only 4 of 12 studies showed positive associations between fat intake and breast cancer risk. However, when all the data were pooled, a significant but weak association was observed for both total and saturated fat in postmenopausal women. Also supporting the same hypothesis, Kushi et al.[24] reported a modest positive association of total fat intake with risk of breast cancer in a study of 34,388 postmenopausal women from Iowa. Another recent, prospective population-based study of dietary fat, calories, and the risk of breast cancer demonstrated that women who developed breast cancer had significantly higher age-adjusted intake of all fats with a stepwise increase in risk across tertiles of intake.[25] However, in the largest prospective cohort study,[26] the Nurses' Health Study, 89,494 women were followed for 8 years and the relative risk for developing breast cancer for the highest quintile of dietary fat intake was only 0.90, indicating no effect of this dietary factor on the risk of developing breast cancer.

E. ANTIOXIDANT VITAMINS (A, C, AND E)

Vitamin A consists of both preformed vitamin A as retinol and retinyl esters, as well as the carotenoids found primarily in fruits and vegetables. A number of case-control studies have examined the role of vitamin A intake and all have found a protective association.[16] Howe et al.[23] reported a significant protective association between total vitamin A and breast cancer in a meta-analysis of nine case-control studies with data on dietary intake of vitamin A. The data are more supportive of carotenoid vitamin A than for the preformed type. In the Nurses' Health Study, Hunter et al.[27] prospectively studied the cohort of 89,494 women and assessed their intake of vitamins A, C, and E from foods and supplements at baseline and in 1984. They found a significant inverse association of vitamin A intake with the risk of breast cancer. They also found that large intakes of vitamin C or vitamin E did not protect the women in this study from breast cancer. In a previous study of postmenopausal women in New York, Graham et al.[22] reported that there was no increase in risk related to the ingested amount of calories, vitamins A, C, or E, dietary fiber, or fat. In a case-control study on women in Buffalo, NY,

Potischman et al.[28] reported that there was no overall association between plasma retinol and breast cancer, but a positive relationship was observed between retinol and breast cancer in the subgroup with low plasma beta-carotene values, suggesting that low plasma carotene may be a risk factor for breast cancer. There have been few published studies linking vitamin E and breast cancer. Three case-control studies have reported protective associations, whereas another two report no effect or a direct effect.[16] In the only prospective study published, as mentioned previously,[27] no protective effect was seen for vitamin E. In Graham et al.'s New York study vitamin C was not found to be protective, but in a subsequent study a protective effect was seen for vitamin C.[29] Howe et al.,[23] in their meta-analysis, observed a significant inverse association for ascorbic acid and breast cancer risk. Hunter et al.,[27] again in the only prospective study on the antioxidant vitamins, reported a weak positive association.

F. SELENIUM

Ecologic studies have demonstrated strong inverse associations between selenium exposure and breast cancer.[30-32] In addition, although the nutrition and cancer literature is represented extensively with animal studies of selenium and its protective effect on mammary carcinogenesis, a substantial body of evidence appears to indicate a lack of any appreciable effect of selenium intake on breast cancer risk, at least within the range of human diets.[33] In a recent case-control study in Sweden,[34] plasma selenium and glutathione peroxidase in erythrocytes were analyzed. In individuals without supplemental selenium intake, a preventive effect for breast cancer was found, increasing with plasma selenium level.[34] This was significant for women over 50 years of age and a nonsignificant effect was seen in women under 50. In a prospective study in the Nurses' Health Study, Hunter et al.[35] collected toenail clippings and determined selenium concentration. The relative risk for selenium concentration from highest to lowest quintile was not different. The authors concluded that selenium intake later in life is not likely to be an important factor in the etiology of breast cancer.[35]

G. VITAMIN D

Although dietary vitamin D deficiency may be a risk factor for mammary carcinogenesis in rodents,[36] and the vitamin in its active form has demonstrated protective effects in experimental models,[37] the only reported study investigating the hypothesis of vitamin D deficiency and cancer of the breast showed no differences between cases and controls in their mean daily intake of the vitamin.[38] Therefore, there is no evidence at this time that vitamin D has any role in the etiology of human breast cancer. However, patients with vitamin D receptor-positive tumors had longer disease-free survival than those with receptor-negative tumors,[37] and vitamin D receptor status has potential as a prognostic indicator.[39]

H. ALCOHOL CONSUMPTION

In recent years, a substantial body of evidence has accumulated to support a positive association between alcohol consumption and breast cancer.[16] Longnecker et al.[40] performed a meta-analysis on 12 case-control studies and concluded that there is an increased relative risk of about 1.4 for each two drinks of alcohol per day. Reichman et al.[41] have reported that in a controlled diet study, alcohol consumption was associated with statistically significant increases in levels of several estrogenic hormones, and that this could be a possible explanation for the positive association seen between alcohol consumption and breast cancer. In a Polish case-control study of breast cancer, smoking and vodka drinking, Pawlega[42] reported that the habit of drinking vodka 20 years earlier significantly increased breast cancer risk in women under 50 years old. In a Canadian study of 56,837 women, Friedenreich et al.[43] reported only a small association of alcohol consumption with breast cancer risk (relative risk of 1.11) and no association at all for postmenopausal women. An Italian case-control study of alcohol and breast cancer risk also reported a moderate increase in risk for the highest quintile of alcohol consumption.[44] Also in a case-control study in Moscow (Russia), Zaridze et al.[45] reported an odds ratio for risk of breast cancer in postmenopausal women of 3.39, thus supporting a hypothetical role of alcohol as an etiologic factor in breast cancer.

I. OTHER DIETARY FACTORS

Caffeine consumption has been examined as a risk factor for breast cancer since elimination of caffeine from the diet has been proposed as a treatment for benign breast disease.[46] However, most case-control studies show no positive association with the disease. In contrast, Hunter et al.[47] observed a weak, but significant inverse association between caffeine consumption and breast cancer risk. The dietary intake of fiber has also been investigated as a potential risk factor for human breast cancer. Van't Veer et al.,[48] in a Netherlands study of the association between dietary fiber, beta-carotene, and breast cancer, reported a statistically significant lower intake of dietary fiber observed in breast cancer cases than in controls. The corresponding odds ratio for intake of dietary fiber was 0.55, but was nonsignificant. The authors suggest that a high intake of cereal products, especially those rich in fiber, may be inversely related to breast cancer risk. Another potential etiological dietary component might be fish. Lund and Bonaa[49] reported reduced breast cancer mortality among fishermen's wives in Norway by comparing death rates and husbands' occupations (fishermen vs. unskilled workers). The authors state that their study supports the hypothesis that fish consumption may be associated with lower breast cancer mortality. Phytoestrogens are another dietary component that may be associated with a protective effect against breast cancer risk. It has been suggested that dietary phytoestrogens, which are present in legumes and grains, provide potential prevention of estrogen-dependent cancers such as breast cancer. Most of the data so far have come from cell culture and animal studies and few human studies have been reported.[50] However, a recent study by Adlercreutz et al.[51] demonstrated that these compounds in the diet (lignans, plant heterocyclic phenols similar in structure to estrogens, and isoflavonoids) may affect uptake and metabolism of sex hormones in post-menopausal women, and thus may inhibit cancer cell growth by competing for estrogen binding sites.

J. PESTICIDES

Recent attention has been drawn to the issue of organochlorine residues and breast cancer. Although this is not specifically a dietary exposure route, Wolff et al.[52] reported that blood levels of organochlorines such as DDT insecticide and PCBs used as fluid insulators of electrical components were higher for breast cancer patients than for controls. These findings suggest that environmental chemical contamination with organochlorine residues may be an important etiologic factor in breast cancer. Given the widespread dissemination of organochlorine insecticides in the environment and the food chain, the implications are that this could be a dietary etiological agent for human breast cancer.

K. SUMMARY

Nutritional factors in the etiology of breast cancer are summarized in Table 1. The data implicating dietary fat in the etiology of breast cancer appear to be weak at best. Hormonal factors such as age at menarche, which is only partially related to diet, seem to be more important than body weight or size. The data on the antioxidant vitamins seem to demonstrate a reasonably consistent protective effect for vitamin A, and a weakly positive protective effect for vitamin C, with not enough data for evaluating vitamin E. The role of selenium as a breast cancer inhibitory agent is inconclusive at this time. Alcohol seems to be gaining momentum as a culprit in the etiology of breast cancer,[40-45] although the increased risk is not substantial. Any other dietary factors do not appear to have enough evidence at this time to draw any conclusions as to their role in breast cancer.

III. CERVICAL CANCER

Although the cervical cancer incidence rates have decreased in the U.S. in the past 40 years, this cancer site remains a significant problem in the lower socioeconomic strata, as well as in other parts of the world.[53] Nutritional influences on the development of cervical cancer have long been of interest. Many nutrients have been studied for a possible relationship to cervical neoplasia, as well as other nondietary factors in this disease. These etiological factors include a number of sexual and reproductive factors, as well as oral contraceptive use and smoking, none of which will be discussed in this review.

TABLE 1
Studies of Nutrients and Breast Cancer Risk

Nutrient	Type of Study/Factor Studied	Ref.
Dietary fat	Descriptive	5–7
	Correlation	8–10
	Nutritionally mediated factors	11–15, 17, 18
	Case-control, cohort	16, 19–26
Vitamin A	Dietary	16, 23, 27–29
Vitamin C	Dietary	16, 23, 27, 28
Vitamin E	Dietary	16, 27
Selenium	Ecologic	30–32
	Dietary	33
	Serologic	34
	Toenails	35
Vitamin D	Dietary	38
	Receptors	37, 39
Alcohol	Consumption	16, 40–45
Other Factors	Caffeine ingestion	46, 47
	Fiber intake	48
	Fish consumption	49
	Phytoestrogens	50, 51
	Pesticide exposure	52

A. VITAMIN A AND CAROTENOIDS

The majority of reports have found no association between the dietary intake of preformed vitamin A and risk of cervical dysplasia, *in situ* cancer, or invasive disease (for an excellent review, see Potischman[53]). Most of the serologic studies agree with the dietary intake studies[53] in concluding that there is no relation between vitamin A and cervical neoplasia. Results from analysis of carotenoid intakes and cervical cancer were mixed, which is not surprising, since this was a very heterogeneous group of studies (Table 2). A recent case-control study conducted in Latin America[54] showed no trend with extent of disease, although stage IV cases had lower carotene values than other cases.

In analyses of carotenoid intakes, seven studies[55-61] found that the cases consumed lower intakes than controls, four[55,62-64] found no difference, and one[65] reported intakes higher for cases than controls. Serologic studies of carotenoid levels were slightly more consistent, with lower levels of carotenoids among cases than controls in 8 [56,61,66-71] out of 12 studies.[66,72-74] To summarize, although there was some indication that carotenoids may be protective, the studies were not consistent.

B. VITAMIN C

Most studies[56-59,61,65,69,75,76] of vitamin C (both dietary and serologic) seemed to be associated with a reduction in risk for cervical neoplasia. There

TABLE 2
Case-Control Studies of Nutrients and Cervical Cancer

Nutrient/Type of Study	Association w/Risk	Ref.
Carotenoids		
Dietary	No difference	55, 62–64
	Inverse	55–61
	Positive	65
Serologic	No difference	66, 72–74
	Inverse	56, 61, 66–71
Vitamin C		
Dietary	No difference	62–64
	Inverse	56, 58, 59, 61, 65, 75
Serologic	No difference	72
	Inverse	69, 76
Vitamin E		
Dietary	No difference	63
	Inverse	58
Serologic	No difference	70, 74
	Inverse	66, 77, 78
Folate		
Dietary	No difference	56, 58, 59, 62, 64
	Inverse	79, 80
Serologic	No difference	82
	Inverse	69, 80, 81

Adapted from Potischman, N., *J. Nutr.,* 123, 424, 1993.

were two studies that only found a protective effect among smokers.[63,64] However, this is not inconsistent, since smoking is a risk factor for this disease and is also related to vitamin C status. Two serologic studies have also suggested that vitamin C may play a protective role in cervical cancer.[69,76]

C. VITAMIN E
Vitamin E has not been studied extensively in terms of cervical neoplasia,[58,63,68,70,74,77,78] however, two serologic studies of cervical dysplasia demonstrated lower levels of vitamin E to be associated with a higher grade lesion, and even lower concentrations in those with invasive cancers.[68,77] Overall, studies with vitamin E and cervical cancer risk showed mixed results with no clear-cut conclusion which could be drawn.

D. FOLATE
The case for folate in the etiology of cervical cancer is probably stronger than for any other nutrient studied.[79-82] Since 1977 several reports have indicated an increased incidence of cervical cancer among oral contraceptive users.[83-86] An early study reported that there were morphologic similarities between megaloblastic anemia and those features present in the cervical cells of oral contraceptive users.[87] Supplementation with folate improved the

cervical dysplasia associated with oral contraceptive use.[88] There is also an association of human papilloma virus (HPV) type 16 prevalence and lowered folate status, which may suggest that folate status may be linked with HPV infection and not with dysplastic progression.[89] In a clinical intervention trial, the data did not confirm the hypothesis that oral folate supplements would improve cervical dysplasia.[89] There were no statistically different rates of normal biopsies between the folate-treated subjects and those receiving placebo. However, as in the case-control study, there was a higher incidence of HPV-16 positives among those cases with low red blood cell folate initially, leading the authors to conclude that folate deficiency may exert a cocarcinogenic effect in the presence of HPV-16 exposure.[90]

E. OTHER

In a study of the associations between cervical cancer and serological markers of nutritional status in Latin America, an inverse trend for cholesterol and triglyceride concentrations was observed with stage of disease, suggesting a clinical effect of cervical cancer on blood lipids.[54] A single study has associated pork intake and HPV-related disease. Schneider et al.[91] reported that international correlations suggest that pork intake is positively associated with incidence of cervical cancer, a disease also related to HPV. Pork meat or dietary factors associated with pork meat consumption may be involved in the development of HPV-related diseases.[91]

F. SUMMARY

In summary, the relation between nutrients and cervical neoplasia appears to be predominantly limited to the effects of folate. Preformed vitamin A did not appear to be related to risk of any preinvasive or invasive cervical lesions, whereas vitamin C has been associated with a reduced risk for dysplasia, *in situ* cancer, and invasive disease, especially among smokers. There was some evidence of reduced risks associated with various carotenoids and vitamin E at all stages of the disease, but the overall results were inconsistent. Folate was the only nutrient that appeared to be protective for dysplastic lesions, but not related to the risk of *in situ* or invasive disease. Red blood cell folate was the best predictor of dysplasia, better than serum or dietary folate. It has also been suggested that more research is needed into the interactions between nutrients and other risk factors for this disease, such as smoking and HPV infection.

IV. ENDOMETRIAL CANCER

Endometrial cancer has been correlated with cancers of the breast, ovary, colon, and rectum.[11] It tends to be more common in the U.S. than in other parts of the world and to be more frequent in Caucasian women of higher socioeconomic status. The only established etiologic cause for this cancer appears to be the use of exogenous estrogens at the high doses commonly prescribed years ago.[1] Obesity has been cited as a risk factor in a number of studies[92-96] and a hormonal mechanism has been postulated for this association. There also appears to be an association between endometrial cancer risk and body fat distribution, with certain studies demonstrating that women with upper body fat have an increased risk of endometrial cancer.[97] A longitudinal population study[98] of 1462 women in Sweden examined adipose tissue distribution and the occurrence of endometrial cancer. Abdominally localized adipose tissue was associated with irregular ovulation and menstruation, as well as an increased risk of endometrial cancer.[98] Additionally, in a case-control study in China,[99] obesity also proved to be a strong risk factor for endometrial cancer, even in a country where supplemental estrogen use is uncommon. However, another study has shown no association between obesity and endometrial cancer. A case-control study of endometrial adenocarcinoma in Athens, Greece investigated the epidemiology of this cancer in a low-risk setting.[100] No relationship was found between weight and endometrial cancer.

In terms of specific dietary factors and endometrial cancer, one of the first studies was performed in Italy,[94] in which a case-control study collected data on the frequency of consumption of selected dietary items. The cases with endometrial cancer reported a greater fat intake, and a less frequent intake of fruits, vegetables, and grains. A subsequent study by the same investigator[101] examined Italian regional diets and their correlation to breast, ovarian, and endometrial cancer rates. Diets high in fat, protein, and calories increased the incidence rates of all three cancers, and diets high in green vegetable and fresh fruit consumption had a protective effect. The relation between diet and endometrial cancer was more recently examined in China.[102] Women in the highest quartile of total caloric intake had a 2.1-fold increased risk of endometrial cancer, and that risk varied according to the source of calories, with the highest risk attributable to caloric intake from fat and protein confined to foods of animal origin. Following adjustment for total calories, no significant association of risk was found with intake of vegetables, dark green/yellow vegetables, or estimated carotene intake, although fruit and allium vegetables were associated with some reduction in risk. These results suggest that animal fat and protein may play a role in the etiology of endometrial cancer.

In a case-control study of diet and endometrial cancer conducted in Birmingham, AL,[103] a high intake of certain micronutrients was found to be associated with a decreased risk of endometrial cancer for those in the upper tertile of carotene and nitrate intake. There was also an inverse association between endometrial cancer and protein consumption, as well as a direct association with cholesterol intake. More frequent consumption of several vegetables and certain dairy products was associated with a statistically significant decreased risk of endometrial cancer, suggesting that diet plays an important role in this cancer. Although the focus of this review of nutrition and women's cancers does not emphasize all of the experimental studies, a recent rodent study of endometrial cancer is worthy of mentioning. The study[104] was conducted to examine the possible inhibiting effect of indole-3-carbinol, a constituent of cruciferous vegetables, on the spontaneous occurrence of endometrial adenocarcinoma in female Donryu rats. The high incidence of endometrial cancer in this rat strain is thought to be related to increased estrogen/progesterone ratio with aging. Dietary indole-3-carbinol significantly decreased the frequency of endometrial carcinoma, preneoplastic lesions, and mammary fibroadenoma, while it increased the 2-hydroxylation of estradiol. These results suggest that cruciferous vegetables may be protective against the development of endometrial cancer.

In summary, endometrial cancer is primarily associated with excess estrogenic stimulation, and obesity may contribute significantly to this risk. Other potential dietary factors have not been established with any certainty, although there appears to be a growing body of evidence linking high fat diets, especially animal fats, to this risk.

V. OVARIAN CANCER

Similar to endometrial cancer, ovarian cancer is more common in the U.S. and other western countries than in Asia and is also correlated with cancers of the breast, colon, and endometrium. There is a greater-than-expected risk of second primary cancers of the corpus uteri, colon, and breast in patients with ovarian cancer.[105] This supports the hypothesis that there are common etiological factors for these cancer sites. Ovarian cancer also tends to occur more frequently in women in the higher socioeconomic groups and less frequently in women who use oral contraceptives.[106-109] In one case-control study, Annegers et al.[110] observed that obesity is not a risk factor for ovarian cancer, and in another there was no effect of height or weight.[111] In terms of dietary influences Cramer et al.[112] found that ovarian cancer cases consumed significantly greater amounts of animal fat and considerable less vegetable fat than did controls. In contrast, Byers et al.[113] found no such association. Most studies of weight and height did not find an association with ovarian cancer risk.[1] Two studies[114,115] have reported an association between coffee drinking and an increased risk of ovarian cancer, and another one[113] did not. Therefore, coffee's role as an etiologic agent in ovarian cancer is not conclusive. Most recently, a study of mortality trends of breast, colorectal, ovarian, and prostate cancer in Spain, Italy, Greece, Yugoslavia, England, and Wales implicated consumption of fat-containing foods in the increase in cancer at these sites in Mediterranean countries,[116] whereas in England and Wales a decrease in ovarian and colorectal cancer among women was observed.[116]

In summary, although the risk for ovarian cancer has been linked inversely to oral contraceptive use, no clear-cut dietary associations have been discerned for this cancer site. Since screening and early detection are not available for this cancer, more research is needed.

VI. SUMMARY AND CONCLUSIONS

In summary, the overwhelming message that emerges from all of the data on nutrition and women's cancers is that there are few nutrients that demonstrate a compelling role in the development of these cancers. The role of dietary fat in breast cancer is far from resolved, and the role of alcohol is just beginning to surface. Vitamin A intake and, to a lesser extent, vitamin C appear to be protective, but that does not mean that their role is causative in nature. More work needs to be undertaken into the mechanisms of the antioxidant vitamins in protection against human breast cancer. As more research into the genetics of breast cancer emerges, it becomes more important to understand the nutritional factors in this disease in the context of the genetic risk factors, and this should become a focus for future research efforts.

In terms of nutritional factors in cervical cancer, folate is the only dietary component that appears to demonstrate any consistent protective effect that can be readily assessed. There is also some promise for a protective role for vitamin C, but this is not compelling. The overwhelming risk factors for cervical cancer appear to be smoking and HPV infection, and we should begin to direct research efforts to the effects of nutritional variables interacting with these risk factors.

Endometrial cancer is primarily associated with excess estrogenic stimulation, but obesity may contribute to this risk. Any future research efforts should perhaps investigate how dietary components actually influence this risk. Ovarian cancer does not appear to have any major dietary factor associated with its etiology, although animal fats may play an obscure role. Ovarian cancer is an enigma in terms of early diagnosis and possible causation, so clearly more research is needed into this cancer.

In conclusion, the implications for women and their risks for cancers unique to women, in terms of what types of diets would potentially protect them, are limited to the same dietary recommendations that have been promoted by all health groups in recent years: maintain ideal body weight, eat plenty of fruits and vegetables, decrease fat and fatty meat consumption, and limit alcohol consumption to modest intakes.

REFERENCES

1. Commitee on Diet and Health, Food and Nutrition Board, Commission on Life Sciences, National Research Council, *Diet and Health, Implications for Reducing Chronic Disease Risk*, National Academy Press, Washington, D.C., 1989, chap. 22.
2. Doll, R. and Peto, R., The causes of cancer: quantitative estimates of avoidable risks in the United States today, *J. Natl. Cancer Inst.*, 66, 1191, 1981.

3. Wynder, E. L. and Gori, G. B., Contribution of the environment to cancer incidence: an epidemiological exercise, *J. Natl. Cancer Inst.*, 58, 825, 1977.

4. MacMahon, B., Cole, P., and Brown, J., Etiology of human breast cancer: a review, *J. Natl. Cancer Inst.*, 50, 21, 1973.

5. Kolonel, L. N., Cancer patterns of four ethnic groups in Hawaii, *J. Natl. Cancer Inst.*, 65, 1127, 1980.

6. Dunn, J. E., Jr., Breast cancer among American Japanese in the San Francisco Bay area, *Natl. Cancer Inst. Monog.*, 47, 157, 1977.

7. Moolgavkar, S. H., Day, N. E., and Stevens, R.G., Two-stage model for carcinogenesis: epidemiology of breast cancer in females, *J. Natl. Cancer Inst.*, 65, 559, 1980.

8. Committee on Diet, Nutrition, and Cancer, Assembly of Life Sciences, National Research Council, *Diet, Nutrition, and Cancer*, National Academy Press, Washington, D.C., 1982, chap. 17.

9. Carroll, K. K. and Khor, H. T., Dietary fat in relation to tumorigenesis, *Prog. Biochem. Pharmacol.*, 10, 308, 1975.

10. Gaskill, S. P., McGuire, W. L., Osborne, C. K., and Stern, M. P., Breast cancer mortality and diet in the United States, *Cancer Res.*, 39, 3628, 1979.

11. Miller, A. B., An overview of hormone-associated cancers, *Cancer Res.*, 38, 3985, 1978.

12. Frisch, R. E., Hegsted, D. M., and Yoshinaga, K., Body weight and food intake at early estrus of rats on a high-fat diet, *Proc. Natl. Acad. Sci. U.S.A.*, 72, 4172, 1975.

13. Frisch, R. E. and McArthur, J. W., Menstrual cycles: fatness as a determinant of minimum weight for height necessary for their maintenance or onset, *Science*, 185, 949, 1974.

14. Miller, A. B., Epidemiology of gastrointestinal cancer, *Compr. Ther.*, 7, 53, 1981.

15. Gray, G. E., Pike, M. C., and Henderson, B. E., Breast cancer incidence and mortality rates in different countries in relation to known risk factors and dietary practices, *Br. J. Cancer*, 39, 1, 1979.

16. Willett, W., Diet and breast cancer, *Contemp. Nutr.*, 18, 1, 1993.

17. London, S. J., Colditz, G. A., Stampfer, M. J., Willett, W. C., Rossner, B., and Speizer, F. E., Prospective study of relative weight and breast cancer, *J.A.M.A.*, 262, 2853, 1989.

18. Hunter, D. J. and Willett, W. C., Diet, body size, and breast cancer, *Epidemiol. Rev.*, 15, 110, 1993.

19. Phillips, R. L., Role of life-style and dietary habits in risk of cancer among Seventh-Day Adventists, *Cancer Res.*, 35, 3513, 1975.

20. Miller, A. B., Kelly, A., Choi, N. W., Matthews, V., Morgan, R. W., Munan, L., Burch, J. D., Feather, J., Howe, G. R., and Jain, M., A study of diet and breast cancer, *Am. J. Epidemiol.*, 107, 499, 1978.

21. Lubin, J. H., Blot, W. J., and Burns, P. E., Breast cancer following high dietary fat and protein consumption, *Am. J. Epidemiol.*, 114, (Abstr.), 422, 1981.

22. Graham, S., Marshall, J., Mettlin, C., Rzepka, T., Nemoto, T., and Byers, T., Diet in the epidemiology of breast cancer, *Am. J. Epidemiol.*, 116, 68, 1982.

23. Howe, G. R., Hirohata, T., Hislop, T. G., Iscovich, J. M., Yuan, J. M., Katsouyanni, K., Lubin, F., Marubini, E., Modan, B., and Rohan, T., Dietary factors and risk of breast cancer: combined analysis of 12 case-control studies, *J. Natl. Cancer Inst.*, 82, 561, 1990.

24. Kushi, L. H., Sellers, T. A., Potter, J. D., Nelson, C. L., Munger, R. G., Kaye, S. A., and Folsom, A. R., Dietary fat and postmenopausal breast cancer, *J. Natl. Cancer Inst.*, 84, 1092, 1992.

25. Barrett-Connor, E. and Friedlander, N. J., Dietary fat, calories, and the risk of breast cancer in postmenopausal women: a prospective population-based study, *J. Am. Coll. Nutr.*, 12, 390, 1993.

26. Willett, W. C., Hunter, D. J., Stampfer, M. J., Colditz, G., Manson, J. E., Spiegelman, D., Rosner, B., Hennekens, C. H., and Speizer, F. E., Dietary fat and fiber in relation to risk of breast cancer, *J.A.M.A.*, 268, 2037, 1992.

27. Hunter, D. J., Stampfer, M. J., Colditz, G. A., Manson, J., Rosner, B., Hennekens, C. H., Speizer, F. E., and Willett, W. C., A prospective study of consumption of vitamins A, C and E and breast cancer risk, *Am. J. Epidemiol.*, 134, 715, 1991.

28. Potischman, N., McCulloch, C. E., Byers, T., Nemoto, T., Stubbe, N., Milch, R., Parker, R., Rasmussen, K. M., Root, M., and Graham, S., Breast cancer and dietary and plasma concentrations of carotenoids and vitamin A, *Am. J. Clin. Nutr.*, 52, 909, 1990.

29. Graham, S., Hellmann, R., Marshall, J., Freudenheim, J., Vena, J., Swanson, M., Zielezny, M., Nemoto, T., Stubbe, N., and Raimondo, T., Nutritional epidemiology of postmenopausal breast cancer in western New York, *Am. J. Epidemiol.*, 134, 552, 1991.

30. Shamberger, R. J., Tytko, S. A., and Willis, C. E., Antioxidants and cancer. VI. Selenium and age-adjusted human cancer mortality, *Arch. Environ. Health*, 31, 231, 1976.

31. Clark, L. C., The epidemiology of selenium and cancer, *Fed. Proc.*, 44, 2584, 1985.

32. Schrauzer, G. D., White, D. A., and Schneider, C. J., Cancer mortality correlation studies. III. Statistical associations with dietary selenium intake, *Bioinorg. Chem.*, 7, 23, 1977.

33. Garland, M., Willett, W. C., Manson, J. E., and Hunter, D. J., Antioxidant micronutrients and breast cancer, *J. Am. Coll. Nutr.*, 12, 400, 1993.

34. Hardell, L., Danell, M., Angqvist, C. A., Marklund, S. L., Fredriksson, M., Zakari, A. L., and Kjellgren, A., Levels of selenium in plasma and glutathione peroxidase in erythrocytes and the risk of breast cancer: a case-control study, *Biol. Trace Elem. Res.*, 36, 99, 1993.

35. Hunter, D. J., Morris, J. S., Stampfer, M. J., Colditz, G. A., Speizer, F. E., and Willett, W. C., A prospective study of selenium status and breast cancer risk, *J.A.M.A.*, 264, 1128, 1990.

36. Jacobson, E. A., James, K. A., Newmark, H. L., and Carroll, K. K., Effects of dietary fat, calcium, and vitamin D on growth and mammary tumorigenesis induced by 7,12-dimethylbenz(a)anthracene in female Sprague-Dawley rats, *Cancer Res.*, 49, 6300, 1989.

37. Colston, K. W., Berger, U., and Coombes, R. C., Possible role for vitamin D in controlling breast cancer cell proliferation, *Lancet*, 28, 188, 1989.

38. Simard, A., Vobecky, J., and Vobecky, J. S., Vitamin D deficiency and cancer of the breast: an unprovocative ecological hypothesis, *Can. J. Public Health*, 82, 300, 1991.

39. Berger, U., McClelland, R. A., Wilson, P., Greene, G. L., Haussler, M. R., Pike, J. W., Colston, K., Easton, D., and Coombes, R. C., Immunocytochemical determination of estrogen receptor, progesterone receptor, and 1,2-dihydroxyvitamin D_3 receptor in breast cancer and relationship to prognosis, *Cancer Res.*, 51, 239, 1991.

40. Longnecker, M., Berlin, J. A., Orza, M. J., and Chalmers, T. C., A meta-analysis of alcohol consumption in relation to risk of breast cancer, *J.A.M.A.*, 260, 652, 1988.

41. Reichman, M. E., Judd, J. T., Longcope, C., Schatzkin, A., Clevidence, B. A., Nair, P. P., Campbell, W. S., and Taylor, P. R., Effects of alcohol consumption on plasma and urinary hormone concentrations in premenopausal women, *J. Natl. Cancer Inst.*, 85, 722, 1993.

42. Pawlega, J., Breast cancer and smoking, vodka drinking and dietary habits: a case-control study, *Acta. Oncol.*, 31, 387, 1992.

43. Friedenreich, C. M., Howe, G. R., Miller, A. B., and Jain, M. G., A cohort study of alcohol consumption and risk of breast cancer, *Am. J. Epidemiol.*, 137, 512, 1993.

44. Ferraroni, M., Decarli, A., Willett, W. C., and Marubini, E., Alcohol and breast cancer risk: a case-control study from northern Italy, *Int. J. Epidemiol.*, 20, 859, 1991.

45. Zaridze, D., Lifanova, Y., Maximivitch, D., Day, N. E., and Duffy, S. W., Diet, alcohol consumption and reproductive factors in a case-control study of breast cancer in Moscow, *Int. J. Cancer*, 48, 493, 1991.

46. Minton, J. P., Foecking, M. K., Webster, D. J., and Matthews, R. H., Response of fibrocystic disease to caffeine withdrawal and correlation of cyclic nucleotides with breast disease, *Am. J. Obstet. Gynecol.*, 135, 157, 1979.

47. Hunter, D. J., Manson, J. E., Stampfer, M. J., Colditz, G. A., Rosner, B., Hennekens, C. H., Speizer, F. E., and Willett, W. C., A prospective study of caffeine, coffee, tea, and breast cancer, *Am. J. Epidemiol.*, 136, 1000, 1992.

48. Van't Veer, P., Kolb, C. M., Verhoef, P., Kok, F. J., Schouten, E. G., Hermus, R. J., and Sturmans, F., Dietary fiber, beta-carotene and breast cancer: results from a case-control study, *Int. J. Cancer*, 45, 825, 1990.

49. Lund, E. and Bonaa, K. H., Reduced breast cancer mortality among fishermen's wives in Norway, *Cancer Causes Control*, 4, 283, 1993.

50. Kurzer, M. S., Diet, estrogen and cancer, *Contemp. Nutr.*, 17, 1, 1992.

51. Adlerkreutz, H., Mousavi, Y., Clark, J., Hockerstedt, K., Hamalainen, E., Wahala, K., Makela, T., and Hase, T., Dietary phytoestrogens and cancer: in vitro and in vivo studies, *J. Steroid Biochem. Mol. Biol.*, 41, 331, 1992.

52. Wolff, M. S., Toniolo, P. G., Lee, E. W., Rivera, M., and Dubin, N., Blood levels of organochlorine residues and risk of breast cancer, *J. Natl. Cancer Inst.*, 85, 648, 1993.

53. Potischman, N., Nutritional epidemiology of cervical neoplasia, *J. Nutr.*, 123, 424, 1993.

54. Potischman, N., Hoover, R. N., Brinton, L. A., Swanson, C. A., Herrero, R., Tenorio, F., de Britton, R. C., Gaitan, E., and Reeves, W. C., The relations between cervical cancer and serological markers of nutritional status, *Nutr. Cancer*, 21, 193, 1994.

55. LaVecchia, C., Decarli, A., Fasoli, M., Parazzini, F., Franceschi, S., Gentile, A., and Negri, E., Dietary vitamin A and the risk of intraepithelial and invasive cervical neoplasia, *Gynecol. Oncol.*, 30, 187, 1988.

56. Brock, K. E., Berry, G., Mock, P. A., MacLennan, R., Truswell, A. S., and Brinton, L. A., Nutrients in diet and plasma and risk of *in situ* cervical cancer, *J. Natl. Cancer Inst.*, 80, 580, 1988.

57. Marshall, J. R., Graham, S., Byers, T., Swanson, M., and Brasure, J., Diet and smoking in the epidemiology of cancer of the cervix, *J. Natl. Cancer Inst.*, 70, 847, 1983.

58. Verreault, R., Chu, J., Mandelson, M., and Shy, K., A case-control study of diet and invasive cervical cancer, *Int. J. Cancer*, 43, 1050, 1989.

59. Herrero, R., Potischman, N., Brinton, L. A., Reeves, W. C., Brenes, M. M., Tenorio, F., deBritton, R. C., and Gaitan, E., A case-control study of nutrient status and invasive cervical cancer. I. Dietary indicators, *Am. J. Epidemiol.*, 134, 1335, 1991.

60. Wylie-Rosett, J. A., Romney, S. L., Slagle, N. S., Wassertheil-Smoller, S., Miller, G. L., Palan, P. R., Lucido, D. J., and Duttagupta, C., Influence of vitamin A on cervical dysplasia and carcinoma in situ, *Nutr. Cancer*, 6, 49, 1984.

61. Van Eenwyk, J., Davis, F. G., and Bowen, P. E., Dietary and serum carotenoids and cervical intraepithelial neoplasia, *Int. J. Cancer*, 48, 34, 1991.

62. Ziegler, R. G., Jones, C. J., Brinton, L. A., Norman, S. A., Mallin, K., Levine, R. S., Lehman, H. F., Hamman, R. F., Trumble, A. C., Rosenthal, J. F., and Hoover, R. N., Diet and the risk of *in situ* cervical cancer among white women in the United States, *Cancer Causes Control, 2,* 17, 1991.

63. Slattery, M. L., Abbott, T. M., Overall, J. C., Robison, L. M., French, T. K., Jolles, C., Gardner, J. W., and West, D. W., Dietary vitamins A, C, and E and selenium as risk factors for cervical cancer, *Epidemiology*, 1, 8, 1990.

64. Ziegler, R. G., Brinton, L. A., Hamman, R. F., Lehman, H. F., Levine, R. S., Mallin, K., Norman, S. A., Rosenthal, J. F., Trumble, A. C., and Hoover, R. N., Diet and the risk of invasive cervical cancer among white women in the United States, *Am. J. Epidemiol.*, 132, 432, 1990.

65. de Vet, H. C., Knipschild, P. G., Grol, M. E. C., Schouten, H. J. A., and Sturmans, F., The role of beta carotene and other dietary factors in the etiology of cervical dysplasia: results of a case-control study, *Int. J. Epidemiol.*, 20, 603, 1991.

66. Harris, R. W. C., Forman, D., Doll, R., Vessey, M. P., and Wald, N. J., Cancer of the cervix uteri and vitamin A, *Br. J. Cancer*, 53, 653, 1986.

67. Palan, P. R., Romney, S. L., Mikhail, M., Basu, J., and Vermund, S. H., Decreased plasma beta-carotene levels in women with uterine cervical dysplasias and cancer, *J. Natl. Cancer Inst.*, 80, 454, 1988.

68. Palan, P. R., Mikhail, M. S., Basu, J., and Romney, S. L., Plasma levels of antioxidant beta-carotene and alpha-tocopherol in uterine cervix dysplasias and cancer, *Nutr. Cancer*, 15, 13, 1991.

69. Orr, J. W., Wilson, K., Bodiford, C., Cornwell, A., Soong, S. J., Honea, K. L., Hatch, K. D., and Singleton, H. M., Nutritional status of patients with untreated cervical cancer. II. Vitamin assessment, *Am. J. Obstet. Gynecol.*, 151, 632, 1985.

70. Potischman, N., Herrero, R., Brinton, L. A., Reeves, W. C., Stacewicz-Sapuntzakis, M., Jones, C. J., Brenes, M. M., Tenorio, F., deBritton, R. C., and Gaitan, E., A case-control study of nutrient status and invasive cervical cancer. II. Serologic indicators, *Am. J. Epidemiol.*, 134, 1347, 1991.

71. Smith, A. H. and Waller, K. D., Serum beta-carotene in persons with cancer and their immediate families, *Am. J. Epidemiol.*, 133, 661, 1991.

72. Basu, J., Palan, P. R., Vermund, S. H., Goldberg, G. L., Burk, R. D., and Romney, S. L., Plasma ascorbic acid and beta-carotene levels in women evaluated for HPV infection, smoking, and cervix dysplasia, *Cancer Detect. Prevent.*, 15, 165, 1991.

73. Lambert, B., Brisson, G., and Bielman, P., Plasma vitamin A and precancerous lesions of cervix uteri: a preliminary report, *Gynecol. Oncol.*, 11, 136, 1981.

74. Heinonen, P. K., Kuoppala, T., Koskinen, T., and Punnonen, R., Serum vitamins A and E and carotene in patients with gynecologic cancer, *Arch. Gynecol. Obstet.*, 241, 151, 1987.

75. Wassertheil-Smoller, S., Romney, S. L., Wylie-Rosett, J., Slagle, S., Miller, G., Lucido, D., Duttagupta, C., and Palan, P. R., Dietary vitamin C and uterine cervical dysplasia, *Am. J. Epidemiol.*, 114, 714, 1981.

76. Romney, S. L., Duttagupta, C., Basu, J., Palan, P. R., Karp, S., Slagle, N. S., Dwyer, A., Wassertheil-Smoller, S., and Wylie-Rosett, J., Plasma vitamin C and uterine cervical dyaplasia, *Am. J. Obstet. Gynecol.*, 151, 976, 1985.

77. Cuzick, J., DeStavola, B. L., Russell, M. J., and Thomas, B. S., Vitamin A, vitamin E and the risk of cervical intraepithelial neoplasia, *Br. J. Cancer*, 62, 651, 1990.

78. Knekt, P., Serum vitamin E levels and risk of female cancers, *Int. J. Epidemiol.*, 17, 281, 1988.

79. McPherson, R. S., Nutritional factors and the risk of cervical dysplasia, *Am. J. Epidemiol.*, 130, 830, 1989.

80. Van Eenwyk, J., Davis, F. G., and Colman, N., Folate, vitamin C, and cervical intraepithelial neoplasia, *Cancer Epidemiol. Biomarkers Prevent.*, 1, 119, 1992.

81. Butterworth, C. E., Hatch, K. D., Macaluso, M., Cole, P., Sauberlich, H. E., Soong, S.-J., Borst, M., and Baker, V. V., Folate deficiency and cervical dysplasia, *J.A.M.A.*, 267, 528, 1992.

82. Potischman, N., Brinton, L. A., Laiming, V. A., Reeves, W. C., Brenes, M. M., Herrero, R., Tenorio, F., deBritton, R. C., and Gaitan, E., A case-control study of serum folate levels and invasive cervical cancer, *Cancer Res.*, 51, 47785, 1991.

83. Peritz, E., Ramcharan, S., Frank, J., Brown, W. L., Huang, S., and Ray, R., The incidence of cervical cancer and duration of oral contraceptive use, *Am. J. Epidemiol.*, 106, 462, 1977.

84. Stern, E., Steroid contraceptive use and cervical dysplasia: increased risk of progression, *Science*, 196, 1460, 1977.

85. Swan, S. H. and Brown, W. L., Oral contraceptive use, sexual activity and cervical carcinoma, *Am. J. Obstet. Gynecol.*, 139, 52, 1981.

86. Vessey, M. P., Lawless, M., McPherson, Y., and Yeates, D., Neoplasia of the cervix uteri and contraception: a possible adverse effect of the pill, *Lancet*, 2, 930, 1983.

87. Whitehead, N., Reyner, F., and Lindenbaum, J., Megaloblastic changes in the cervical epithelium. Association with oral contraceptive therapy and reversal with folic acid, *J.A.M.A.*, 226, 1421, 1973.

88. Butterworth, C. E., Jr., Hatch, K. D., Gore, H., Mueller, H., and Krumdieck, C. L., Improvement in cervical dysplasia associated with folic acid therapy in users of oral contraceptives, *Am. J. Clin. Nutr.*, 35, 73, 1982.

89. Butterworth, C. E., Jr., Hatch, K. D., Soong, S.-J., Cole, P., Tamura, T., Sauberlich, H. E., Borst, M., Macaluso, M., and Baker, V., Oral folic acid supplementation for cervical dysplasia: a clinical intervention trial, *Am. J. Obstet. Gynecol.*, 166, 803, 1992.

90. Borst, M., Butterworth, C. E., Jr., Baker, V., Kuykendall, K., Gore, H., Soong, S., and Hatch, K. D., Human papillomavirus screening for women with atypical papanicolaou smears, *J. Reprod. Med.*, 36, 95, 1991.

91. Schneider, A., Morabia, A., Papendick, U., and Kirchmayr, R., Pork intake and human papillomavirus-related disease, *Nutr. Cancer*, 13, 209, 1990.

92. Elwood, J. M., Cole, P., Rothman, K. J., and Kaplan, S. D., Epidemiology of endometrial cancer, *J. Natl. Cancer Inst.*, 59, 1055, 1977.

93. Henderson, B. E., Casagrande, J. T., Pike, M. C., Mack, T., and Rosario, I., The epidemiology of endometrial cancer in young women, *Br. J. Cancer*, 47, 749, 1983.

94. LaVecchia, C. A., Decarli, M., Fasoli, M., and Gentile, A., Nutrition and diet in the etiology of endometrial cancer, *Cancer*, 57, 1248, 1986.

95. Lew, E. A. and Garfinkel, L., Variations in mortality by weight among 750,000 men and women, *J. Chronic Dis.*, 32, 563, 1979.

96. Wynder, E. L., Escher, G. C., and Mantel, N., An epidemiological investigation of cancer of the endometrium, *Cancer*, 19, 489, 1966.

97. Schapira, D. V., Nutrition and cancer prevention, *Prim. Care*, 19, 481, 1992.

98. Lapidus, L., Helgesson, O., Merck, C., and Bjorntorp, P., Adipose tissue distribution and female carcinomas. A 12-year follow-up of participants in the population study of women in Goteborg, Sweden, *Int. J. Obesity*, 12, 361, 1988.

99. Shu, X.-O., Brinton, L. A., Zheng, W., Gao, Y. T., Fan, J., and Fraumeni, J. F., A population based case-control study of endometrial cancer in Shanghai, China, *Int. J. Cancer*, 49, 38, 1991.

100. Koumantaki, Y., Tzonou, A., Koumantakis, E., Kaklamani, E., Aravantinos, D., and Trichopoulos, D., A case-control study of cancer of the endometrium in Athens, *Int. J. Cancer*, 43, 795, 1989.

101. LaVecchia, C., Nutritional factors and cancers of the breast, endometrium and ovary, *Eur. J. Cancer Clin. Oncol.*, 25, 1945, 1989.

102. Shu, X. O., Zheng, W., Potischman, N., Brinton, L. A., Hatch, M. C., Gao, Y. T., and Fraumeni, J. F., A population-based case-control study of dietary factors and endometrial cancer in Shanghai, People's Republic of China, *Am. J. Epidemiol.*, 137, 155, 1993.

103. Barbone, F., Austin, H., and Partridge, E. E., Diet and endometrial cancer: a case-control study, *Am. J. Epidemiol.*, 137, 393, 1993.

104. Kojima, T., Tanaka, T., and Mori, H., Chemoprevention of spontaneous endometrial cancer in female Donryu rats by dietary indole-3-carbinol, *Cancer Res.*, 54, 1446, 1994.

105. Reimer, R. R., Hoover, R., Fraumeni, J. F., and Young, R. C., Second primary neoplasms following ovarian cancer, *J. Natl. Cancer Inst.*, 61, 1195, 1978.

106. Casagrande, J. T., Louie, E. W., Pike, M. C., Roy, S., Ross, R. K., and Henderson, B. E., "Incessant ovulation" and ovarian cancer, *Lancet*, 2, 170, 1979.

107. Cramer, D. W., Hutchison, G. B., Welch, W. R., Scully, R. E., and Knapp, R. C., Factors affecting the association of oral contraceptives and ovarian cancer, *N. Engl. J. Med.*, 307, 1047, 1982.

108. Nasca, P. C., Greenwald, P., Chorost, S., Richart, R., and Caputo, T., An epidemiologic case-control study of ovarian cancer and reproductive factors, *Am. J. Epidemiol.*, 119, 705, 1984.

109. Weiss, N. S., Lyon, J. L., Liff, J. M., Vollmer, W. M., and Daling, J. R., Incidence of ovarian cancer in relation to the use of oral contraceptives, *Int. J. Cancer*, 28, 669, 1981.

110. Annegers, J. F., Strom, H., Decker, D. G., Dockerty, M. B., and O'Fallon, W. M., Ovarian cancer: incidence and case-control study, *Cancer*, 43, 723, 1979.

111. Hildreth, N. G., Kelsey, J. L., LiVolsi, V. A., Fischer, D. B., Holford, T. R., Mostow, E. D., Schwartz, P. E., and White, C., An epidemiologic study of epithelial carcinoma of the ovary, *Am. J. Epidemiol.*, 114, 398, 1981.

112. Cramer, D. W., Welch, W. R., Hutchinson, G. B., Willett, W., and Scully, R. E., Dietary animal fat in relation to ovarian cancer risk, *Obstet. Gynecol.*, 63, 833, 1984.

113. Byers, T., Marshall, J., Graham, S., Mettlin, C., and Swanson, M., A case-control study of dietary and nondietary factors in ovarian cancer, *J. Natl. Cancer Inst.*, 71, 681, 1983.

114. La Vecchia, C., Franceschi, A., Decarli, A., Gentile, P., Liata, M., Regello, M., and Togoni, G., Coffee drinking and risk of epithelial ovarian cancer, *Int. J. Cancer*, 33, 559, 1984.

115. Trichopoulos, D., Papapostolou, M., and Polychronopoulou, A., Coffee and ovarian cancer, *Int. J. Cancer*, 28, 691, 1981.

116. Serra-Majem, L., La Vecchia, C., Ribas-Barba, L., Prieto-Ramos, F., Lucchini, F., Ramon, J. M., and Salleras, L., Changes in diet and mortality from selected cancers in southern Mediterranean countries, *Eur. J. Clin. Nutr.*, 47, S25, 1993.

Chapter 12

NUTRITION GUIDELINES DURING PREGNANCY AND LACTATION

Mary Story and Irene Alton

CONTENTS

0-8493-8502-4/96/$0.00+$.50
© 1996 by CRC Press, Inc.

I. NUTRITION GUIDELINES DURING PREGNANCY AND LACTATION

A woman's dietary intake and nutritional status prior to conception and during pregnancy profoundly influence embryonic and fetal development and the course and outcome of pregnancy. After delivery, dietary practices affect lactational performance and postpartum recovery. Promoting the positive nutritional status of women throughout the childbearing years will reduce the incidence of perinatal death, low birth weight, and developmental disabilities as well as improve maternal health and well-being. This chapter reviews the major preconceptional and periconceptional nutrition issues.

II. PRECONCEPTIONAL NUTRITION ISSUES

There is increasing evidence that prepregnancy and interpregnancy nutritional health significantly impact the outcome of a subsequent pregnancy. For example, data from the Special Supplemental Food Program for Women, Infants, and Children (WIC) have indicated a decreased incidence of low birth weight, a higher mean birth weight, and improved iron status in subsequent pregnancies of women who received postpartum WIC benefits.[1] Food shortages at the time of conception have been associated with perinatal mortality, congenital malformations, and low birth weight.[2]

Adequate nutrient stores and intakes at the time a woman enters pregnancy will help to assure normal embryonic and fetal development. Conversely, nutritional deficiencies as well as excesses (e.g., preformed vitamin A) may result in congenital malformations or spontaneous abortion. A large proportion of U.S. women of childbearing age, particularly those of low income, have been found in national surveys to have dietary intakes of several major nutrients which are significantly below recommended levels.[3] For example, 60% of women below the poverty level and 43% of higher income women had calcium intakes less than 70% of the recommended dietary allowances (RDA) for nonpregnant women. Only 10% of women met the RDA for iron and zinc, while 60 to 70% had iron intakes of less than 70% of the RDA. Nearly 40% of poor and 20% of higher income women had folate intakes less than 70% of recommended intake.[4] In addition, more than 50% of U.S. women consumed diets which may provide insufficient energy, protein, vitamins, and minerals. Thus they may enter pregnancy with inadequate diets.[5,6]

A. FOLATE AND NEURAL TUBE DEFECTS

The development of the central nervous system is especially sensitive to the nutritional environment during the first few weeks of gestation, before a woman is aware of her pregnancy.[7] This is dramatically demonstrated by the role of folate insufficiency in the etiology of both recurrent and first occurrence neural tube defects (NTDs) (i.e., spina bifida, anencephaly, encephalocele). In a large, randomized, double-blind trial, supplementation with 4.0 mg of folate, prior to and during early gestation, was demonstrated to have a 71% protective effect against the recurrence of NTDs in the offspring of women who had a previously affected pregnancy.[8] While women who have had an infant or fetus with a NTD are at greater risk for these birth defects in subsequent pregnancies, 95% of NTD cases are first occurrences.[9] A more recent Hungarian study (also randomized and double-blind in design) has provided conclusive evidence that folate supplementation (in this study, 0.8 mg/d for 1 month prior to conception and during early pregnancy) can reduce the risk of NTD occurrence.[10] Since the portion of the neural tube primarily affected by NTDs closes by the 20th day after conception,[11] adequate folate prior to pregnancy is essential to prevent malformations. The U.S. Public Health Service has thus recommended that all U.S. women of childbearing age who are capable of becoming pregnant consume 400 µg of folate per day, a level more than twice that of the RDA. This recommendation is expected to avert more than 50% of the 2000 to 3000 NTD cases which occur in the U.S. per year.[12]

It is not yet clear whether folate deficiency or a defect in the metabolism of folic acid is the cause of folate-related NTD cases,[13] nor is it clear what minimum dosage of folate is effective in preventing NTD cases or whether improved dietary intakes, fortification of certain foods, and/or vitamin supplementation is the best mode of achieving the recommended folate intake.

The current level of folate in the diets of U.S. women is approximately 180 µg/d. Careful selection of foods consistent with the Daily Food Guide Pyramid[14] (Table 1) can result in folate intakes of 400 µg/d, particularly if fortified breakfast cereals are included. Major dietary sources of folate include fortified cereals, dried beans, greens, broccoli, asparagus, spinach, and orange juice.

B. WEIGHT STATUS

Weight status, reflected by body mass index (BMI = wt/ht^2) is a major determinant of fetal growth and infant size. Women who enter pregnancy with a low BMI (<19.8) are at increased risk for delivering infants who are of low birth weight or small for gestational age (SGA). Underweight gravida may also be more likely to experience pregnancy complications such as infection, premature rupture of membranes, or anemia.[3,15] Women with eating disorders (anorexia nervosa or bulimia nervosa) who become pregnant are at increased risk for pregnancy complications including inadequate weight gain, hyperemesis, premature delivery, low birth weight, and perinatal mortality.[1,16]

TABLE 1
Daily Food Guide for Women

Food Group	Pre/Interpregnancy Servings/Day	Pregnancy/Lactation Servings/Day	Serving Size
Breads, fortified cereals, rice, pasta	6–11	6–11	1 slice bread 1 oz (3/4 to 1 cup) dry cereal 1/2 cup cooked rice, pasta, grits, or cereal 1/2 bun, bagel, or English muffin 1 6-in. tortilla 3 or 4 small plain crackers
Vegetables	3–5[a]	3–5[a]	1 cup raw leafy vegetables 1/2 cup of other kinds 3/4 cup vegetable juice
Fruits	2–4[b]	2–4[b]	1 medium apple, banana, or orange 1/2 cup of small or diced fruit 3/4 cup of fruit juice
Dairy products	2–3	3	1 cup of milk or yogurt 1-1/2 oz of cheese 2 oz of processed cheese
Meats, poultry, fish, dry beans and peas, eggs and nuts	2–3	3	2–3 oz of cooked lean meat, poultry, or fish 1/2 cup of cooked dry beans, 1 egg or 2 Tbsp of peanut butter = 1 oz of lean meat
Fats, oils and sweets	Use sparingly		

[a]   Include vitamin A source (broccoli, carrot, greens, spinach, squash, sweet potato).
[b]   Include vitamin C source (citrus/fortified juice, orange, grapefruit, cantaloupe, peppers, strawberries).

Modified from U.S. Department of Agriculture, Human Nutrition Information Service, The Food Guide Pyramid, Home and Garden Bulletin, No. 252 (HG-249), Hyattsville, MD, 1992.

Women with a very high BMI (>29.0) at conception are at greater risk for gestational diabetes, hypertension, operative delivery, large-for-gestational-age infants, and perinatal morbidity.[17] In addition, both low and high BMIs may adversely affect fertility.[1,2] Both weight change and resolution of eating disorders require long-term effort. To optimize fetal growth and pregnancy outcome in these high-risk women, weight control counseling and intervention in eating disorders must begin long before pregnancy is planned.

C. SUBSTANCE USE

Currently, approximately 30% of U.S. women smoke cigarettes, 20% are moderate to heavy drinkers, and 10% use illicit drugs.[5] Women who heavily use or abuse these substances prior to conception are likely to enter pregnancy with a low BMI and depleted nutrient stores. Since chemical dependency (particularly of cocaine) often requires long-term treatment, identification and management of substance abuse, as well as smoking cessation efforts prior to conception, will reduce the risk of fetal exposure and improve the woman's nutritional status as she enters pregnancy.

D. MEDICAL CONDITIONS

Iron deficiency anemia during pregnancy has been related to higher rates of prematurity and the delivery of low-birth-weight infants.[5] A recent study, however, has observed these adverse outcomes when anemia occurred in the first trimester only, rather than in later pregnancy.[18] Correction of anemia (hgb <12.0 g/dl) and replacement of iron stores prior to conception should thus reduce the likelihood of anemia in early gestation and lessen the risk of prematurity and low birth weight in a subsequent pregnancy. Improved iron status may also increase fertility.[1]

Good blood glucose control at the time of conception and during the early weeks of pregnancy when organogenesis is occurring will reduce the risk of spontaneous abortion and congenital anomalies in infants of diabetic women who are planning a pregnancy.[19] Adherence to a diet resulting in lowered blood phenylalanine levels in women with phenylketonuria (PKU) before conception will reduce the risk of microcephaly, mental retardation, and craniofacial and cardiac defects in their offspring.[7] Women with acquired immune deficiency syndrome (AIDS) may have a severely compromised nutritional status including protein-calorie malnutrition and deficiencies of vitamins and minerals such as zinc, calcium, vitamin A, vitamin C, and vitamin B_6.[5] Those who become pregnant are thus at extremely high nutritional risk. Women with long-term oral contraceptive use may have decreased blood levels of folate, vitamin C, vitamin B_6, vitamin B_{12}, and beta-carotene. These nutrient levels may not normalize until 4 months after discontinuing the pill.[5]

E. BREASTFEEDING PROMOTION

Most women make the decision to breastfeed prior to becoming pregnant. Educating women about the benefits of breastfeeding and breastfeeding promotion efforts in the preconceptional period are thus likely to improve breastfeeding rates and ultimately infant health.

F. NUTRITION SERVICES

To assure good pregnancy outcome, nutrition assessment and counseling of all women of childbearing age must be an integral part of preventive health care, family planning visits, and infertility care. Risk conditions which warrant nutrition management are included in Table 2.

TABLE 2
Indicators of Nutrition Risk

Risk Condition	Pre/Interpregnancy	Pregnancy	Lactation
Young maternal age	X	X	X
Poverty/homelessness	X	X	X
Complete vegetarianism	X	X	X
Anemia	X	X	X
AIDS	X	X	X
Gastrointestinal disorders	X	X	X
Phenylketonuria	X	X	X
Diabetes	X	X	X
Gestational diabetes		X	X
Eating disorders	X	X	X
Rigid dieting	X	X	X
Low/high BMI	X	X	X
Excessive/inadequate gestational weight gain		X	X
High parity/closely spaced pregnancy	X	X	X
Suspected IUGR		X	
Hyperemesis		X	
Long-term oral contraceptive use	X		
Excessive vitamin/mineral supplement use	X	X	X

III. PERICONCEPTIONAL NUTRITION ISSUES

Nutritional status during pregnancy is well recognized as a major and modifiable factor influencing maternal and newborn health. Dietary intake, hemoglobin level, and gestational weight gain are all key indicators of maternal nutritional status.

During pregnancy, energy and nutrient requirements are increased to support the growth and maintenance of maternal, placental, and fetal tissue. Higher rates of low birth weight have been associated with maternal diets low in energy and/or in several nutrients, including energy, protein, folate, iron, zinc, magnesium and B vitamins.[2] The higher nutrient needs of pregnancy are met primarily by increased dietary intakes, as well as alterations in nutrient absorption and/or metabolism and use of maternal stores.[3] Energy and nutrient needs during pregnancy are influenced by conditions such as adolescent growth, high levels of physical activity, multiple gestation, and substance abuse.

A. ENERGY

Sufficient energy in pregnancy is essential for optimal fetal growth and efficient utilization of protein, vitamins, and minerals. The energy cost of pregnancy is related to tissue synthesis, an increase in basal metabolism to support new tissue, and maternal fat stores. Recently, it has been demonstrated that both basal metabolism and fat storage are influenced by maternal energy status before and during pregnancy.[20] Total energy needs are thus variable and dependent on prepregnancy BMI, body composition, stage of pregnancy, and composition and amount of weight gain, as well as physical activity level and growth. The RDA for energy in pregnancy is 300 additional kilocalories per day during the second and third trimesters, based on theoretical changes in energy metabolism and maternal fat gain.[20,21] More recently, energy needs have been estimated to be as low as 150 kcal/d for some women.[22] It now appears that energy needs are lowest in underweight women and highest in obese women.[20] Younger adolescents have also been recently demonstrated to have higher energy needs to support adequate fetal growth than older adolescents or adults.[23]

Severe energy restriction in the first trimester has been related to higher rates of prematurity, perinatal mortality, and central nervous system (CNS) malformations.[24] Fetal growth retardation appears to be the primary effect of energy deficiency during the second and third trimesters. Less severe energy restriction may result in inadequate maternal weight gain and utilization of dietary protein as an energy source. In addition, fat mobilization resulting in ketonemia, which has recently been demonstrated to have adverse effects on infant behavioral and intellectual development, may occur.[25]

Since energy needs are highly variable and individual, no single value can be applied to all pregnant women. The best indicators of adequate energy intakes are maternal appetite and satisfactory weight gain.

B. PROTEIN

Additional protein is required for maternal, placental, and fetal tissue synthesis. Approximately 8.5 g of protein per day are needed to support peak fetal growth. Assuming a 70% efficiency of utilization, the RDA for protein is 10 additional grams or a total of 60 g/d.[21] Previous higher recommended intakes were based on erroneous estimates of protein storage during pregnancy. Average U.S. dietary intakes of protein are approximately 75 to 100 g/d, and inadequate intakes during pregnancy are infrequently reported.[26] Complete vegetarians who exclude all animal products or women with low energy intakes, as well as those with hyperemesis or eating disorders, may be at risk for low protein intakes. High protein supplements could potentially increase the risk of premature delivery and are not recommended during pregnancy.[27]

C. VITAMINS AND MINERALS

Tissue synthesis, increased metabolic demands, and fetal storage increase the need for most vitamins and minerals during pregnancy. Studies on dietary intakes of U.S. pregnant women indicate that mean intakes of several vitamins and minerals are consistently below the RDAs, including those of vitamin D, folate, vitamin B_6, iron, zinc, and calcium.[27] These nutrients are of special importance during pregnancy. Maternal vitamin D deficiency may have adverse effects on fetal growth, bone ossification, dental enamel formation, and neonatal calcium homeostasis.[28] Women who do not consume vitamin

D-fortified dairy products and do not get adequate sunlight exposure are at risk for vitamin D deficiency.[28] Vitamin B_6 deficiency has been associated with adverse effects on fetal growth and neonatal behavior.[29] The need for folate, required for nucleic acid synthesis, is higher in response to maternal and fetal tissue growth and increased erythropoiesis.[13] The RDA for folate is 400 µg, more than double that of the nonpregnant woman. Possible effects of folate insufficiency during pregnancy include fetal growth retardation, preterm delivery, spontaneous abortion, and congenital malformations.[27,30] The association of folate with NTDs is discussed in the preconceptional and supplement sections. Malabsorption syndromes, substance abuse, and the use of folate-antagonistic drugs place women at risk for folate deficiency.

Tissue growth, fetal stores, and maternal red cell mass expansion increase iron needs to nearly 6 mg/d during the second and third trimesters.[31] Despite enhanced absorption of dietary iron, insufficient intakes and marginal iron stores make iron deficiency anemia relatively common in pregnancy. At highest risk are adolescents, African Americans, and/or Hispanics, and women with high parity, short interpregnancy interval, multiple gestation, and low dietary intakes of meat or ascorbic acid.[27] According to 1990 pregnancy nutrition surveillance data, the prevalence of iron deficiency anemia is 25% in U.S. pregnant women as defined by the CDC criteria listed in Table 3. Higher rates were observed in African Americans (46%) and adolescents (37%).[31]

TABLE 3
Criteria for Anemia in Women

	Hemoglobin (g/dl) Below	Hematocrit (%) Below
Pre/interpregnancy	12.0	36
Pregnancy		
Trimester 1	11.0	33
Trimester 2	10.5	32
Trimester 3	11.0	33
Lactation	12.0	26

Note: Cigarette smoking raises cutoff (0.3 g/dl hb; 1.0% hct at 10 to 20 cigarettes per day and 0.5 g/dl hb; 1.5% hct at 20 to 40 per day) Altitude raises cutoff (e.g., 0.5 g/dl hb; 1.5% hct at 5,000 ft). Values in African Americans are approximately 0.5 g/dl hb; 1.5% hct.

Modified from Institute of Medicine, *Nutrition During Pregnancy and Lactation. An Implementation Guide.* National Academy of Sciences, Food and Nutrition Board, National Academy Press, Washington, D.C., 1992.

Several studies have found maternal iron deficiency anemia to significantly increase (by two- to threefold) the risk for prematurity and low birth weight, particularly in underweight women.[32,33] Recently, iron deficiency was found to be associated with these adverse outcomes only when it occurred in early pregnancy.[18] Decreased fetal iron stores may be an additional risk of maternal iron deficiency.[34]

The pregnancy RDA for iron is 30 mg/d, twice that for nonpregnant women.[21] Iron supplementation is necessary to achieve this level. Iron status can also be improved by increased consumption of meat, fish, poultry, and ascorbic acid, which enhance dietary iron absorption from nonheme sources.

The bone calcium content of the fetus is approximately 28 g, deposited primarily during the last trimester when skeletal growth is maximal. Changes in calcium metabolism as well as a nearly twofold increase in dietary calcium absorption help meet fetal needs while protecting maternal bone stores. There is some concern, however, that insufficient dietary calcium intakes may compromise maternal bone health or decrease fetal bone density. To support fetal bone mineralization and maintain maternal bone stores, the RDA during pregnancy is 1200 mg of calcium per day, 400 mg above the nonpregnant levels.[21] Higher calcium intakes (e.g., 1600 mg/d) may be desirable for adolescents.[35] Sufficient calcium intakes are especially important in those who are under age 25, since peak bone mass development is thought to occur prior to this age. Dairy products comprise more than 50% of dietary calcium intakes. Women with lactose intolerance, which improves during pregnancy, can usually tolerate small servings of milk as well as aged cheese, yogurt with live cultures, and enzyme-treated milk. Calcium-fortified orange juice can also provide significant amounts of this mineral (300 mg/8 oz).

The need for zinc increases in pregnancy in response to its role in protein and nucleic acid metabolism and cell replication. The zinc content of maternal, placental, and fetal tissue accumulation as well as expanded blood volume is approximately 300 mg and estimated needs are 2.6 mg/d during the second half of pregnancy.[36] While the pregnancy RDA for zinc is 15 mg/d, significantly lower intakes have been observed.[21,37] Although inconclusive, several studies have associated low maternal plasma or tissue zinc levels with pregnancy complications including hypertensive disorders, intrauterine growth retardation, prematurity, and congenital malformations, as well as prolonged labor, intrapartum hemorrhage, and maternal infections.[36] Risk conditions for zinc deficiency in pregnancy include complete vegetarianism, heavy tobacco or alcohol use, hyperemesis, inflammatory bowel disease, pica, and excessive iron or folate intakes.

D. VITAMIN AND MINERAL SUPPLEMENTS

Although national surveys have noted dietary intakes below the RDAs for several vitamins and minerals among U.S. pregnant women, food selection consistent with the Daily Food Guide Pyramid[14] can meet the nutrient needs of pregnancy (see Table 1). The exception is iron, which must be supplemented to prevent iron deficiency and maintain maternal iron stores. When it is necessary to use nutrient supplements, the practitioner and the woman should realize that supplements do not substitute for nutrition education and counseling, nor reduce the need for dietary improvement. To lessen the risk of nutrient excesses, imbalances, or fetal teratogenicity, women should be assessed for and cautioned against self-prescribed nutrient supplements or dosages. High doses of vitamin A (e.g., >10,000 IU/d), associated with CNS and renal anomalies, and vitamin D (>800 IU/d), associated with craniofacial anomalies in the offspring, are of particular concern.[6]

1. Iron

The Institute of Medicine (IOM) has recommended that all women routinely receive 30 mg of elemental iron per day during the second and third trimesters of pregnancy, when iron needs are greatest.[27] Recovery of iron stores in women who do not take iron supplements may take up to 2 years.[38]

The hemoglobin or hematocrit level should be determined at the first prenatal visit and periodically throughout pregnancy. If iron deficiency anemia is diagnosed (hemoglobin <11.0 g/dl during the first and third trimesters, and < 10.5 g/dl during the second trimester, when hemodilution is greatest [see Table 3]), supplementation with 60 to 120 mg of elemental iron is indicated until the anemia is resolved. A multivitamin-mineral supplement containing 15 mg zinc and 2 mg copper is also indicated when therapeutic doses of iron are used, because iron at this level may compete with zinc absorption and increased zinc intakes may compromise copper absorption and utilization.[27] The iron contained in the multivitamin-mineral supplement is not considered when treating anemia because the calcium, phosphate, and magnesium content of these supplements may inhibit iron absorption. Moreover, iron supplements should not be taken within 1 h of taking multivitamin-mineral supplements nor other inhibitors of iron absorption such as calcium supplements, dairy products, antacids, bran, whole grains, coffee, or tea.[40]

Poor compliance with iron supplementation in pregnancy is common, particularly among adolescents,[31] and may be related to gastrointestinal discomfort, difficulty swallowing tablets, or difficulty remembering to take them. Discussing the benefits of iron supplements for maternal well-being and infant health, suggestions to minimize gastrointestinal discomforts (e.g., taking with meals and gradually increasing the dosage), and ways to incorporate taking the supplement into daily activities may help improve compliance. Liquid iron can be used for those who cannot swallow tablets. If the hemoglobin does not improve after 2 to 4 weeks of iron therapy (which the woman has complied with), the diagnosis of iron deficiency should be confirmed by determining the serum ferritin level before iron therapy is continued. Values <20 μg indicate depleted iron stores, while higher levels suggest other causes of deficient hemoglobin level, such as infection or excess hemodilution. In the future, determining the serum transferrin receptor concentration will provide a more sensitive method of determining iron stores in pregnancy because its values are not affected by hemodilution or inflammation.[41]

2. Calcium

A supplement of 600 mg of elemental calcium per day, taken with meals to maximize acidity and solubility, is recommended when dietary intakes fail to supply 600 mg/d (eg., two servings of dairy products).[27] Although the calcium needs of pregnancy are relatively low (2 to 5% of average bone stores), calcium intakes below 600 mg/d have been associated with negative calcium balance in adults.[27] When vitamin D-fortified dairy products are not consumed and sunlight exposure is inadequate (e.g., those in northern climates during winter months), vitamin D supplementation of 5 μg/d may also be indicated.[27]

High doses of calcium supplements may increase the risk of kidney stones as well as adversely affect iron and zinc status and should be used with caution. Although the etiology of leg cramps associated with pregnancy is unknown, it is believed by some to be related to blood calcium levels. Because supplementation with 2 g of calcium in a double-blind study did not prove beneficial in relieving leg cramps,[42] the use of calcium supplements for this purpose does not appear to be warranted. Some studies have suggested that supplementation with 2 g calcium per day may reduce the incidence of gestational hypertension.[43] However, more evidence is needed before high levels of calcium supplements can be recommended to prevent hypertensive disorders of pregnancy.[27]

3. Folate

Based on a three- to fivefold protective effect of folic acid against the recurrence of NTDs noted by the Multivitamin Research Council study,[8] as well as other findings, the CDC and IOM have recommended folic acid supplementation for women with a history of a NTD-affected pregnancy. The recommended dose of 4.0 mg/d for at least 1 month prior to conception and during the first 12 weeks of gestation (based on the level used in the MRC study) must be taken under the supervision of a physician.

4. Multivitamin-Mineral Supplements

Routine use of relatively high doses of multivitamin-mineral supplements have been a long-accepted practice in obstetrical care. In low risk women consuming a nutritionally adequate diet, this may be unnecessary. The IOM has recommended the assessment of dietary practices and risk conditions and the use of a low-dose supplement when indicated.[40] Conditions warranting vitamin/mineral supplementation include failure to regularly consume a nutritionally adequate diet, multiple gestation, heavy cigarette smoking (20 or more per day), alcohol or drug abuse, complete vegetarianism, and/or treatment of anemia with therapeutic doses of iron.[27]

E. WEIGHT GAIN

Weight gain during pregnancy is a strong predictor of fetal growth and health, particularly during the second and third trimesters. Low gestational weight gains have been associated with higher rates of low birth weight, small-for-gestational-age infants, prematurity, and perinatal morbidity and mortality. The degree of effect gestational weight gain has on infant size is modified by prepregnancy weight status: a low prepregnancy weight increases the effect, and a high prepregnancy weight lessens it.[27] Thus, women who enter pregnancy with a low BMI, particularly if weight gain is inadequate, are at greater risk for adverse pregnancy outcome. Conversely, obese women tend to deliver infants of higher birth weight, despite lower gestational weight gain. Regardless of degree, however, gestational weight gain is linearly correlated with infant birth weight in women of all prepregnant weight categories, including the very obese.[44] Moreover, weight gains below 16 lb in obese women have been associated with higher rates of small-for-gestational-age infants and higher perinatal mortality rates.[17,45,46]

There is increasing evidence that gestational weight gain in younger adolescents has a greater effect on infant birth weight than in older adolescents or adults.[23,47,48] Young adolescents have been shown to require higher gestational weight gains to produce infants of birth weight comparable to those of older controls. Recently, in spite of higher weight gain, younger adolescents have been found to produce smaller infants and retain a larger proportion of gestational weight gain after delivery.[23]

Recommendations for gestational weight gain as well as observed mean weight gains during pregnancy have increased over the years, with a corresponding decreased incidence of low birth weight and perinatal morbidity and mortality. However, according to National Natality Survey data, African American women and adolescents (those at highest risk for delivering a low-birth-weight infant) were more likely to receive inappropriately low weight-gain advice.[49]

Based on the influence of prepregnancy weight status on fetal growth and a wide range of weight gains associated with good pregnancy outcomes, the IOM in 1990 recommended a range of gestational weight gains for four prepregnant weight categories (see Table 4).[27] Weight gains at the higher end of the range are recommended for young adolescents and African American women, and those at the lower end of the range are for women with heights under 62 in. The recommended weight gain for a twin pregnancy is approximately ten additional pounds.

In addition to total weight gain, the rate and pattern of weight gain have been shown to influence fetal growth and length of gestation. In adults, Abrahms found weight gains <270 g/week to be associated with a nearly threefold increase in the incidence of small-for-gestational-age infants,[50] while a similar low rate of gain during the second half of pregnancy resulted in higher rates of preterm delivery.[51] In adolescents, despite adequate total weight gains, early inadequate gains (<4.3 kg by 24 weeks gestation) were associated with increased rates of small-for-gestational-age infants, while late inadequate weight gain (<400/week after 24 weeks) resulted in higher rates of preterm deliveries.[52] Recommended rates of weight gain are listed in Table 5. Weight gains of less than 1 kg/month in women of normal prepregnancy BMI or less

TABLE 4
Recommended Weight Gain during Pregnancy

Prepregnant BMI	Weight Gain (lb)
Low (<19.8) (underweight)	28–40
Normal (19.8–26.0)	25–35
High (26.1–29.0) (overweight)	15–25
Very High (>29) (obese)	≥15

From Institute of Medicine, *Nutrition During Pregnancy and Lactation. An Implementation Guide,* National Academy of Sciences, Food and Nutrition Board, National Academy Press, Washington, D.C., 1992.

than 0.5 kg/month in women of high BMI, as well as gains in excess of 3 kg/month, warrant evaluation.[40] Potential causes of inadequate weight gain include insufficient energy intakes, high levels of physical activity or physically demanding employment, psychosocial stress, gastrointestinal or dental problems, chemical abuse, limited food access, carbohydrate intolerance, dieting, and eating disorders. Excessive weight gain may be related to high fat or energy intakes, infrequent large meals, or a low level of physical activity. High weight gains associated with fluid retention or following a recent rapid weight loss or cessation of smoking or chemical use should be differentiated from other causes and the woman should be reassured.

TABLE 5
Recommended Weight Gain Rate during Pregnancy

Prepregnant BMI	Trimester 1 (total lb.)	Trimester 2, 3 (lb/week)
Low	5	1 or more
Normal	3	1
High	2	0.66
Very high	1.5	0.5

From Institute of Medicine, *Nutrition During Pregnancy: Part I. Weight Gain, Part II. Nutrient Supplements,* Committee on Nutrition Status During Pregnancy and Lactation, Food and Nutrition Board, National Academy Press, Washington, D.C., 1990.

F. SUBSTANCE USE

In addition to direct, adverse effects on the fetus, the nutrition-related consequences of tobacco, alcohol, and drug use can further compromise pregnancy outcome. Potential effects of chemical use on maternal nutritional status include decreased nutrient intake, reduced nutrient absorption, increased nutrient losses, or altered nutrient metabolism and utilization.

Cigarette smoking has been associated with lower gestational weight gains, which may be the result of alterations in energy metabolism, and decreased placental transfer of zinc.[53,54] Smokers tend to have poorer eating habits than nonsmokers, including breakfast-skipping and lower dietary intakes of protein, zinc, iron, and B-complex vitamins.[5] Moreover, smokers have been observed to have decreased plasma levels of several nutrients including vitamin C, folate, beta carotene, and vitamins B_6 and E. Tobacco use may alter the metabolism of nutrients and result in increased requirements.[5]

High intakes of alcohol may result in altered metabolism and utilization of amino acids, folate, zinc, and vitamin B_6. Alcohol increases zinc excretion, reduces placental amino acid transport, and interferes with enzyme activity related to nucleic acid synthesis.[5] Illicit drug use, particularly of cocaine, has been associated with poor dietary habits. Lower serum ferritin levels as well as lower blood levels of folate and vitamin C have been observed in women who used drugs during pregnancy.[5]

G. MEDICAL CONDITIONS

To achieve normal fetal size and good pregnancy outcome, strict maternal blood glucose control is essential in pregnancies complicated by diabetes. Women with PKU require rigid dietary adherence to prevent elevated blood phenylalanine level and increased risk of mental retardation in the infant. Women with AIDS are likely to have multiple nutrition problems, including protein-calorie malnutrition, vitamin and mineral deficiencies, and inadequate weight gain, and thus require intensive nutrition management.

H. NUTRITION SERVICES

The IOM has recommended that all women receive nutrition assessment and individualized care during pregnancy, regardless of level of nutrition risk, socioeconomic status, health status, or type of care provider.[55] Nutrition services have demonstrated to be not only effective in improving pregnancy outcome, but cost effective. Recently, it has been observed that women who did not receive advice on vitamin use, dietary intake, weight gain, and avoidance of tobacco, alcohol, and drugs were 1.3 times more likely to deliver a low-birth-weight infant.[56] Women at high risk for nutrition problems will require intensive nutrition services and care (see Table 2).

IV. LACTATION

An adequate volume of breast milk of appropriate nutrient composition can be produced despite suboptimal dietary intakes by drawing on maternal nutrient stores and tissue reserves. Nutrient levels maintained at maternal expense include those of protein, fat, carbohydrate, folate, and most minerals, including calcium. In contrast, low dietary intakes of most vitamins, particularly of vitamin B_6, A, and D, are reflected in decreased breast milk levels.[56,57] If the woman has experienced long-term dietary inadequacies, nutrient stores may be depleted and breast milk composition of all nutrients may be altered. Severe maternal malnutrition may interfere with breast milk production, secretion, and possibly immunologic properties.[56]

Nutrient needs are increased during lactation in accordance with the volume of breast milk produced and the duration of breastfeeding. Recommended intakes of nutrients are higher than those of pregnancy, with the exception of folate, calcium, phosphorus, iron, and vitamins D, K, and B_6.[21] Nutrient RDAs for lactation are highest during the first 6 months, when breast milk volume is approximately 20% higher, than during the second 6 months.[21]

A. ENERGY

The energy cost of lactation is influenced by the volume of milk produced and maternal energy reserves, activity level, and growth status. Based on an estimated 80% efficiency in converting dietary energy to breast milk energy, 80 kcal are needed to produce 1 ml of breast milk containing 70 kcal/ml. The energy needed to exclusively breastfeed a single infant during the first 6 months of lactation would thus be approximately 640 kcal/d, and during the second 6 months, 510 kcal/d. The RDA of an additional 500 kcal/d throughout lactation assumes the availability of approximately 2 to 3 kg of fat deposited during pregnancy to support breast milk production. Women who are underweight, who gained weight inadequately during pregnancy, or who are highly active physically, as well as younger adolescents, will require higher energy intakes (e.g., 650 kcal/d) while lactating.[56,57]

Energy intakes of 2600 kcal/d were found in one study to be too high to facilitate weight loss, while those of 2200 kcal/d appeared to be consistent with successful lactation and gradual weight reduction. The IOM recommends an energy intake of at least 1800 kcal/d to assure adequate milk production and cautions against intakes of less than 1500 kcal/d.[56] Chronically low energy intakes (e.g., <1500 kcal/d) may decrease milk volume to a level of clinical significance to the infant.[57]

B. PROTEIN

Based on the average protein content of breast milk (1.1 g/dl) and a 70% efficiency in converting dietary protein to breast milk protein, the RDA for lactation is 15 g of additional protein per day.[21] U.S. women tend to have ample dietary protein intakes and usually do not require additional amounts to achieve this recommended intake. Complete vegetarians or women with eating disorders may be at risk for insufficient protein intakes. Failure to consume the RDA for protein may result in significant mobilization of a woman's lean tissue stores. For example, a 60-kg woman of 25% body fat could lose approximately 20% of tissue protein to support 6 months of breastfeeding.[56]

C. VITAMINS AND MINERALS

Although dietary intake data on U.S. lactating women are limited, several nutrients (e.g., calcium, magnesium, zinc, folate, and vitamin B_6) are estimated to be below the RDAs based on average nutrient density per 1000 kcal. Some women appear to be at higher risk for suboptimal nutrient intakes. For example, low vitamin A intakes have been observed in low-income women; low calcium, magnesium, and vitamin A levels in African American women; and low iron intakes in adolescents.[56]

Energy intakes consistent with the RDA (e.g., 2700 kcal/d) are also likely to provide recommended intakes of vitamins and minerals with the exception of calcium and zinc. Lower energy intakes are likely to supply insufficient quantities of several nutrients. The vitamin content of breast milk is reflective of maternal intakes. Low intakes of vitamins A, D, B_6, riboflavin, and niacin have been observed to result in lower breast milk levels of these nutrients. Very low maternal intakes of vitamins B_{12} and thiamin have been associated with clinical deficiencies in the infant. Excessive maternal dosages of vitamins A and D may expose the infant to toxic levels of these vitamins.[56] The folate content of breast milk appears to be higher than previously thought (85 vs. 50 μg/dl).[56] The IOM thus recommends an intake of 320 μg/d, which is higher than the RDA of 280 μg/d. Folate stores can be drawn upon to maintain breast milk folate levels, but are quickly depleted.

While breast milk levels of calcium, iron, and zinc are maintained with maternal stores if dietary intakes are low, depletion of stores may occur within a few months, particularly among low-income women or young adolescents. Insufficient dietary calcium intakes may result in mobilization of up to 8% of maternal calcium stores during 6 months of breastfeeding.[56] The long-term effect of this bone loss on maternal bone density is unknown. The RDA for calcium during lactation is 1200 mg/d.[21] Higher intakes (e.g., 1600 mg) may be desirable for young adolescents.[35] The iron demands of lactation are not significant (0.15 to 0.3 mg/d), particularly if menstruation has not resumed.[21] However, depletion of maternal iron stores may occur if dietary intakes have been marginal. The RDA for iron is not increased over prepregnant levels during lactation.

D. VITAMIN AND MINERAL SUPPLEMENTS

The nutrient demands of lactation can be met by the selection of foods according to the Daily Food Guide Pyramid (Table 1).[14] Routine vitamin or mineral supplementation of breastfeeding women is thus not indicated. Complete vegetarians will require supplementation of vitamin B_{12} (2.6 μg/d) and possibly vitamin D (10 μg/d) if sunlight exposure is minimal (IOM). Supplementation with calcium (600 mg/d elemental) may be indicated in women who are unable to consume at least 600 mg of calcium per day. Women with restricted energy intakes may also require multivitamin-mineral supplementation. Women should be cautioned against excessive doses of vitamins and minerals, particularly of vitamins A and D, to avoid exposure of the infant to toxic levels of nutrients.

E. WEIGHT STATUS

For approximately 80% of women, the energy demands of lactation typically result in weight losses of 0.5 to 1.0 kg during the first 4 to 6 months, followed by a slower rate of loss.[56] Lactation is not affected by gradual weight loss or moderate physical activity.[57,58] Overweight women should be counseled to lose 1 to 2 kg/month through increased physical activity and a balanced diet low in fat and sugars after lactation is well established. Rigid dieting and weight loss medications or products are contraindicated.[56] Weight loss is especially important in women who had gestational diabetes (because they are at greater risk for developing type II diabetes mellitus than the general population) as well as those who experienced excessive weight gain during pregnancy.

F. SUBSTANCE USE

Nicotine, alcohol, illicit drugs, and caffeine are excreted in breast milk and have adverse effects on the infant. In addition, breast milk volume can be reduced by cigarette smoking, which inhibits prolactin levels, and by alcohol, which interferes with the milk ejection reflex. Breastfeeding women should be advised to avoid tobacco and illicit drugs and to avoid or limit alcohol intake to <0.5 kg of body weight (12 oz beer = 13 g; 3.5 oz wine = 10 g; 1.5 oz liquor = 15 g alcohol) and to limit caffeine-containing beverages to one to two servings per day.[56]

G. NUTRITION SERVICES

All breastfeeding women should receive nutrition assessment, education, and counseling. To achieve optimal infant growth and development and maternal health, those conditions indicating the need for intensive nutrition follow-up are listed in Table 2.

V. SUMMARY

During pregnancy there is an increased need for nutrients. Women who enter pregnancy undernourished and/or who have an inadequate diet during pregnancy have an increased risk of adverse fetal development and also delivering a low-birth-weight infant. Well-nourished women during pregnancy generally give birth to healthier, heavier babies. Poorly nourished women who eat well and gain adequate weight can greatly improve their chances of giving birth to healthier infants.

Emphasis on remedying preconceptional nutrition problems may also reduce the risk of a poor pregnancy outcome. There is increased evidence that prepregnancy and interpregnancy nutritional health may positively impact pregnancy outcome.

The post-partum period is important to reestablish nutrient reserves and modify body weight if needed. This is also a nutritionally important time for women who choose to breastfeed, as an adequate quality and quantity of food intake is needed for both maternal health and quantity of milk production. Clearly, a focus on maternal nutrition is required during all phases of reproductive life to maximize maternal and fetal health.

REFERENCES

1. Brown, J. E., Preconceptional nutrition and reproductive outcome, *Ann. N. Y. Acad. Sci.,* 67, 286, 1993.
2. Wynn, A., Crawford, M., Doyle, W., and Wynn, S., Nutrition in women in anticipation of pregnancy, *Nutr. Health*, 7, 69, 1991.
3. Abrahms, B. and Berman, C., Women, nutrition and health, *Curr. Probl. Obstet. Gynecol. Fertil.*, 3, 1993.
4. Block, G. and Abrahms, B., Vitamin and mineral status of women of childbearing potential, *Ann. N.Y. Acad. Sci.,* 678, 244, 1993.
5. Bendich, A., Lifestyle and environmental factors that can adversely affect maternal and nutritional status and pregnancy outcomes, *Ann. N.Y. Acad. Sci.*, 678, 255, 1993.
6. Schaeffer, D. M., Maternal nutritional factors and congenital anomalies: a guide for epidemiological investigation, *Ann. N.Y. Acad. Sci.,* 678, 205, 1993.
7. Sulik, K. K. and Sadler, T. W., Postulated mechanisms underlying the development of neural tube defects, *Ann. N.Y. Acad. Sci.,* 678, 8, 1993.
8. MRC Vitamin Study Research Group, Prevention of neural tube defects: results of the Medical Research Council vitamin study, *Lancet,* 338, 131, 1991.
9. Wald, N., Folic acid and the prevention of neural tube defects, *Ann. N.Y. Acad. Sci.,* 678, 112, 1993.
10. Czeizel, A. and Dudas, I., Prevention of the first occurrence of neural tube defects by periconceptional vitamin supplementation, *N. Engl. J. Med.,* 327, 1832, 1992.
11. Hine, J., Folic acid: contemporary clinical perspective, *Perspect. Appl. Nutr.,* 1, 3, 1993.
12. Centers for Disease Control, Use of folic acid for prevention of spina bifida and other neural tube defects, 1983–1991, *Morbid. Mortal. Wkly Rep.*, 40, 513, 1991.
13. Shorah, C. J., Habibzadeh, N., Wild, J., and Smithells, R. W., Possible abnormalities of folate and vitamin B_{12} metabolism associated with neural tube defects, *Ann. N.Y. Acad. Sci.,* 678, 81, 1993.
14. USDA: Food Guide Pyramid, Home and Garden Bulletin #252, U.S. Department of Agriculture, Hyattsville, MD, 1992.
15. Edwards, L. E., Alton, I. R., Barrada, I., and Hakanson, E. Y., Pregnancy in the underweight woman. Course, outcome and growth patterns of the infants, *Am. J. Obstet. Gynecol.*, 135, 297, 1979.
16. Franko, D. and Walton, B., Pregnancy and eating disorders: a review and clinical implications, *Int. J. Eating Disorders*, 13, 41, 1993.
17. Edwards, L. E., Dickes, W. F., Alton, I., and Hakanson, E. Y., Pregnancy in the massively obese. Course, outcome and obesity prognosis in the infant, *Am. J. Obstet. Gynecol.*, 131, 479, 1978.
18. Scholl, T. O. and Hediger, M. L., Anemia and iron-deficiency anemia: compilation of data on pregnancy outcome, *Am. J. Clin. Nutr.*, 59(Suppl.), 492S, 1994.

19. Jovanovic-Peterson, L. and Peterson, C. M., Abnormal metabolism and the risk for birth defects with emphasis on diabetes, *Ann. N.Y. Acad. Sci.,* 678, 228, 1993.

20. King, J. C., Butte, N. F., Bronstein, M. N., Kopp, L. E., and Lindquist, S. A., Energy metabolism during pregnancy: influence of maternal energy status, *Am. J. Clin. Nutr.,* 59(Suppl.), 439S, 1994.

21. National Research Council, *Recommended Dietary Allowances,* 10th ed., National Academy Press, Washington, D. C., 1989.

22. Durnin, J. V., Energy requirements of pregnancy, *Diabetes,* 40(Suppl. 2), 151S, 1991.

23. Scholl, T. O., Hediger, M. L., Schall, J., and Fischer, R. L., Maternal growth during pregnancy and the competition for nutrients, *Am. J. Clin. Nutr.,* in press.

24. Keen, C. L. and Zidenberg-Cherr, S., Should vitamin-mineral supplements be recommended for all women with childbearing potential?, *Am. J. Clin. Nutr.,* 59(Suppl.), 532S, 1994.

25. Rizzo, T., Metzger, B., Burns, W., and Burns, K., Correlations between antepartum maternal metabolism and intelligence of offspring, *N.Engl. J. Med.,* 325, 911, 1991.

26. U.S. Department of Health and Human Services, *The Surgeon General's Report on Nutrition and Health,* U.S. Public Health Service, Washington, D.C., 1988.

27. Institute of Medicine, *Nutrition During Pregnancy: Part I. Weight Gain, Part II. Nutrient Supplements.* Committee on Nutrition Status During Pregnancy and Lactation, Food and Nutrition Board, National Academy Press, Washington, D.C., 1990.

28. Specker, B. L., Do North American women need supplemental vitamin D during pregnancy or lactation?, *Am. J. Clin. Nutr.,* 59(Suppl.), 484S, 1994.

29. Kirksey, A. and Wasynczuk, A. Z., Morphologic, biochemical, and functional consequences of vitamin B6 deficits during central nervous system development, *Ann. N.Y. Acad. Sci.,* 678, 62, 1993.

30. Goldenberg, R., Tamura, T., Cliver, S., Cutter, G., Hoffman, H., and Copper, R., Serum folate and fetal growth retardation: a matter of compliance?, *Obstet. Gynecol.,* 79, 719, 1992.

31. Beard, J. L., Iron deficiency: assessment during pregnancy and its importance in pregnant adolescents, *Am. J. Clin. Nutr.,* 59(Suppl.), 502S, 1994.

32. Lieberman, E., Ryan, K. J., Monson, R. R., and Schoenbaum, S. C., Association of maternal hematocrit with premature labor, *Am. J. Obstet. Gynecol.,* 159, 107, 1988.

33. Scholl, T. O., Hediger, M. L., Fischer, R. L., and Shearer, J. W., Anemia vs. iron deficiency: increased risk of preterm delivery in a prospective study, *Am. J. Clin. Nutr.,* 55, 985, 1992.

34. Puolakka, J., Janne, O., Pakarinan, A., and Vihko, R., Evaluation by serum ferritin assay of the influence of maternal iron stores on the iron status of newborns and infants, *Acta Obstet. Gynecol. Scand.,* 95, 53, 1980.

35. Matkovic, V., Fontana, D., Tominac, C., and Goel, P., Factors that influence peak bone mass formation: a study of calcium balance and the inheritance of bone mass in adolescent females, *Am. J. Clin. Nutr.,* 52, 878, 1990.

36. Jameson, S., Zinc status in pregnancy: the effect of zinc therapy on perinatal mortality prematurity, and placental ablation, *Ann. N.Y. Acad. Sci.,* 678, 178, 1993.

37. Keen, C. L., Taubeneck, M. W., Daston, G. P., Rogers, J. M., and Gershwin, M. E., Primary and secondary zinc deficiency as factors underlying abnormal CNS development, *Ann. N.Y. Acad. Sci.,* 678, 37, 1993.

38. Taylor, D., Mallen, C., McDougall, N., and Lind, T., Effect of iron supplementation on serum ferritin levels during and after pregnancy, *Br. J. Obstet. Gynecol.,* 89, 1011, 1982.

39. Centers for Disease Control, CDC criteria for anemia in children and childbearing age women, *Morbid. Mortal.Wkly. Rep.,* 38, 400, 1989.

40. Institute of Medicine, *Nutrition During Pregnancy and Lactation. An Implementation Guide,* National Academy Press, Washington, D.C., 1992.

41. Carriaga, M. T., Skikne, B. S., Finley, B., Cutler, B., and Cook, J. D., Serum transferrin receptor for the detection of iron deficiency in pregnancy, *Am. J. Clin. Nutr.,* 54, 1077, 1991.

42. Hammar, M., Berg, G., Solheim, F., and Larsson, L., Calcium and magnesium status in pregnant women. A comparison between treatment with calcium and vitamin C in pregnant women with leg cramps, *Int. J. Vitam. Nutr. Res.*, 57, 179, 1987.

43. Prentice, A., Maternal calcium requirements during pregnancy and lactation, *Am. J. Clin. Nutr.,* 59(Suppl.), 477S, 1994.

44. Seidman, D. S., Ever-Hadani, P., and Gale, R., The effect of maternal weight gain in pregnancy on birth weight, *Obstet. Gynecol.*, 74, 240, 1989.

45. Parker, J. D. and Abrams, B. F., Prenatal weight gain advice: an examination of the recent prenatal weight gain recommendations of the Institute of Medicine, *Obstet. Gynecol.*, 79, 664, 1992.

46. Naeye, R. L., Weight gain and the outcome of pregnancy, *Am. J. Obstet. Gynecol.*, 135, 3, 1979.

47. Frisancho, A. R., Matos, J., and Flegel, P., Maternal nutritional status and adolescent pregnancy outcome, *Am. J. Clin. Nutr.*, 38, 739, 1983.

48. Haiek, L. and Lederman, S. A., The relationship between maternal weight for height and term birth weight in teens and adult women, *J. Adolesc. Health Care,* 10, 16, 1989.

49. Taffel, S. M., Keppel, K. G., and Jones, G. K., Medical advice on maternal weight gain and actual weight gain: results of the 1988 national maternal and infant health survey, *Ann. N.Y. Acad. Sci.,* 678, 293, 1993.

50. Abrahms, B. F. and Newman, V., Small for gestational age birth: maternal predictors and comparison with risk factors of spontaneous preterm delivery in the same cohort, *Am. J. Obstet. Gynecol.*, 164, 785, 1991.

51. Abrams, B. F., Newman, V., Key, T., and Parker, J. D., Maternal weight gain and preterm delivery, *Obstet. Gynecol.,* 74, 577, 1989.

52. Hediger, M. L., Scholl, T. O., Belsky, D. H., Ances, I. G., and Salmon, R. W., Patterns of weight gain in adolescent pregnancy: effects on birth weight and preterm delivery, *Obstet. Gynecol.*, 74, 6, 1989.

53. Kuhnert, B., Kuhnert, P., Groh-Wargo, S., Erhard, P., and Leaebnik, N., Smoking alters the relationship between maternal zinc intake and biochemical indices of fetal zinc status, *Am. J. Clin. Nutr.,* 55, 981, 1992.

54. National Research Council, *Nutrition Services in Perinatal Care*, 2nd ed., National Academy Press, Washington, D.C., 1992.

55. Kogan, M., Alexander, G., Kotelchuck, M., and Nagey, D., Relation of the content of prenatal care to the risk of low birth weight: maternal reports of health behaviors advice and initial prenatal care procedures, *J.A.M.A.*, 271, 1340, 1994.

56. National Research Council, *Nutrition During Lactation*, National Academy Press, Washington, D.C., 1991.

57. Butte, N. F., Garza, C., Stuff, J. E., O'Brian, Smith, E., and Nichols, B. L., Effect of maternal diet and body composition on lactational performance, *Am. J. Clin. Nutr.*, 39, 296, 1984.

58. Dewey, K. G. and McCrory, M. A., Effects of lactation and physical activity on pregnancy and lactation, *Am. J. Clin. Nutr.*, 59(Suppl.), 446S, 1994.

Chapter 13

NUTRITIONAL CONCERNS OF THE FEMALE RECREATIONAL ATHLETE

Catherine G. Ratzin Jackson

CONTENTS

I. INTRODUCTION — DEFINING THE FEMALE RECREATIONAL ATHLETE

A. INCIDENCE IN THE POPULATION AND DIFFICULTY OF STUDY

Although true numbers are difficult to estimate, it has been reported that almost 40% (37.7%) of the adult female population of the U.S., those who are over 18 years old, claim they exercise or play sports regularly.[1] Projecting this to the estimated number of adult American women in 1995, this represents approximately 48 million exercisers. The activity she chooses to do most is "exercise walking", which represents about 37% of this population. The other most chosen activities in descending order are swimming (30%), bicycle riding (23%), aerobic exercise and camping (18%), and exercising with equipment (17%).[1] However, this vast population receives virtually no notice in scientific studies related to nutrition and performance. There are also no clear definitions of recreational athletes, but recreational activities usually involve an element of choice and the desire for a pleasureable experience or fun.[2] The recreational female athlete is sometimes defined as someone who does not receive coaching, but many women exercise at relatively high levels with no coach; they follow suggestions found in the popular press and hints from other exercisers. This vast population must rely on extrapolated nutrition and exercise information from high-performance female athletes who comprise a very small percentage of the population, about whom there is yet another dearth of data, since a much smaller number of studies have been completed on women athletes compared to men. A nutrition book designated specifically for the recreational athlete has only recently been published.[3]

It is of some interest that the reason sometimes given for this lack of attention is that females have only "recently" begun all this exercise, but the personal experiences of many women belie this concept. There has been an explosive growth of women in sport over the last 25 years; prior to that women have been exercising as long as men have, only they have called it work. Women have only "recently" been recognized. A more cogent explanation understood by many female nutritionists and exercise physiologists is that the population of convenience for numerous studies is the college-age male, about whom we have more information than any other human group on earth, who is chosen partially because there is a large data base with which to compare results and partially because research is done at colleges and universities which they attend. Research done on females often uses small numbers of subjects and has few, if any, studies with which to compare findings, thereby making the research more difficult and frustrating. It is also sometimes necessary to discount the influence of menstrual cycle on findings, thereby making it somewhat more complicated. However, the current trend is to at least recognize that this work needs to be done, thereby greatly improving the chances that the recreational female athlete data base will be expanded.

B. STEREOTYPES

When females are studied there is a heightened focus on psychological aberrations, as has been shown to be prevalent in the medical treatment of women for quite some time. Physiological explanations for results are not as apparent and sometimes discounted. This bias can be found in the most fundamental areas of study, as illustrated in one of the most respected texts used in medical schools.[4] After the author concluded that most data have been collected on young males and that females have lower relative values in performance indicators and higher values for body fat, which suggest that women will not be as fast or strong but might have more endurance, it was stated:

> Finally, one cannot neglect the effect of the sex hormones on temperament. There is no doubt that testosterone promotes aggressiveness and that estrogen is associated with a more mild temperament. Certainly a large part of competitive sports is the aggressive spirit that drives a person to maximum effort, often at the expense of judicious restraint.

The author of that comment probably never met a female recreational fencer with a weapon in her hand. The result of these stereotypes is that women recreational athletes are virtually forgotten and are frequently mentioned almost as an afterthought in studies where they are sometimes listed as "active", perhaps suggesting a level of physical exercise above comatose. If the woman happens to be in the little-studied generation of 40 to 50, she most certainly finds that she is treated as if she does not exist, but becomes reestablished as a sentient being when she becomes postmenopausal. Therefore, this chapter must use information gleaned from studies of female athletes who tend to participate for reasons other than enhancement of health and fun and from studies where the recreational athlete has not been the major focus of the research.

II. DIETARY CONCERNS

A. ENERGY METABOLISM

In order to understand an activity and how to best meet dietary needs, it is first important to determine whether it is nonaerobic, anaerobic, aerobic, or some combination of types. There are many misconceptions about nutrition and exercise which can be traced directly back to a poor understanding of energy metabolism. Not all dietary practices should be used for all activities, as there now emerges the concept of specificity of nutritional practice, as has been recognized for some time in types of exercise.[5] It is not the intent of this chapter to explore this issue in detail and the reader is directed to texts in exercise physiology and other nutrition books for detailed information.

In general, short term and highly intense activities are nonaerobic and do not depend to a great extent on anything other than stores of ATP immediately available in the exercising muscle. The dietary practices of the exerciser under these circumstances would have little effect on energy availability. When exercise progresses in time to 1 to 3 min, always considering that intensity will change the time frame, an activity stresses the lactic acid system and there is a high reliance on carbohydrate stores for energy production. Should activity progress at least 5 min, the activity is characterized by aerobic metabolism and, while carbohydrate stores are necessary for the process to continue, the muscle can now use fat and protein for energy production. While the contribution of fat and carbohydrate is somewhat understood, the amount of energy delivery from protein is still not clear, but it is thought that a person who exercises aerobically uses it to a greater degree than one who exercises anaerobically.

B. GENERAL DIETARY ISSUES

Energy or caloric intake needs to be adequate to meet not only the needs for basal metabolism, which is the greatest need for calories in the body, but the additional activity must be covered. It is not known how the female recreational athlete would be categorized for energy intake purposes, but it is stated that approximately 26% of the female population of the U.S. self-reports that they are 20% or more over desirable weight standards.[1] Self-reporting and other methods of diet assessment may not produce completely accurate information, but they are useful to follow trends where there is concern for the prevention of disease.[6] While there is a concern for obesity, on one hand, and the need to lower fat and cholesterol in the diet for concerns about cardiovascular disease, there is another concern when caloric intake is reduced without making appropriate food choices to cover the needs of the body. The American diet in general has been changing and healthier patterns are developing, but the latest data show that the majority of women 19 to 50 years old failed to consume recommended amounts of iron, calcium, magnesium, zinc, vitamin B_6, vitamin A, and folacin.[7] This occurred in conjuction with the report that about six out of ten women take supplements in addition to their normal diet. Fat intakes have been decreasing, although they are not yet low enough, and carbohydrate intakes have been increasing. Dietary fiber intakes are not yet high enough to eliminate concerns about cancer.[7] The implications become clear that sound nutrition advice is extremely important for the recreational female athlete.

C. MACRONUTRIENT RECOMMENDATIONS

It is difficult to recommend general guidelines for energy intake and individual needs should be carefully assessed, but certain patterns emerge. There are concerns that particular groups of female athletes are at risk for diet-related health problems if they consume too few calories and make poor food choices.[8,9] While competitive athletes seem to have difficulty, it is thought that recreational athletes fare better in dietary practices than their inactive counterparts, but continue to have lower than recommended intakes of iron and calcium.[10] The ideal diet for an individual athlete or sport is still uncertain but is similar to recommendations made for the general population with higher carbohydrate intake required. It has been suggested that athletes consume 10 to 15% protein, 30 to 35% fat, and 50 to 60% carbohydrate.[11] There are sport-specific recommendations,[12] but, in general, recreational athletes would do well to have a nutritional analysis done to determine exactly what their particular pattern has become and then modify their diets to match the aforementioned suggestions for macronutrients.

The macronutrient which will have the greatest effect in the recreational athlete is water. It is not the intent of this chapter to explore this issue, but it can be stated that one of the greatest affectors of performance is the hydration state of the athlete. The less conditioned the individual the greater the reliance on hydration state for the proper functioning of the body with respect to the sweat response and for the maintainance of proper blood volume. In general, if an individual is thirsty she is already dehydrated. The reader is directed to other sources for detailed information on this topic written specifically for the recreational athlete[13] and for more detail in nutrition for women athletes.[14,15]

D. WEIGHT CONTROL

Conditioning changes much of the physiology of the body and not all is known as to how this affects weight control. The physiology of the obese individual may be altered in some way to maintain the obesity, since it has been shown that fat calories may be stored preferentially in obese women who reduce their weight, thereby assuring resumption of the weight lost.[16] Obese individuals also consume higher amounts of dietary fat and added sugar than lean individuals, even when energy intakes are the same.[17] Exercise has a positive effect in metabolizing the lipids in the diet if they are consumed.[18] The regional distribution of fat may also play a role in the ease with which weight may be maintained or lost; upper body obesity in females is more closely associated with abnormalities in metabolism than lower body obesity.[19] Diet composition and activity patterns seem to have a greater association with the amount of body fat than the number of calories consumed.[17] In normal individuals, exercise combined with diet has been shown to be the most effective way to keep weight stable, a practice which is considered the most healthy.[20,21] The recidivism rate for weight loss is very high and is lowered when exercise practices developed during weight loss are maintained as part of the life-style.[22] Dieting alone has serious consequences in loss of muscle protein and changes in metabolism associated with not being able to maintain the weight loss for long periods of time.[23] Exercise may also subtly change appetite and brain regulation, which has the effect of placing the individual in caloric deficit and ultimate weight loss.[24]

E. MICRONUTRIENT RECOMMENDATIONS

As previously stated, women in the U.S. show that they consume levels of iron, calcium, magnesium, zinc, vitamin B_6, vitamin A, and folacin below the recommended dietary allowance (RDA).[7] It is recognized that intakes below the RDA do not necessarily indicate that deficiencies exist. The RDAs are allowance levels for large population groups and are intentionally set high to cover the needs of almost everyone within a specific category. With respect to athletes, vitamin and mineral supplements are commonly used and deficiencies usually coexist with restricted food intake.[25] The reports of deficiencies appear to be specific to the groups investigated, but it is usually recognized that, as seen in the general population, female athletes usually have low intakes of calcium, iron, and zinc.

Vitamin and mineral supplements are generally safe unless large doses are consumed and caution should be used in self-administered megadose therapy where the supplement achieves pharmacological status. Since vitamin and mineral supplements are more commonly used by females, some attention will be given to safety of their use. Fat-soluble vitamins are generally more toxic than water-soluble vitamins and recent information indicates several concerns.[26-29] Two fat-soluble vitamins are associated with high dosage problems. Vitamin A intoxication has commonly been reported at levels of approximately 25,000 $IU \cdot d^{-1}$.[26-29] Some of the symptoms of toxicity include abdominal pain, anorexia, blurred vision, headache, drowsiness, muscle weakness, nausea, and vomiting. Vitamin E seems to have no side effects unless 300 $IU \cdot d^{-1}$ is exceeded. Symptoms of toxicity include nausea, fatigue, headache, elevation of serum lipids and double vision; high intakes also interfere with vitamin K activity.[27]

Water-soluble vitamins were thought to be very safe, but this has proved to be untrue in some cases. Pyridoxine (vitamin B_6) is neuroactive and produces symptoms of sensory neuropathy. The level shown to produce symptoms has consistently with time been reported lower and lower in the literature and the toxicity threshold for some individuals may be as low as 300 to 500 $mg \cdot d^{-1}$. The controversy over vitamin C continues, but several of the widely reported effects have proved unfounded. Conditioned scurvy has not been substantiated, oxalate kidney stones have not been seen, and vitamin B_{12} destruction was probably an artifact of the test used to measure vitamin C. Other effects have been substantiated and they include gastrointestinal distress (nausea, abdominal pain, diarrhea) with doses as low as 1000 mg, probably due to the acidity, not the vitamin itself; oxygen demand of tissue is increased and problems may ensue if one ascends altitude; dental enamel may be eroded if chewable tablets are used daily; copper intake may be decreased; and, rarely, some individuals develop a rash showing delayed hypersensitivity allergy.[27]

The two major minerals of concern, iron and calcium, are covered in subsequent sections. Deficiencies of vitamin A, iron, and zinc are most often associated with protein deficiency, which is commonly seen in high-performance athletes. Zinc is identified as a concern for athletes[30] and toxicity levels are difficult to determine due to its association with copper, iron, and phytates. One of the most toxic trace minerals is copper and its supplementation should be discouraged. Selenium in excess can cause extensive tissue damage but its threshold is not known. Manganese may present a problem in individuals whose iron status is compromised.[27] As an individual ages there is often a change in vitamin status and deficiencies in one or more of the B vitamins develop.[31] Vitamin B_6 has been investigated in female athletes and observed changes show that there are effects of training status and age.[32] It becomes clear that there should be a minimum reliance on supplementation; however, supplementation is often warranted for iron and calcium.

III. THE TRACE MINERAL IRON

A. ACTION WITHIN THE BODY

Iron, a trace mineral present in all body cells, has long been recognized as an essential component of the diet. It is related directly to the proper functioning of many biochemical reactions where oxygen is metabolized and in DNA synthesis. Iron acts in metabolic pathways where oxygen is transported and is vital in synthesis of oxygen-carrying proteins such as myoglobin in muscle and hemoglobin in blood. Iron is also a fundamental component of the electron transport system where cytochromes, which contain iron, are used to cycle electrons and hydrogens in the synthesis of the energy carrier molecule of the body, ATP. Therefore iron is directly related to energy production within the body.[33] The fact remains, however, that iron deficiency might be the most common nutritional deficiency in the world.[34]

B. GENERAL REQUIREMENTS

The 1989 RDA for women between the ages of 11 and 50 is 15 mg·d^{-1}.[35,36] This represents a lower value than suggested in earlier RDAs and has provoked some controversy that these recommended levels are now too low. Over 50 years of age the value drops to 10 mg·d^{-1}. Values for pregnant women are double the 11- to 50-year-old recommendation.[36] It is clear that these intakes depend on caloric or energy intake, but it is difficult to determine exactly how much iron may be consumed by an average person. In order to cover the iron needs of adult menstruating women and recognizing the fact that only about 15% of the iron consumed can be absorbed, 2.84 mg·d^{-1} should be provided. Women using anovulatory drugs have lower needs which are met by 1.89 mg·d^{-1} or 12.6 mg available iron, 6.3 mg of iron for every 1000 kcal if 2000 kcal·d^{-1} is consumed. Therefore, the average American diet for the woman not on anovulatory drugs should contain 9.45 mg of iron for every 1000 kcal if 2000 kcal·d^{-1} is consumed,[37] but this may not represent the diet of a female athlete. Calculations done by Manore et al.[38] showed that an average of 6 mg/1000 kcal was ingested by female long distance runners, who also tend toward vegetarian eating habits due to the persistent quest for carbohydrate in the diet. If this represents female recreational athletes as well, it would be difficult for them to consume enough iron if the RDA is followed. A caloric intake of 2200 is the RDA for 11 to 50 year olds and they would then consume 13.2 mg·d^{-1}, below the RDA. If caloric intake is increased to 2500, then the RDA for iron is met but the cost might be excess body fat, which creates a dilemma. The woman over 50 will consume slightly more than the RDA with the recommended energy intake of 1900 kcal.

C. STUDIES OF IRON STATUS IN WOMEN WHO EXERCISE

The understanding of the relationships among dietary iron intake, voluntary supplementation, and performance in high-performance female athletes is not clear and is confounded by lack of standardized criteria and terminology for normal and deficiency states. Studies in female athletes tend to focus on the role of menstruation in blood loss as a major concern and rarely consider other issues.[34] There are few studies which even mention the category of recreational female athlete, who tends to be identified quite by accident when activity patterns are noted.

In a study by Newhouse et al.[39] it was reported that, as a group, females do not consume adequate iron in their diets. Although the assessment of activity level was not the purpose of the study and those engaging in regular exercise were not identified by number, it was stated that the "majority" of the 111 female subjects between the ages of 18 and 40 trained regularly three times per week at three fourths maximal effort for at least 120 min, thereby indicating that over half of the randomly selected women were recreational athletes. Of the total number of women 40% were either iron depleted (43 subjects had serum ferritin below 20 µg·l^{-1}) or iron deficient (4 subjects had hemoglobin below 120 g·l^{-1}). Two women fit both criteria; energy intake was not assessed. Iron supplementation (320 mg ferrous sulfate or 100 mg elemental iron per day taken for 12 weeks) was successful in bringing values to normal and did not affect serum copper, calcium, zinc, or magnesium levels, a concern when iron supplementation occurs.

Female endurance athletes who run distance are often recognized as having low energy (caloric) intakes[40] which are thought to be too low in many cases to support the proper balance of vitamins and minerals; low intake of calories in all women will result in iron deficiency.[37] The assumption by many has been that increased caloric intakes ensure adequate vitamin and mineral intakes as well. In a brief communication Green et al.[41] observed that this was not the case. Triathletes who competed and were surveyed did consume adequate amounts of calories, but they still had low intakes of six minerals and three vitamins. Included were low intakes of iron. The recommendaton was that athletes needed more accurate nutrition information in order to make better food choices. However, female recreational athletes tend to fare somewhat better nutritionally. In a study by Pate et al.[10] it was observed that female recreational runners, defined as those who ran regularly but were not competitive, had diets much closer to recommendations for optimum dietary regimens given by public health officials. They consumed more carbohydrate and less fat than their inactive counterparts, while protein intake was less. Although these dietary practices are considered healthy, there still persisted the fact that iron intakes were as low as in the inactive women. Also observed was low calcium intake.

Iron status may be altered by prolonged periods of conditioning or training in females and it has been reported consistently that female athletes who run may have difficulty getting enough iron in the diet.[38] The issue becomes more complex when it is also reported that female athletes in sports other than running and nonathletes may present almost identical levels of iron deficiency, strongly suggesting that the number of athletes representing iron deficiency is no more than the level found in the general female population.[42] This in no way discounts the seriousness of impaired performance which can occur if the depletion results in anemia. However, it appears that not all recreational female athletes should be concerned. Also observed was the fact that some female athletes who are initially normal develop iron deficiency during the course of a season of conditioning, suggesting that they may require more iron than an inactive woman.[42] A long-term study which followed collegiate female field hockey players over a period of three consecutive competitive years found that body iron stores and iron reserves tended to become progressively more depleted after consecutive seasons.[43] The reasons for the observations found in the previous studies were linked to dietary practices, as it has been reported that activity per se does not necessarily lead to depletion in the mineral status of iron, copper, and zinc when intakes are adequate.[44]

D. EFFECT OF PROTEIN INTAKE

When females exercise they are often given advice about elevating their level of carbohydrate to levels sometimes exceeding 60% of caloric intake. Simple calculations would suggest that levels of fat and protein would concomitantly be reduced and therefore so would the nutrients supplied by these sources. Telford et al.[45] reported that iron status may have a greater association with percentage protein intake than overall energy intake as is frequently suggested, thereby corroborating the concept that when one approaches vegetarian dietary practices iron intake should be monitored, with this advice not being restricted to athletes.

E. DEFICIENCY

Symptoms of iron deficiency are vague and include fatigue, decreased appetite, headache, heartburn, shortness of breath, or excessive menstrual discharge. If deficiency does occur it is in progressive stages, the last of which is iron deficiency anemia defined as <12 g·dl⁻¹ circulating hemoglobin in adult women. These values, however, must be judged in light of exercise-induced plasma volume expansion which dilutes hemoglobin and red blood cell concentration.[46] During exercise itself there is a hemoconcentration which is compensated after exercise by hormone changes which increase plasma volume. These effects are seen most accutely in aerobic exercise, with the endurance athlete often presenting as a slightly anemic individual when blood is analyzed.

True iron deficiency anemia, even if mild, will impair performance[47] and iron therapy is suggested (325 mg three times per day for 2 months). It should be pointed out that this level of supplementation may be successful in raising serum ferritin levels in prelatent/latent iron deficiency but may not be associated with significant improvements in work capacity.[48] Iron deficiency may also predispose females to impaired thermogenesis and thermoregulatory responses, thereby decreasing their ability to withstand cold exposure.[49] Women who are mildly iron deficient have also been shown to be less satisfied with their performance than women who were normal, but treatment did not change performance or "mood".[42] The cause in women, whether or not they are recreational athletes, is predominantly insufficient iron in the diet, although other mechanisms such as loss of iron in urine and the gastrointestinal tract,[50] menstrual losses, and hemolysis during high levels of conditioning[45] play a role. Iron is also lost in sweat and the degree of loss is the same in males and females; however, these losses coupled with low dietary intake may contribute to negative iron balance.[51] Women who exercise tend to favor a modified vegetarian dietary regimen,[52] although the definition and degree of vegetarianism is often not clear, since "vegetarian" was defined as one who consumed milk, eggs, fish, poultry, and very little, <100 g·week⁻¹, or no red meat. Decreased iron in the diet may lead to iron deficiency without anemia; however, vegetarianism alone may not be responsible for low iron intake.[53] Female athletes who wish to become vegetarians, or who are already practicing, are directed to become knowledgeable about this dietary practice and are referred to information written specifically for the recreational athlete.[53]

F. SOURCES AND TOXICITY

Iron in the diet is found as heme iron from meats, poultry, and fish and is more readily absorbed than nonheme iron from plant sources. Acids in the meal tend to aid nonheme iron absorption, which is why beverages such as orange juice, for its ascorbic acid content, are suggested for inclusion in meals high in nonheme iron. However, the degree of nonheme iron inhibition associated with the composition of the meal is not clear, as calcium content should also interfere with absorption but does so in unpredictable ways.[54]

Iron status is so often reported as low in females that an awareness in the population has been developed, as it has been shown that many women are heeding the warnings since iron is the most common supplement taken in the greatest amounts compared to other nutritional support. It cannot, however, be recommended that iron supplementation become routine unless it has been shown, through blood analysis, to be necessary. Seldom reported to the public are problems due to iron toxicity which can occur with chronic iron overload.[55] While enhanced growth of infectious agents is a major concern for iron-deficient individuals, there are significant direct alterations in immune function with iron overload.[27] However, the threshold for adverse effects of supplemental iron is not known; it probably depends on intakes of other substances such as manganese, zinc, ascorbic acid, and protein, and it is thought to be around 100 to 200 mg/d.[27] Lead toxicity can also cause a rare apparent iron deficiency which in turn enhances lead absorption, again suggesting the need for evaluation before treatment is undertaken.[55]

G. TESTING

The only accurate way to determine iron status is to have it tested by blood analysis. It is also recommended that this be done on more than one occasion, since iron status may be misinterpreted if a single blood sample is collected because of day-to-day variation in the indicators used for assessment.[56] Currently, hematological tests include hematocrit, hemoglobin concentration, mean corpuscular volume, red cell distribution, marrow iron stain, and zinc/protoporphyric/heme. Biochemical tests include serum iron concentration, total iron-binding capacity, transferrin saturation, transferrin receptor concentration, serum ferritin concentration, and liver iron concentration. Of all of these measures, the "gold standard" has long been serum ferritin concentration since this is an absolute measure of depleted iron stores. However, low serum ferritin concentration does not necessarily mean that peripheral tissues are being deprived of iron.[55] Regardless of this fact, mild iron deficiency is difficult to assess in the clinical chemistry laboratory.[54]

H. RECOMMENDATIONS

Since iron and calcium represent two major nutritional deficiencies in the population of women in the U.S. today, they will also represent problems for recreational athletes. If both iron and calcium supplementation are chosen then it is important to coordinate their consumption. Calcium carbonate should be used and both minerals should be consumed between meals. Calcium tends to inhibit nonheme iron absorption when both are consumed in the same meal, but the degree is unpredictable.[54]

Female recreational athletes should consume adequate amounts of calories in their diets to assure good iron availability, since the cause of iron deficiency is most likely due to a low intake of iron.[14,57,58] If iron deficiency is suspected the athlete should have her blood tested before embarking on an aggressive self-prescribed program of iron supplementation. The physician should be chosen who understands athletic pseudoanemias and has experience interpreting the blood values of exercisers. Heme iron sources and protein intake should be monitored for adequacy and if a vegetarian diet is chosen the recreational athlete is directed to learn the best way to proceed which does not mean that one just gives up flesh foods. Acidic beverages such as orange juice consumed at meals and consumption of meats, poultry, and fish enhance absorption.[59] Inhibitors of absorption are known to be tea, coffee and wheat bran.[35,37] If calcium supplements are also used then both the iron and calcium in carbonate form should be taken between meals. If weight loss is also desired the female recreational athlete should follow the recommendations of the American College of Sports Medicine[60] which suggests that caloric deficit be matched equally with dietary caloric restriction and weight loss proceeds in a gradual manner. The recommendations for cardiovascular fitness will not necessarily result in weight loss and this should be carefully determined.

IV. DISORDERED EATING

A. PREVALENCE

Much research on exercising female populations points to the fact that low iron status and many other indicators of poor nutrition are highly associated with low caloric intake.[8,9] The intake can become so low in certain groups that life-threatening disorders can result. Since the incidence in the population of recreational female athletes is unknown, it would be a reasonable assumption to expect these disorders to be found in similar percentages as the general population. While the term eating disorders has become quite recognizable over the last decade, the clinical diagnosis of anorexia nervosa and bulimia nervosa is difficult. Additionally, estimates of incidence vary widely, but an acceptable approximation is 1% and 1 to 3% of the U.S. population, respectively.[61] The self-imposed starvation of primarily young women is difficult to diagnose accurately until a myriad of physiological aberrations has already occurred.[62] Although the etiology is unknown, psychological, social, cultural, and biological factors are thought to interact. The externally imposed pressure to become thin and to succeed becomes internalized with potentially fatal results.

Excessive physical activity is a common observation in these disorders to the extent that is has been proposed that obligatory running in males is a correlate of anorexia nervosa in females, as some have found common basic personality traits between the two groups.[63] Blumenthal and colleagues[62] refute this concept and found little empirical evidence to substantiate the theory. Habitual runners in this study found running to be a form of adaptive behavior which served to enhance physical and psychological functions rather than promote self-destruction. Support that running is not an analog of anorexia was given by Weight and Noakes,[64] who found that running did not attract persons with anorexic personalities. These two conflicting opinions point to the controversial nature of analyzing these behaviors.

In females, attention has focused on eating disorders in certain categories of activity which focus on endurance activity or appearance of the body. Estimates of prevalence are difficult due to varying criteria and the sport analyzed. Female dancers are frequently identified as at risk for eating disorders, but their prevalence may be no greater than nondancers. In a study by Holderness et al.,[65] the previous observation was coupled with the conclusion that women dancers showed fewer tendencies to substance use and abuse (amphetamines, barbiturates, tranquilizers, hallucinogens, and cocaine) than nondancers, thereby suggesting that even when at risk for eating disorders an exercising population still maintains some positive health behaviors.

Pathogenic weight control behaviors are commonly found in competitive adolescent female gymnasts[66] and in female college varsity level athletes.[67] However, others[68] suggest that athletes as a group may actually have a lower active incidence rate than other females in their age categories.

In a broader perspective, there is the recognition of disordered eating which may not be as severe as the above-mentioned syndromes, but is a problem in female exercising populations and presents the risk for developing full disorder.[69] The spectrum of eating difficulties is defined on a continuum from normal concerns about body weight to diagnosable eating disorders, with vast numbers of women prone to the category of disordered eating. Largely confined to women it is thought to be the perpetual cultural reinforcement of the notion that a woman should be lithe and slim. The biological reality of the female body is somehow not recognized either in the population or in sports.

B. INFLUENCE OF MISINFORMATION ABOUT BODY COMPOSITION

Difficulties arise when athletes are influenced by coaches and others not knowledgeable in assessment of body fat percentages and its appropriate use. All methods of assessing body composition have errors and the realistic way to use these techniques is to monitor progress over time rather than focus on specific criteria for percentage body fat. The association between a specific body fat percentage and performance has never been made, as all performance combines physiological characteristics with psychological attributes which are difficult to measure. Coaches and others such as role models and parents may not possess current nutrition information which may compound the problem when they try to give advice to the female athlete. There is also an almost absolute refusal on the part of American culture to recognize the fact that a normal female body ranges between 18 and 33% body fat in the optimal health range, with a minimal weight of 14% below which it is risky for a female to go.[70] Ideal fitness ranges between 16 and 25%. Part of the difficulty is encountered when the majority of females portrayed in the media hovers around 10% body fat, a level associated with eating disorders, amenorrhea, and early osteoporosis. Young females and their male peers who admire these airbrushed symbols do not know what a normal healthy female of perhaps 25% body fat looks like. In my own experience teaching body composition classes to university kinesiology majors, it was found that education does not necessarily change these impressions. At the end of each semester, after assessing body composition at least ten different ways, my students are asked to list the percent body fat which they would like to have. In the most recent semester, male (n = 43) responses indicated that 70% wanted to lose body fat, 16% were satisfied, and 14% wanted to gain body fat. Female (n = 42) responses indicated that 83% wanted to lose body fat, 7% were satisfied, and 10% wanted to gain body fat. All but two of these individuals were in male and female categories of optimal health and all had exams to pass to assure that they understood the concepts of body composition.[71] Disordered eating becomes a reality when cultural influences outweigh education.

C. SEASONAL VARIATION

It has been observed that the dietary practices of female athletes show seasonal variation related to exercise patterns and that dieting may occur when they are not participating in as much activity.[72] Others have suggested that disordered eating is confined to the season of athletic participation[69] and that problems are readily reversible on termination of the athletic activity. This is not necessarily true if the female recreational athlete progresses to amenorrhea and restricts calcium intake. There has been recognition of a combination of disorders found in adolescent and young adult female athletes designated the female athlete triad.[73] The triad is composed of disordered eating, amenorrhea, and osteoporosis. Usually beginning with disordered eating in the exercising female it progresses to amenorrhea, although menstrual irregularities can occur in the absence of an eating disorder. The amenorrhea is a sign of decreased estrogen production which can then can lead to bone loss, which in some individuals is comparable to that seen in postmenopausal women. This bone loss may not be reversible. It is absolutely crucial that recreational female athletes be aware of this syndrome. A task force has been formed by the American College of Sports Medicine which provides current information concerning this issue.[74]

V. MENSTRUAL CYCLE FUNCTION

A. EXERCISE EFFECTS

In a very thorough review of known issues and mechanisms to date, Loucks[75] presented effects of exercise training on the menstrual cycle. The existence of delayed menarche was acknowledged in athletes, but evidence could not support that it is the actual training which is responsible for the delay. Athletic amenorrhea appears to be related to abrupt initiation of high volume aerobic conditioning in some women predisposed by a yet-to-be identified mechanism. Luteal suppression, lack of ovulation, in regularly menstruating athletes may represent an end point of successful acclimation to training in robust individuals. However, temperature regulation during endurance exercise done at the luteal phase is adversely affected as elevated core temperatures have been observed.[76] Mechanisms are currently obscure often due to lack of clarity in studies with numerous confounding variables and lack of full scientific inquiry bringing to bear the most current tests available. The fact is that this research area has greatly piqued the interest of exercise physiologists, because disruption of cycle may have an adverse effect on the maintainance of bone density; therefore, it shows promise for immediate and future study.[75]

B. DIET AND EXERCISE EFFECTS COMBINED

It has been recognized that menstrual cycle function is affected by diet and exercise habits.[77] It has also been reported that the diet habits of women are concomitantly affected by phases of the menstrual cycle.[78] Observations of 14 women over a period of 1 year produced a sinusoidal regression curve phenomenon which showed regulatory and behavioral phenomenon-relating phases of the menstrual cycle to food selection and consumption.[79] Energy intake was elevated in the 10 d prior to menses with a preference shown for fat, although protein and carbohydrate intakes were also nonsignificantly elevated. Basal metabolic rate was also elevated during this time. Post menses energy intake and basal metabolic rate dropped for 10 d and began to reverse upward to repeat the cycle. Activity patterns may also reflect similar changes, as women have been noted to be more active during the periods of increased food intake.[80] Observations such as these have implications for treating eating disorders, obesity, and premenstrual syndrome.

Menarche can be delayed with high levels of physical activity, but the reasons are not currently clear. While low-percentage body fat has been proposed as a causative factor,[81] it has also been refuted.[82] When amenorrheic runners were compared to eumenorrheic runners, populations in which menstrual irregularities or secondary amenorrhea have consistently been observed, it was found that percent body fats were not different.[83] The observation has, however, been made that certain categories of females whose difficulties may begin very early in life, such as those who participate in ballet, may become predisposed to eating disorders and early osteoporotic changes leading to more bone injuries at early ages.[84] Menstrual disturbances are invariably seen in these groups which can persist into adult life. Eating problems are an important etiologic consideration in the pathogenesis of amenorrhea in athletes, but it is also clear that the difficulty is multidimensional.[85] The pattern of increased musculoskeletal injuries is also seen in adult premenopausal women who have menstrual irregularities.[86]

Normal hormonal patterns of the menstrual cycle can be altered by reproductive status, prior menstrual and exercise history, stress, nutrition, and body composition changes, all of which can be influenced by exercise.[87-93] Menstrual dysfunction secondary to active exercise participation is well documented, but not all who exercise are affected. Low resting metabolic rate which may be the result of caloric restriction[94] is implicated.[95] The average adult woman consumes approximately 1700 kcal/d[96] and women who exercise are known to consume less. Dieting alone can induce menstrual cycle disturbances. It was shown that a 1000-kcal, vegetarian, high carbohydrate diet produced measurable changes which were more pronounced in females below the age of 25.[97]

In the one study found which actually identified female recreational athletes, menstrual function and eating behavior were evaluated in recreational weight lifters and competitive body builders.[98] One hundred three female weight lifters were compared to a control sample of 92 women who did not weight train. All subjects were classified by menstrual cycle (eumenorrheic, oligomenorrheic, amenorrheic) and a subgroup of women who weight lifted were classified as competitive. The average percent body fat for all lifters was 20%, while competitive lifters were 17.7%. Two percent were amenorrheic. Eighteen percent were oligomenorrheic which was considered high and an indication of menstrual dysfunction; the combined percentage is similar to that found in runners. Although there appeared to be an excessive concern with food and weight loss the behaviors were not those of disordered eating. The authors expressed concern that these women were at risk due to their preoccupation with weight; close to a third of weight lifters and the majority of competitive body builders self-reported menstrual dysfunction. Energy intakes were not assessed.

Thus it is important for recreational female athletes to consume adequate calories in their diets and notice changes in menstrual cycle activity which may be associated with abrupt changes in volume of aerobic conditioning. The resulting changes in menstrual function are not just gynecological concerns, but should be thoroughly evaluated for nutritional status as well.

VI. BONE STATUS

An inevitable consequence of aging is loss of bone with the end result of osteoporosis, a disorder of epidemic proportions in the U.S. Partly to blame may be the current trend of Americans who attempt to reduce caloric and cholesterol consumption by lowering intake of dairy products which contain the calcium bone needs. The loss of calcium from the skeleton predisposes bone to fractures and compressions of the spine leading to deformity. It is possible that the concern for reducing risk factors for cardiovascular disease may be increasing the risk for osteoporosis. We are just beginning to understand that the integrity of bone requires a complex integration of the hormones estrogen and testosterone, diet, and exercise and that focusing on one parameter at a time is too simplistic. A special chapter devoted to this subject is found elsewhere in this volume.

The recreational female athlete most assuredly should become aware of the affectors of bone remodeling and should do what she can to protect the density of her bones. Bone mineral describes bone mass and is measured by the amount of calcium phosphate crystal present in bone.[99] Bone mineral density describes the amount of bone mineral found in a specific measured bone area.[99] A dynamic tissue, bone constantly adapts to the stresses which are either placed on or removed from the skeleton, but the process is long and slow.

The highest bone density values are found in male weight lifters, thus suggesting that there is also an interaction of muscle mass which places stress on bone and forces it to adapt.[100] It was thought for some time that "weight bearing" exercise would be the best type of stimulus in the female to protect bone integrity, which is compromised by age, immobility, corticosteroid use, and premenopausal loss of the ability to produce estrogen. The exercises proposed and evaluated were running and swimming. Heinrich and co-workers[101] found that weight training or resistance training may provide a better stimulus for increasing bone mineral content due to increased muscle weight.

The interactions of exercise, hormones, diet, and bone density are complex in the female. While it is not certain when the greatest bone mass is achieved, it is known that bone is gained during adolescence, plateaus perhaps in the third decade where is it somewhat stable, although decline has been observed, until approximately age 50, after which there is a gradual and progressive loss.[99] In females, this coincides with menopause and the loss of bone density within the first 5 years after this event is dramatic.[102] Thus, if a line were drawn throughout a lifetime it would show progressive decline after the third decade with the angle of decline modified by diet, exercise, and hormone balance. While much attention has been placed recently on understanding how to slow this loss, the fact remains that 75% of the variance may be hereditary and only 20% may be modifiable by activity or strength interventions.[99] Thus, a female recreational athlete who has a mother or grandmother with osteoporosis should become as educated as possible in intervention and should take an active role in preserving her bone density throughout her lifetime.

Much attention has been given in recent years to studying the interaction of amenorrhea and bone density.[103] It has been shown that amenorrheic athletes, who are characterized by the absence of menstrual cycles accompanied by persistent low circulating endogenous estrogen,[104] have low bone mineral density in the lumbar spine.[105] The comparison to bone mineral densities found in postmenopausal osteoporosis has been made.[103]

Amenorrhea was long thought to be a benign side effect of high levels of endurance exercise, but this finding suggests a much more serious consideration.[106] Often accompanying this syndrome is the finding that these women have low daily energy intake.[105] In the past it was proposed that the low caloric intake led to a low percent body fat (<17%) and that the body fat level initiated the difficulties,[107] but this has been disputed[83, 108] by investigators who have found amenorrheic runners whose body fats were not below 17%. It was also suggested that vegetarian diet may predispose a female to amenorrhea and therefore low bone mineral density, but this has also been challenged.[109] It has, however, been shown that diet has a strong effect on bone status, since stress fractures are more common in dancers with restrictive diets than those whose diets are more liberal.[110] Exercise and load on the bone also have a strong association and a thorough review was written by Dalsky.[111] Oral contraceptive use seems to give some protective effect.[112] Although not all of the answers are known, it has been shown that athletes with menstrual dysfunction who reduce the amount of exercise and gain weight may become eumenorrheic and recover some bone mineral content. However, it is not yet known if full recovery is possible.[104,113]

In summary, it is known that bone status is probably most affected by female estrogen status. Diet and exercise are also important. Therefore estrogen status should be maintained as long as possible, calcium intake should be high throughout the lifetime, and the female should adopt a life-style which includes exercise, the exact type, frequency, intensity, and duration of which is yet to be determined. Adult females (25–50 years; postmenopausal women on estrogen replacement therapy) should consume 1000 mg·calcium·d^{-1} [114] which should be increased to 1500 mg·d^{-1} if she is postmenopausal and not on estrogen therapy. The RDA is probably still too low in recommending 800 mg·d^{-1} for women 25 to 50; the RDA for 19- to 24-year-old women is 1200 mg·d^{-1}. If estrogen therapy cannot or will not be considered, calcitonin-salmon injections can be used in women in high-risk categories. A female recreational athlete who suspects a strong genetic predisposition to osteoporosis should become as well informed about bone health as early in life as possible and should obtain information from the National Osteoporosis Foundation.[115]

VII. CONCLUSIONS

In conclusion, it has been shown that the female recreational athlete leads a healthier life-style than her inactive counterpart. While it is not prudent to focus on what can go wrong, it is wise to become attuned to her body and pay attention to signs that exercise levels may be too intense. She should become educated in sound nutritional practices and eat a varied diet based on current recommendations found in the food pyramid concept for normal mixed and vegetarian diets.[116,117] While one can never guarantee a greater quantity of life, the quality of her life will be greatly enhanced by following the recommendations made in this and other chapters of this book.

REFERENCES

1. U.S. Bureau of the Census, Statistical Abstract of the U.S.: 1993, 113th ed., Washington, D.C., 1993.
2. Van Dinter, N. R., Introduction: competitive vs. recreational athletes: an American recreational and cultural perspective, in *Nutrition for the Recreational Athlete,* Jackson, C. G. R., Ed., CRC Press, Boca Raton, FL, 1995.
3. Jackson, C. G. R., *Nutrition for the Recreational Athlete,* CRC Press, Boca Raton, FL, 1995.
4. Guyton, A. C., Ed., Sports physiology, in *Textbook of Medical Physiology,* W. B. Saunders, Philadelphia, 1991, 940.

5. Jackson, C. G. R. and Simonson, S., The relationships between human energy transfer and nutrition, in *Nutrition for the Recreational Athlete,* Jackson, C. G. R., Ed., CRC Press, Boca Raton, FL, 1995.

6. Mertz, W., Tsui, J. C., Judd, J. T., Reiser, S., Hallfrisch, J., Morris, E. R., Steele, P. D., and Lashley, E., What are people really eating? The relationship between energy intake derived from estimated diet records and intake determined to maintain body weight, *Am. J. Clin. Nutr.,* 54, 291, 1991.

7. Welsh, S. and Guthrie, J. F., Changing American diets, in *Micronutrients in Health and in Disease Prevention,* Bendich, A. and Butterworth, C. E., Eds., Marcel Dekker, New York, 1991.

8. Brownell, K. D., Nelson Steen, S., and Wilmore, J. H., Weight regulation practices in athletes: analysis of metabolic and health effects, *Med. Sci. Sports Exerc.,* 19, 546, 1987.

9. Chen, J. D., Wang, J. F., Li, K. J., Zhao, Y. W., Wang, S. W., Jiao, Y., and Hou, X. Y., Nutritional problems and measures in elite and amateur athletes, *Am. J. Clin. Nutr.,* 49, 1084, 1989.

10. Pate, R. R., Sargent, R. G., Baldwin, C., and Burgess, M. L., Dietary intake of women runners, *Int. J. Sports Med.,* 11, 461, 1990.

11. Grandjean, A. C., Macronutrient intake of U.S. athletics compared with the general population and recommendations made for athletes, *Am. J. Clin. Nutr.,* 49, 1070, 1989.

12. Grandjean, A. C., Nutrition for swimmers, *Clin. Sport Med.,* 5, 65, 1986.

13. Frye, S., Fluids, hydration and performance concerns of all recreational athletes, in *Nutrition for the Recreational Athlete,* Jackson, C. G. R., Ed., CRC Press, Boca Raton, FL., 1995.

14. Ruud, J. S. and Grandjean, A. C., Nutritional concerns of female athletes, in *Nutrition in Exercise and Sport,* 2nd ed., Wolinsky, I. and Hickson, J.F., Jr., Eds., CRC Press, Boca Raton, FL, 1994, 347.

15. Somer, E., *Nutrition for Women, The Complete Guide,* Henry Holt, New York, 1993.

16. Yost, T. J. and Eckel, R. H., Fat calories may be preferentially stored in reduced-obese women: a permissive pathway for resumption of the obese state, *J. Clin. Endocrinol. Metab.,* 67, 259, 1988.

17. Miller, W. C., Lindeman, A. K., Wallace, J., and Niederpruem, M., Diet composition, energy intake, and exercise in relation to body fat in men and women, *Am. J. Clin. Nutr.,* 52, 426, 1990.

18. Goldberg, L. and Elliot, D. L., The effect of exercise on lipid metabolism in men and women, *Sports Med.,* 4, 307, 1987.

19. Campaigne, B. N., Body fat distribution in females: metabolic consequences and implications for weight loss, *Med. Sci. Sports Exerc.,* 22, 291, 1990.

20. Angotti, C. M. and Levine, M. S., Review of five years of a combined dietary and physical fitness intervention for control of serum cholesterol, *J. Am. Diet. Assoc.,* 94, 634, 1994.

21. Hagan, R. D., Upton, S. J., Wong, L., and Whittam, J., The effects of aerobic conditioning and/or caloric restriction in overweight men and women, *Med. Sci. Sports Exerc.,* 18, 87, 1986.

22. Haus, G., Hoerr, S. L., Mavis, B., and Robison, J., Key modifiable factors in weight maintenance: fat intake, exercise, and weight cycling, *J. Am. Diet. Assoc.,* 94, 409, 1994.

23. Grubbs, L., The critical role of exercise in weight control, *Nurse Pract.,* 18, 20, 1993.

24. Staten, M. A., The effect of exercise on food intake in men and women, *Am. J. Clin. Nutr.,* 53, 27, 1991.

25. Haymes, E. M., Vitamin and mineral supplementation of athletes, *Int. J. Sport Nutr.,* 1, 146, 1991.

26. Cerny, L. and Cerny, K., Can carrots be addictive: an extraordinary form of drug dependence, *Br. J. Addict.,* 87, 1195, 1992.

27. Hathcock, J. N., Safety of vitamin and mineral supplements, in *Micronutrients in Health and in Disease Prevention,* Bendich, A. and Butterworth, C. E., Eds., Marcel Dekker, New York, 1991.

28. Hathcock, J. N., Hattan, D. G., Jenkins, M. Y., Mcdonald, J. T., Sundaresan, P. R., and Wilkening, V. L., Evaluation of vitamin A toxicity, *Am. J. Clin. Nutr.*, 52, 183, 1990.

29. van Dam, M. A., The recognition and treatment of hypervitaminosis A, *Nurse Pract.*, 14, 28, 1989.

30. Deuster, P. A., Day, B. A., Singh, A., Douglass, L., and Moser-Veillon, P. B., Zinc status of highly trained women runners and untrained women, *Am. J. Clin. Nutr.*, 49, 1295, 1989.

31. Miller, W. C., Niederpruem, M. G., Wallace, J. P., and Lindeman, A. K., dietary fat, sugar, and fiber predict body fat content, *J. Am. Diet. Assoc.*, 94, 612, 1994.

32. Manore, M. M. and Leklem, J. E., Effect of carbohydrate and vitamin B$_6$ on fuel substrates during exercise in women, *Med. Sci. Sports Exerc.*, 20, 233, 1988.

33. Ponka, P., Schulman, H. M., and Woodworth, R. C., *Iron Transport and Storage,* CRC Press, Boca Raton, FL, 1990.

34. Haymes, E.M., Trace minerals and exercise, in *Nutrition in Exercise and Sport,* Wolinsky, I. and Hickson, J. F., Eds., CRC Press, Boca Raton, Fl, 1994, 223.

35. Monsen, E. R., The 10th edition of the Recommended Dietary Allowances: what's new in the 1989 RDAs?, *J. Am. Diet. Assoc.*, 89, 1748, 1989.

36. Food and Nutrition Board, *Recommended Dietary Allowances,* 10th ed., National Academy of Sciences, Washington, D.C., 1989.

37. Hallberg, L. and Rossander-Hulten, L., Iron requirements in menstruating women, *Am. J. Clin. Nutr.*, 54, 1047, 1991.

38. Manore, M. M., Besenfelder, P. D., Wells, C. L., Carroll, S. S., and Hooker, S. P., Nutrient intakes and iron status in female long-distance runners during training, *J. Am. Diet. Assoc.*, 89, 257, 1989.

39. Newhouse, I. J., Clement, D. B., and Lai, C., Effects of iron supplementation and discontinuation on serum copper, zinc, calcium, and magnesium levels in women, *Med. Sci. Sports Exerc.*, 25, 562, 1993.

40. Haymes, E. M. and Spillman, D. M., Iron status of women distance runners, sprinters, and control women, *Int. J. Sports Med.*, 10, 430, 1989.

41. Green, D. R., Gibbons, C., O'Toole, M., and Hiller, W. B. O., An evaluation of dietary intakes of triathletes: are RDAs being met?, *J. Am. Diet. Assoc.*, 89, 1653, 1989.

42. Risser, W. L., Lee, E. J., Poindexter, H. B. W., West, M. S., Pivarnik, J. M., Risser, J. M. H., and Hickson, J. F., Iron deficiency in female athletes: its prevalence and impact on performance, *Med. Sci. Sports Exerc.*, 20, 116, 1988.

43. Diehl, D. M., Lohman, T. G., Smith, S. C., and Kertzer, R., Effects of physical training and competition on the iron status of female field hockey players, *Int. J. Sports Med.*, 7, 264, 1986.

44. Lukaski, H. C., Hoverson, B. S., Gallagher, S. K., and Bolonchuk, W. W., Physical training and copper, iron, and zinc status of swimmers, *Am. J. Clin. Nutr.*, 51, 1093, 1990.

45. Telford, R. D., Cunningham, R. B., Deakin, V., and Kerr, D. A., Iron status and diet in athletes, *Med. Sci. Sports Exerc.*, 25, 796, 1993.

46. Eichner, E. R., Sports anemia, iron supplements, and blood doping, *Med. Sci. Sports Exerc.*, 24, S315, 1992.

47. Clarkson, P. M., Vitamins and trace minerals, in *Perspectives in Exercise Science and Sports Medicine, Ergogenics,* Lamb, D. R., and Williams, M. H., Eds., Brown & Benchmark, Dubuque, IA, 1991.

48. Newhouse, I. J., Clement, D. B., Taunton, J. E., and McKenzie, D. C., The effects of prelatent/latent iron deficiency on physical work capacity, *Med. Sci. Sports Exerc.*, 21, 263, 1989.

49. Lukaski, H. C., Hall, C. B., and Nielsen, F. H., Thermogenesis and thermoregulatory function of iron-deficient women without anemia, *Aviat. Space Environ. Med.*, 61, 913, 1990.

50. Lampe, J. W., Slavin, J. L., and Apple, F. S., Iron status of active women and the effect of running a marathon on bowel function and gastrointestinal blood loss, *Int. J. Sports Med.*, 12, 173, 1991.

51. Lamanca, J. J., Haymes, E. M., Daly, J. A., Moffatt, R. J., and Waller, M. F., Sweat iron loss of male and female runners during exercise, *Int. J. Sports Med.,* 9, 52, 1988.

52. Snyder, A. C., Dvorak, L. L., and Reopke, J. B., Influence of dietary iron source on measures of iron status among female runners, *Med. Sci. Sports Exerc.,* 21, 7, 1989.

53. Ratzin, R. A., Nutritional concerns for the vegetarian recreational athlete, in *Nutrition for the Recreational Athlete,* Jackson, C. G. R., Ed., CRC Press, Boca Raton, FL, 1995.

54. Cook, J. D., Dassenko, S. A., and Whittaker, P., Calcium supplementation: effect on iron absorption, *Am. J. Clin. Nutr.,* 53, 106, 1991.

55. Labbe, R. F., Iron status: from deficiency to toxicity, *Clin. Chem. News,* September, 24, 1993.

56. Borel, M. J., Smith, S. M., Derr, J., and Beard, J. L., Day-to-day variation in iron-status indices in healthy men and women, *Am. J. Clin. Nutr.,* 54, 729, 1991.

57. Strand, S. M., Clarke, B. A., Slavin, J. L., and Kelly, J. M., Effects of physical training and iron supplementation on iron status of female athletes, *Med. Sci. Sports Exerc.,* 16, 161, 1984.

58. Monsen, E. R., Hallberg, L., Layrisse, M., Hegsted, D. M., Cook, J. D., Mertz, W., and Finch, C. A., Estimation of available dietary iron, *Am. J. Clin. Nutr.,* 31, 134, 1978.

59. Layrisse, M., Martinez-Torres, C., and Roche, M., Effect of interaction of various foods on iron absorption, *Am. J. Clin. Nutr.,* 21, 1175, 1968.

60. *Proper and Improper Weight Loss Programs,* American College of Sports Medicine Position Stand, P.O. Box 1440, Indianapolis, IN, 46206–1440.

61. Fairburn, C. G., Phil, M., and Beglin, S. J., Studies of the epidemiology of bulimia nervosa, *Am. J. Psychiatry,* 147, 401, 1990.

62. Blumenthal, J., Rose, S., and Chang, J. L., Anorexia and exercise: Implications from recent findings, *Sports Med.,* 2, 237, 1985.

63. Yates, A., Leehey, K., and Shisslak, C., Running: an analogue of anorexia?, *N.Engl. J. Med.,* 308, 251, 1983.

64. Weight, L. M., and Noakes, T. D., Is running an analog of anorexia?: a survey of the incidence of eating disorders in female distance runners, *Med. Sci. Sports Exerc.,* 19, 213, 1987.

65. Holderness, C. C., Brooks-Gunn, J., and Warren, M. P., Eating disorders and substance use: a dancing vs a nondancing population, *Med. Sci. Sports Exerc.,* 26, 297, 1994.

66. Loosli, A. R., Benson, J., Gillien, D. M., and Bourdet, K., Nutrition habits and knowledge in competitive adolescent female gymnasts, *Phys. Sportsmed.,* 14, 118, 1986.

67. Rosen, L. W., McKeag, D. B., Hough, D. O., and Curley, V., Pathogenic weight control behavior in female athletes, *Phys. Sportsmed.,* 14, 79, 1986.

68. Kurtzman, F. D., Yager, J., Landsverk, J., Wiesmeier, E., and Bodurka, D. C., Eating disorders among selected female student populations at UCLA, *J. Am. Diet. Assoc.,* 89, 45, 1989.

69. Wilson, G. T. and Eldredge, K. L., Pathology and development of eating disorders: implications for athletes, in *Eating, Body Weight, and Performance in Athletes, Disorders of Modern Society,* Brownell, K. D., Rodin, J., and Wilmore, J. H., Eds., Lea & Febiger, Philadelphia, 1992, 115.

70. Lohman, T. G., ACSM Tutorial: *Body Composition Assessment,* presented at the ACSM annual meeting, handout, June 1989.

71. Jackson, C. G. R., unpublished results, 1994.

72. Nutter, J., Seasonal changes in female athletes' diets, *Int. J. Sport Nutr.,* 1, 395, 1991.

73. Yeager, K. K., Agostini, R., Nattiv, A., and Drinkwater, B., The female athlete triad: disordered eating, amenorrhea, osteoporosis, *Med. Sci. Sports Exerc.,* 25, 775, 1993.

74. American College of Sports Medicine Public Information Department, P. O. Box 1440, Indianapolis, IN, 46206-1440; phone (317)637-9200; FAX (317)634-7817.

75. Loucks, A. B., Effects of exercise training on the menstrual cycle: existence and mechanisms, *Med. Sci. Sports Exerc.,* 22, 275, 1990.

76. Pivarnik, J. M., Marichal, C. J., Spillman, H. T., and Morrow, J. R., Menstrual cycle phase affects temperature regulation during endurance exercise, *Med. Sci. Sports Exerc.,* 22, S119, 1990.

77. Puhl, J. L. and Brown, C. H., *The Menstrual Cycle and Physical Activity,* Human Kinetics Publishers, Champaign, IL, 1986.

78. Gong, E. J., Garrel, D., and Calloway, D. H., Menstrual cycle and voluntary food intake, *Am. J. Clin. Nutr.,* 49, 252, 1989.

79. Tarasuk, V. and Beaton, G. H., Menstrual-cycle patterns in energy and macronutrient intake, *Am. J. Clin. Nutr.,* 53, 442, 1991.

80. Webb, P., 24-Hour energy expenditure and the menstrual cycle, Am. *J. Clin. Nutr.,* 44, 614, 1986.

81. Frisch, R. E., Wyshakr, G., and Vincent, L., Delayed menarche and amenorrhea in ballet dancers, *N. Engl. J. Med.,* 303, 17, 1980.

82. Plowman, S. A., Liu, N. Y., and Wells, C., Body composition and sexual maturation in premenarcheal athletes and nonathletes, *Med. Sci. Sports Exerc.,* 23, 23, 1991.

83. Sanborn, C. F., Albrecht, B. H., and Wagner, W. W., Athletic amenorrhea: lack of association with body fat, *Med. Sci. Sports Exerc.,* 19, 207, 1987.

84. Benson, J. E., Geiger, C. J., Eiserman, P. A., and Wardlaw, G. M., Relationship between nutrient intake, body mass index, menstrual function, and ballet injury, *J. Am. Diet. Assoc.,* 89, 58, 1989.

85. Brooks-Gunn, J., Warren, M. P., and Hamilton, L. H., The relation of eating problems and amenorrhea in ballet dancers, *Med. Sci. Sports Exerc.,* 19, 41, 1987.

86. Lloyd, T., Triantafyllou, S. J., Baker, E. R., Houts, P. S., Whiteside, J. A., Kalenak, A., and Stumpf, P. G., Women athletes with menstrual irregularity have increased musculo-skeletal injuries, *Med. Sci. Sports Exerc.,* 18, 374, 1986.

87. Baker, E. R., Mathur, R. S., Kirk, R. F., and Williamson, H. O., Female runners and secondary amenorrhea: correlation with age, parity, mileage and plasma hormonal and sex-hormone-binding globulin concentrations, *Fertil. Steril.,* 36, 183, 1981.

88. Brooks, S. M., Sanborn, C. F., Albrecht, B. H., and Wagner, W. W., Diet in athletic amenorrhea, *Lancet,* 3, 559, 1984.

89. Carlberg, K. A., Buckman, M. T., Peake, G. T., and Riedesel, M. L., Body composition of oligo/amenorrheic athletes, *Med. Sci. Sports Exerc.,* 15, 215, 1983.

90. Dale, E. and Goldberg, D. L., Implications of nutrition in athletes with menstrual cycle irregularities, *Can. J. Appl. Sport Sci.,* 7, 74, 1982.

91. Loucks, A. B. and Horvath, S. M., Exercise induced stress responses of amenorrheic and eumenorrheic runners, *J. Clin. Endocrinol. Metab.,* 59, 1109, 1984.

92. Schwartz, B., Cumming, D. C., Biordan, E., Selye, M., Yen, S. C., and Rebar, R. W., Exercise associated amenorrhea: a distinct entity, *Am. J. Obstet. Gynecol.,* 141, 622, 1981.

93. Warren, M. P., Effect of undernutrition on reproductive function in the human, *Endocr. Rev.,* 4, 363, 1983.

94. Shetty, P. S., Adaptive changes in basal metabolic rate and lean body mass in chronic undernutrition, *Hum. Nutr. Clin. Nutr.,* 38C, 443, 1984.

95. Myerson, M., Gutin, B., Warren, M. P., May, M. R., Contento, I., Lee, M., Pi-Sunyer, F. X., Pierson, R. N., Jr., and Brooks-Gunn, J., Resting metabolic rate and energy balance in amenorrheic and eumenorrheic runners, *Med. Sci. Sports Exerc.,* 23, 15, 1991.

96. Nationwide Food Consumption Continuing Survey of Food Intakes by Individuals. Women 19–50 Years and Their Children 1–5 Years, 1 Day, U.S. Department of Agriculture, NFCS CSFII Report No. 85, 1985.

97. Schweiger, U., Laessle, R., Pfister, H., Hoehl, C., Schwingenschloegel, M., Schweiger, M., and Pirke, K.-M., Diet-induced menstrual irregularities: effects of age and weight loss, *Fertil. Steril.,* 48, 746, 1987.

98. Walberg, J. L. and Johnston, C. S., Menstrual function and eating behavior in female recreational weight lifters and competitive body builders, *Med. Sci. Sports Exerc.,* 23, 30, 1991.

99. Snow-Harter, C. and Marcus, R., Exercise, bone mineral density, and osteoporosis, in *Exerc. Sport Sci. Rev.,* 19, 351, 1991.

100. Block, J. E., Genant, H. K., and Black, D., Greater vertebral bone mineral mass in exercising young men, *West. J. Med.,* 145, 39, 1986.

101. Heinrich, C., Going, S. B., Pamenter, R. W., Perry, C. D., Boyden, T. W., and Lohman, T. G., Bone mineral content of cyclically menstruating female resistance and endurance trained athletes, *Med. Sci. Sports Exerc.,* 22, 558, 1990.

102. Meema, H. E. and Meema, S., Cortical bone mineral density vs. cortical thickness in the diagnosis of osteoporosis: a roentgenological-densitometric study, *J. Am. Geriatric Soc.,* 17, 120, 1969.

103. Drinkwater, B. D., Nelson, K. L., Chesnutt, C. S., Bremner, Q. J., Shainholtz, S., and Southworth, M. B., Bone mineral content of amenorrheic and eumenorrheic athletes, *N. Engl. J. Med.,* 311, 277, 1984.

104. Drinkwater, B., Nilson, K., Ott, S., and Chesnut, C. H., III, Bone mineral density after resumption of menses in amenorrheic athletes, *J.A.M.A.,* 256, 380, 1986.

105. Nelson, M. E., Fisher, E. C., Catsos, P. D., Meredith, C. N., Turksoy, R. N., and Evans, W. J., Diet and bone status in amenorrheic runners, *Am. J. Clin. Nutr.,* 43, 910, 1986.

106. Drinkwater, B., Amenorrheic athletes: at risk for premature osteoporosis, *Proc. 1st IOC World Congress on Sports Sciences, Colorado Springs, CO,* U.S. Olympic Committee, 1989.

107. Frisch, R. E. and McArthur, J. W., Menstrual cycles: fatness as a determinant of minimum weight for height necessary for their maintenance or onset, *Science,* 185, 949, 1974.

108. Howat, P. M., Carbo, M. L., Mills, G. Q., and Wozniak, P., The influence of diet, body fat, menstrual cycling, and activity upon the bone density of females, *J. Am. Diet. Assoc.,* 89, 1305, 89.

109. Hunt, I. F., Murphy, N. J., Henderson, C., Clari, V. A., Jacobs, R. M., Johnston, P. K., and Coulson, A. H., Bone mineral content in postmenopausal women: comparison of omnivores and vegetarians, *Am. J. Clin. Nutr.,* 50, 517, 1989.

110. Frusztajer, N. T., Dhuper, S., Warren, M. P., Brooks-Gunn, J., and Fox, R. P., Nutrition and the incidence of stress fractures in ballet dancers, *Am. J. Clin. Nutr.,* 51, 779, 1990.

111. Dalsky, G., Effect of exercise on bone: permissive influence of estrogen and calcium, *Med. Sci. Sport Exerc.,* 22, 281, 1990.

112. Myburgh, K., Hutchins, J., Fataar, A., Bewerunge, L., Boltman, G., and Noakes, T. D., Higher bone density and fewer stress fractures in athletes using oral contraceptives, *Med. Sci. Sports Exerc.,* 22, S77, 1990.

113. Lindberg, J. S., Powell, M. R., Hunt, M. M., Ducey, D. E., and Wade, C. E., Increased vertebral bone mineral in response to reduced exercise in amenorrheic runners, *West. J. Med.,* 146, 39, 1987.

114. National Institutes of Health Consensus Development Conference Statement, Optimal Calcium Intake, June 6–8, 1994; NIH Office of Medical Applications of Research, Bethesda, MD.

115. National Osteoporosis Foundation, 301 E. 57th St., 3rd floor, Dept. NU, New York, NY, 10022.

116. *Food Guide Pyramid,* Human Nutrition Info. Service, Home and Garden Bulletin, No. 249, U.S. Department of Agriculture, 1992.

117. *Food Guide Pyramid for Vegetarians,* The General Conference Nutrition Council, The Health Connection, Phone: 1-800-548-8700 or (301)790-9735.

Chapter 14

NUTRITION ISSUES OF WOMEN IN THE U.S. ARMY*†

Nancy King and Eldon W. Askew

CONTENTS

I. INTRODUCTION

Although the stereotypical image of military life is that of soldiers eating in large mess halls, the majority of peacetime American soldiers have the option of consuming their meals away from the military environment, at home,

---

* The views, opinions, and/or findings in this report are those of the authors and should not be construed as an official Department of the Army position, policy, or decision, unless so designated by other official documentation.

† Work performed at the U.S. Army Research Institute of Environmental Medicine, Natick, MA.

or in public establishments. However, some soldiers (e.g., basic trainees) are required to subsist in military dining facilities for certain extended time periods during their training. Periodically, all soldiers eat military rations* in the field environment during training or field operations. The type of ration provided in the dining facility or the field is contingent upon the unit's missions, tactical scenarios, and availability of cooks and rations. Although nutritionally adequate military rations are provided, the soldiers pick and choose the ration components they eat based on what is available, their food preferences, and what they think is good for them. This fact underscores the important role played by nutritional surveys of actual food consumption, which serve to determine true nutrient intake.

A small number of women have participated in military nutritional surveys.[1-6] The results from these studies suggest that nutritional problems encountered by women in the U.S. Army are not greatly different from those faced by their civilian counterparts. However, nutritional problems of female soldiers may be exacerbated by physical performance demands imposed by military training and by the need to meet weight for height and body fat standards.

II. HISTORICAL PERSPECTIVE ON ACTIVE DUTY MILITARY WOMEN

With over 203,000 female members on active duty in U.S. military services,[7] women have become an integral part of the Armed Forces. For some time, the quota of women serving in any of the military services was set at 2%. In 1967, Public Law 90-130 lifted this ceiling. In the U.S. Army alone, between 1970 and 1980, the percentage of women escalated from 1.46 to 9.85%, almost a sevenfold increase.[8] As of June 30, 1993, women composed 12.3% of the U.S. Army active-duty personnel (71,640 women).[7]

Most women serving in the U.S. military before World War II were nurses. During World War II, women's jobs consisted mainly of nursing, administration, and clerical; a few had jobs in naval intelligence and communications. Shortly after the war, women's positions were returned to the "traditional female jobs" of clerks, secretaries, and routine communications. Military positions available to women today are diverse and not as traditional.[9] For instance, female officers in the U.S. Army may serve in executive positions, tactical operations, intelligence, engineering/maintenance, scientific/professional, medical, administrative, and supply/logistics. Military Occupational Specialties for enlisted females include infantry gun crew/seamanship, electronic equipment repair, communications/intelligence, medical/dental, technical specialist, functional support/administration, electrical/mechanical equipment repair, crafts, and service/supply.

---

* Generally, a ration is the nutritionally adequate food to subsist one person for 1 d, while a meal is a specified quantity of food provided to one person during one scheduled serving period. Thus, a ration in the dining hall setting consists of three meals.

III. PROFILE OF U.S. ARMY WOMEN

Anthropometric characteristics of U.S. Army women are depicted in Table 1. These data were provided by an anthropometric survey of 2208 U.S. Army women in 1988.[10]

TABLE 1
Anthropometric Survey of
U.S. Army Women in 1988

Sample size	2208
Ethnicity (%)	
White	51.6
Black	41.8
Hispanic	2.6
Asian/Pacific	1.4
American Indians	0.6
Mixed/other	1.9
Age groups (%)	
≤20 years	16.4
21–24 years	29.8
25–30	32.0
≥31 years	21.7
Height, mean/range (cm)	162.9/142.8–187.0
Body weight, mean/range (kg)	62.0/41.3–96.7

From Gordon, C. C., Churchill, T., Clauser, C. E., Bradtmiller, B., McConville, J.T., Tebbetts, I., and Walker, R.A., *1988 Anthropometric Survey of U.S. Army Personnel: Summary Statistics Interim Report,* Technical Report NATICK/TR-89/027, U.S. Army Natick Research, Development and Engineering Center, Natick, MA, 1989.

For the female soldier, body weight and composition (thinness) denotes more than just appearance (esthetics) and health, since they have an impact upon retention in the service and the continuation of a woman's military career (Tables 2 and 3).[11,12] Body composition is related to physical fitness in that a high percentage of body fat correlates negatively to aerobic fitness capacity.[13] Thus, body composition is an integral part of physical fitness and essential for maintaining physical readiness. In a recent Health Risk Appraisal Assessment,[14] 34% of 13,078 female soldiers reported exceeding the U.S. Army weight for height standards. Results from a body composition research project[15] conducted in 1984 indicated that female soldiers had a mean body fat of 28% with a range of 5 to 50%. In this study, body fat in 260 women from different ethnic backgrounds, aged 17 to 40 years, was assessed by hydrostatic weighing.[15]

Pregnant and post-partum military women have a particular concern about the requirement to meet the body weight/fat standards and the physical fitness

TABLE 2
Height/Weight Standards for U.S. Army Women

Height (in.)	Maximum Allowable Weight (lb), by Age Category			
	17–20	21–27	28–39	40 and over
58	112	115	119	122
59	116	119	123	126
60	120	123	127	130
61	124	127	131	135
62	129	132	137	139
63	133	137	141	144
64	137	141	145	148
65	141	145	149	153
66	146	150	154	158
67	149	154	159	162
68	154	159	164	167
69	158	163	168	172
70	163	168	173	177
71	167	172	177	182
72	172	177	183	188
73	177	182	188	193
74	183	189	194	198
75	188	194	200	204
76	194	200	206	209
77	199	205	211	215
78	204	210	216	220
79	209	215	220	226
80	214	220	227	232

From *The Army Weight Control Program,* Army Regulation 600-9 (update change 1), Headquarters, Department of the Army, Washington, D.C., 1994; Friedl, K.E., *Body Composition and Physical Performance,* Marriott, B.M. and Grumstrup-Scott, J., Eds., National Academy Press, Washington, D.C., 1992, chap. 3 and appendix E.

test 135 d after delivery (42 d of convalescence leave and 90 d of restricted physical activity).[16,17] This adds an unusual amount of stress, which may encourage some of these women to limit their food intake during pregnancy as well as during lactation.

Army soldiers are required biannually to pass a physical fitness test, which consists of pushups, situps, and a 2-mi run, with passing scores adjusted for age.[17] Because of this requirement, female soldiers may be more physically active than their civilian counterparts. Fifty-seven percent of the female participants (n = 13,078) surveyed in an Army Health Risk Appraisal Assessment reported doing aerobic exercise three or more times a week.[14] Women assigned to operational units or undergoing initial entry or specialty training are probably more physically active on average than other women in the U.S. Army.

TABLE 3
Percent Body Fat Standards
for U.S. Army Women

Age (years)	Percent Body Fat
17–20	30
21–27	32
28–39	34
>40	36

From *The Army Weight Control Program,* Army Regulation 600-9 (Update Change 1), Headquarters, Department of the Army, Washington, D.C., 1994; Friedl, K.E., *Body Composition and Physical Performance,* Marriott, B.M. and Grumstrup-Scott, J., Eds., National Academy Press, Washington, D.C., 1992, chap. 3 and appendix E.

IV. MILITARY NUTRITIONAL SURVEYS

A. DESCRIPTION OF MILITARY NUTRITIONAL SURVEYS

Only five military nutritional studies have included subjects from both genders,[1-5] and only one study (n = 49) has been specifically designed to determine the nutritional intake of female soldiers.[6] This last study was part of a larger research project (n = 158) that assessed the health, performance, and nutritional status of army women during the initial entry (U.S. Army Basic Combat Training).[18] In two of these six studies, soldiers were fed solely at a field site, while in the other four studies, soldiers were fed mostly at a dining facility. A description of these nutritional surveys is presented in Table 4.

B. MILITARY RATIONS

The ration served in the dining hall studies was the A-Ration, whereas the soldiers participating in the field studies received one or two "Meal, Ready-to-Eat" (MRE) with either B-Ration or Tray Packs (T-Ration).

The A-ration consists of perishable foods and is used in the dining facility setting or when cooking and refrigeration equipment are available in the field. The MRE is an individually packed meal used in the field when the mission and tactical scenario do not permit group feeding. The components are heat processed in retortable pouches (flexible containers). B-Ration components are mostly canned and dehydrated foods, centrally prepared by cooks and then distributed. The B-Ration is used in the field when cooking, but no refrigeration equipment is available. The components of the T-Ration are thermally processed, shelf-stable foods, packaged in hermetically sealed, half-size steam table containers. This ration is ready to heat and serve, thus fewer cooks are required to prepare and serve T-Rations compared to B-Rations. The T-Ration

TABLE 4
Description of Military Nutritional Surveys

Type	Location	When	Duration	Ration	Soldiers Total	Soldiers Females	Age[a]	Ref.
Field	Hawaii	August 1985	44 d	MRE/T	240	40[b]	23	2
	Bolivia[c]	July 1990	15 d	MRE/B[d]	80	13[e]	24	4
Dining hall	West Point	1980	5 d	A	190	54[f]	20	1
	Ft. Jackson	August 1988	7 d[g]	A[h]	81	40[i]	20	3
	West Point	March 1990	7 d	A	205	86[f]	20	5
	Ft. Jackson	April 1993	7 d	A	49	49[i]	21	6

[a]   Mean age of female soldiers.
[b]   Combat service support.
[c]   Elevation 11,500 ft.
[d]   Plus a carbohydrate supplement (125 g).
[e]   50% medical, 33% engineer, 17% other.
[f]   Officer candidates.
[g]   Nonconsecutive.
[h]   MREs served 2 d of field exercise.
[i]   Soldiers-in-training.

Adapted from King, N., Fridlund, K. E., and Askew, E. W., *J. Am. Coll. Nutr.*, 12, 344, 1993. With permission.

is used in the field for group feeding when neither cooking nor refrigeration are possible. A detailed description of each of the military rations has been delineated elsewhere.[19,20]

Military rations are produced according to nutritional standards, thus ensuring that the Military Recommended Dietary Allowances (MRDA) can be met.[21] The MRDA are established jointly by all military services, in concurrence with the Food and Nutrition Board of the National Research Council. The 1985 MRDA are based on the 1980 Recommended Dietary Allowances (RDA),[22] with an increased requirement of some nutrients due to increased physical activity, and therefore increased energy requirement, of soldiers compared to their more sedentary civilian counterparts (Table 5). The MRDA are currently being revised to reflect the 1989 RDA.[23]

The rations are designed to meet the energy and nutritional requirements of both male and female soldiers. Therefore, in certain instances, because male soldiers require and consume more energy per day, nutrient density of the menu (unit of nutrient per 1000 kcal) is not always optimal for the female soldier; depending on energy consumption of the female soldier, intake of some nutrients may be inadequate. Specifically, considering an MRDA of 2400 kcal for energy, the female soldier would have to consume approximately 129% of her energy requirement to meet the calcium MRDA of 1200 mg or 138% energy to meet the iron MRDA of 18 mg.

TABLE 5
The Military Recommended Dietary
Allowances Versus the Recommended
Dietary Allowances

Nutrient	Unit	MRDA[a]	RDA[b]
Energy	kcal	2000–2800	2000–2100
Protein	g	80	44
Vitamin A	mcg RE	800	800
Vitamin D	mcg	5–10	5
Vitamin E	mg TE	8	8
Ascorbic acid	mg	60	60
Thiamin	mg	1.2	1.0–1.1
Riboflavin	mg	1.4	1.2–1.3
Niacin	mg NE	16	13–14
Vitamin B$_6$	mg	2.0	2
Folic acid	mcg	400	400
Vitamin B$_{12}$	mcg	3.0	3.0
Calcium	mg	800–1200	800
Phosphorus	mg	800–1200	800
Magnesium	mg	300	300
Iron	mg	18	18
Zinc	mg	15	15
Iodine	mcg	150	150
Sodium	mg	<4100	—

[a] MRDA for moderately active military women ages
17–50 years old.[21]
[b] RDA for women 19–50 years old.[22]

C. NUTRITIONAL INTAKES

Table 6 shows the mean nutrient intake of female soldiers participating in the six aforementioned military nutritional surveys.[1-6] Data on these 278 women indicate a generally lower nutrient intake in the field than in dining halls. The women in the Hawaii and Bolivia field studies did not meet their MRDA for energy (76 and 70% of the MRDA, respectively), protein (84 and 85%), calcium (58 and 66%), and iron (66 and 65%). (Male soldiers in the Hawaii and Bolivia field studies also had lower intakes than the dining hall participants. However, perhaps due to the difference in body size, men still consumed enough food to meet the MRDA for all nutrients, except energy.) From the data available, it cannot be determined if the low intake was a result of field conditions, extreme environment (high terrestrial altitude, as in Bolivia), or type of rations served.

Less than optimal nutrient intakes were observed in the dining hall studies. In the 1993 Fort Jackson study, the intakes of vitamin B$_6$, folic acid, calcium, magnesium, iron, and zinc were at 75, 65, 73, 89, 90, and 73% of their MRDA, respectively.[6] Folic acid and iron intakes were also suboptimal in the 1980 West Point study, meeting only 85 and 90% of the MRDA, respectively.[1] Zinc

TABLE 6
Mean Nutrient Intake of Female Soldiers

		Field		Dining hall			
Nutrient	MRDA[a]	Hawaii 1985 (n = 36)	Bolivia 1990 (n = 13)	West Point 1980 (n = 54)	Ft. Jackson 1988 (n = 40)	West Point 1990 (n = 86)	Ft. Jackson 1993 (n = 49)
Energy (kcal)	2000–2800	1834	1668	2454[b]	2467	2314	2592
Protein (g)	80	67	68	84	96	79	82
Carbohydrate (g)	330	235	218	284	318	325	365
Fat (g)	<93	70	57	107	94	81	94
Cholesterol (mg)	<300	—[c]	235	—	418	234	466
Vitamin A (mcg RE)	800	1602	1030	—	1690	1250	1390
Ascorbic acid (mg)	60	142	107	147	165	172	89
Thiamin (mg)	1.2	4.0	2.0	11.6	2.0	2.8	1.8
Riboflavin (mg)	1.4	1.6	1.5	9.3	2.2	3.0	2.0
Niacin (mg NE)	16	16.5	19.4	37.3	27	30	20
Vitamin B_6 (mg)	2	—	1.5	—	—	2.6	1.5
Folic acid (mcg)	400	—	178	339	—	428	261
Vitamin B_{12} (mcg)	3.0	—	2.1	4.7	3.7	6.2	5.6
Calcium (mg)	800–1200	577	664	954	907	1001	728
Phosphorus (mg)	800–1200	1065	1059	1347	1600	1391	1296
Magnesium (mg)	300	—	218	—	—	315	267
Iron (mg)	18	11.9	11.7	16.2	18.4	28	16.2
Zinc (mg)	15	—	5	11	—	14	11
Sodium (mg)	<4100	3343	3819	2764	4420	3703	3994

[a] MRDA for moderately active military women ages 17–50 years old.[21]

[b] 3% of kilocalories provided by alcohol intake.

[c] Data not recorded during the survey denoted by "—".

Adapted from King, N., Fridlund, K. E., and Askew, E. W., *J. Am. Coll. Nutr.*, 12, 344, 1993. With permission.

intakes were also suboptimal in the 1980 and the 1990 West Point studies, 73 and 93%, respectively.[1,5] The intake of some nutrients was not assessed (vitamin B_6 and magnesium for the 1980 West Point and 1988 Fort Jackson studies; folic acid and zinc for the 1988 Fort Jackson study).

The macronutrient distribution of the field and dining hall studies is shown on Table 7.[1-6] The similarity of the macronutrient distribution among the studies suggests that food consumption was qualitatively similar but quantitatively lower.

TABLE 7
Caloric Distribution

Nutrient	Field		Dining hall			
	Hawaii 1985	Bolivia 1990	West Point 1980	Ft. Jackson 1988	West Point 1990	Ft. Jackson 1993
Energy[a] (kcal)	1834	1668	2454[b]	2467	2314	2592
Protein[c] (%)	14.6	16.3	13.7	15.6	13.7	12.7
Carbohydrate[c] (%)	51.3	52.3	46.3	51.6	56.2	56.3
Fat[c] (%)	34.4	30.9	39.2	34.3	31.5	32.6

[a] Kilocalories consumed during the study period.

[b] 3% of kilocalories provided by alcohol intake.

[c] Percentage of energy from macro-nutrients; percentages were rounded and may not add up to 100%.

Adapted from King, N., Fridlund, K. E., and Askew, E. W., *J. Am. Coll. Nutr.*, 12, 344, 1993. With permission.

National nutrition surveys, Second National Health and Nutrition Examination Survey (NHANES II) and Continuing Survey of Food Intakes by Individuals (CSFII), have also reported low intakes of vitamin B_6, folic acid, calcium, magnesium, iron, and zinc in the general female population in that age group (20 to 29 years old) in the U.S.[24] (Table 8). This suggests that nutritional problems encountered by female soldiers are similar to those encountered by their civilian counterparts and, therefore, the military setting and type of ration are not the exclusive determinants of low intakes.

V. NUTRITION ISSUES

Nutrient density of military rations presents a subtle problem. While military menus appear nutritionally adequate (providing well above 100% of the MRDA for all nutrients), when the nutrient composition of the menu is expressed in terms of amount of nutrient per 1000 kcal, it is evident that female soldiers are at a disadvantage. Female soldiers may not be able to eat as much as male soldiers. In the 1993 Fort Jackson study, the two main reasons given for not eating the entire portion were (1) not being hungry and (2) being too

TABLE 8
Nutrient Intake of U.S. Female Population

| | | Nutrition monitoring | |
| | | NHANES II[b] | CSFII[c] |
Nutrient	RDA[a]	1976–1980	1985–1986
Energy (kcal)	2000–2100	1675	1674
Protein (g)	44	64	65
Carbohydrate (g)	—	195	198
Fat (g)	—	67	68
Cholesterol (mg)	—	270	302
Vitamin A (mcg RE)	800	841	1048
Ascorbic acid (mg)	60	95	86
Thiamin (mg)	1.0–1.1	1.09	1.17
Riboflavin (mg)	1.2–1.3	1.49	1.51
Niacin (mg NE)	13–14	16.2	17.3
Vitamin B_6 (mg)	2	—	1.2[d]
Folic acid (mcg)	400	—	197[d]
Vitamin B_{12} (mcg)	3	—	4.5[d]
Calcium (mg)	800	662	691
Phosphorus (mg)	800	1117	1065
Magnesium (mg)	300	—	204[d]
Iron (mg)	18	10.7	11.1
Zinc (mg)	15	—	8.8[d]
Sodium (mg)	—	2404	2593

[a] RDA for women 19–50 years.
[b] Second National Health and Nutrition Examination Survey, women 20–29 years (1 d).
[c] Continuing Survey of Food Intakes by Individuals for 1985, women 20–29 years (1 d).
[d] Continuing Survey of Food Intakes by Individuals for 1985, women 20–29 years (4 d).

From Food and Nutrition Board, *Recommended Dietary Allowances,* 9th ed., National Academy of Sciences, Washington, D.C., 1980; Life Sciences Research Office, Federation of American Societies for Experimental Biology, *Nutrition Monitoring in the United States — An Update Report on Nutrition Monitoring,* DHHS Publ. No. (PHS) 89-1255, U.S. Department of Health and Human Services, Washington, D.C., 1989.

full.[6] Furthermore, it would be difficult for most female soldiers to consume the amount of energy required to meet their calcium and iron requirements without gaining weight.

Although the impact of sporadic, low nutrient intakes may be inconsequential, this is not the case when inadequate intake occurs repetitively due to participation in multiple field training exercises. This impact may be even greater if experienced for longer periods of time during extended deployments. Furthermore, since this pattern of low intakes is typical of the general female population in the U.S.,[23] it may be the usual eating pattern of military women (independent of ration or circumstance), and the low nutrient intakes may occur frequently instead of occasionally. Likewise, the efforts of the female soldier toward meeting and maintaining body weight standards, even after childbirth, undoubtedly have a negative impact on what and how much that female soldier chooses to eat.

A low calcium intake during the first three decades of life has been associated with an increased risk of osteoporosis later in life.[25] Although the main contributor to bone density is genetics, it is generally recognized that low calcium intake during adolescence jeopardizes the optimization of peak bone mass. This issue of bone mineral density is of particular concern to the military because of the high incidence of stress fractures and stress reaction injuries in young military women.[26-28]

As part of the 1993 Fort Jackson study and before the beginning of the 8-week training course, we collected historical calcium intake and bone-mineral density data from 111 female soldiers (ages: 17 to 33 years; mode: 19) to determine if there was a correlation between these two variables. Their usual calcium intakes were assessed using the Health Habits and Diet History Questionnaire developed and validated by Block.[29,30] This questionnaire contains an open-ended food frequency section of 60 food items. The soldiers were asked to answer these questions based on their usual eating habits over the past year. Bone-mineral density was determined by dual-energy X-ray absorptiometry[31] using a LUNAR DPX-Plus scanner with the version 3.6 software (LUNAR Corporation, Madison, WI).

Usual calcium intakes ([mean ± SD] 830 ± 413 mg/d, ranging from 268 to 2112 mg/d) and bone-mineral densities ($1.21 ± 0.08$ g/cm², ranging from 1.0 to 1.42 g/cm²) did not correlate significantly ($r = 0.069, p > 0.05$).[32] Dividing the group into whites, blacks, hispanics, and others (American Indians and Alaska Natives [n = 2]) also yielded no association (Whites [n = 67]: r = 0.02; Blacks [n = 27]: r = 0.26; Hispanics [n = 15]: r = 0.40).

A stepwise, multiple-regression analysis was completed using bone-mineral density as the dependent factor and considering other factors that may influence bone-mineral density such as ethnicity, family history of osteoporosis, age, pregnancy history, smoking history, body mass index, protein intake, sodium intake, caffeine consumption, and fiber intake. This analysis revealed that the only factors significantly ($p < 0.01$) related to bone-mineral density for this group of female soldiers were body mass index, ethnicity, and family history of osteoporosis.[32] A history of amenorrhea was not included in the analysis since only 1 out of these 111 women reported having an amenorrhea history. (Incidentally, irregularities of menstrual cycle, including amenorrhea, is one of the disqualifiers for enlistment in the military;[16] this may explain the relatively low reported incidence of this disorder in this particular study.)

Negative iron balance has been associated with decrements in physical performance and has also been related to various neurologic, cognitive, and immunologic problems.[33,34] Therefore, suboptimal intakes of dietary iron are of concern to military women. Hematological values from the two West Point studies and the 1993 Fort Jackson study are shown in Table 9.[35-37] Friedl et al. reported increasing levels of iron deficiency: 36.6% of the female cadets (n = 41) had ferritin levels of less than 12 ng/ml, 22% had iron saturation levels of less than 16%, and 4.9% had hemoglobin levels of less than 12 g/dl.[35] Nevertheless, serum markers of iron status for the 1990 West Point study were not significantly affected by dietary iron intakes.[5] Westphal et al. observed that 63.3% of the soldiers-in-training (n = 49) had ferritin levels of less than 12 ng/mL, 42.9% had iron saturation levels of less than 16%, and 24.5% had hemoglobin levels of less than 12 g/dl.[36] Though these mean hematological values were lower than those reported in the other two studies, serum markers of iron status for the 1993 Fort Jackson study were also not significantly associated with iron intakes.[36]

TABLE 9
Hematological Values[a] of Female Soldiers-in-Training

	Normal Range	West Point 1980 (n = 30–72[b])	West Point 1990 (n = 22[c])	Ft. Jackson 1993 (n = 49[d])
Hemoglobin (g/dl)	12–16	13.3 ± 1.2	12.5 ± 1.0	12.6 ± 0.2
Hematocrit (%)	37–47	39.1 ± 2.3	37.8 ± 2.4	37.4 ± 0.4
Serum iron (mcg/dl)	65–175	80.0 ± 38.0	72.0 ± 41.0	69.2 ± 6.0
TIBC (mcg/dl)	300–360	344.0 ± 44.0	326.0 ± 46.0	334.1 ± 6.8
Iron saturation (%)	20–55	23.0 ± 11.2	22.1 ± 13.3	20.4 ± 1.8
Ferritin (ng/ml)	22–447	25.0 ± 11.0	18.0 ± 13.0	10.6 ± 1.7
RCB folate (ng/ml)	169–707	431.0 ± 138.0	309.0 ± 65.0	157.2 ± 53.3
Serum folate (ng/ml)	2.2–17.3	11.7 ± 6.2	9.3 ± 3.7	3.6 ± 0.3

[a] Mean ± SD.
[b] Reference 37.
[c] Females that did not donate blood the week prior to testing and did not use iron or general vitamin-mineral supplements.[35]
[d] Soldiers that participated on nutrition intake data only; blood drawn 10 d after nutrient intake data collection.[36]

Adapted from King, N., Fridlund, K. E., and Askew, E. W., *J. Am. Coll. Nutr.*, 12, 344, 1993. With permission.

Low intakes of folic acid have been associated with neural tube defects; thus, folic acid is of particular concern to pregnant women.[38] It has been suggested that adequate folic acid intake is essential from at least 4 weeks before conception through the first 3 months of pregnancy.[39] Since most female soldiers are of childbearing age[10] and not all pregnancies are planned in advance (many conceptions occur upon returning from field training exercises or deployments, when folic acid intake has been potentially at its worst for several days), inadequate intakes of folic acid becomes an important issue for military women as well. It has been estimated that, in the early 1980s, approximately 10% of active-duty military female personnel were pregnant at any given time.[40] However, few, if any, studies have assessed the incidence of birth defects among military women.[40]

Red blood cell and serum folate levels for the two West Point studies and the 1993 Fort Jackson study are shown in Table 9.[35-37] Except for red blood cell folate from the 1993 Fort Jackson study, the mean values were within normal limits. The 1993 Fort Jackson study data reveal a significant ($p < 0.05$) but weak ($r = 0.37$) correlation between folic acid intake and serum folate.[36]

VI. MILITARY NUTRITION INITIATIVES

Of the ten leading causes of death in the U.S. (heart diseases, cancers, strokes, unintentional injuries, chronic obstructive lung diseases, pneumonia and influenza, diabetes mellitus, suicide, chronic liver disease and cirrhosis, and atherosclerosis), five have been associated with diet (coronary heart disease, some types of cancer, stroke, diabetes mellitus, and atherosclerosis) and another three (cirrhosis of the liver, accidents, and suicide) have been associated with excessive alcohol intake.[41] Furthermore, high blood pressure, obesity, dental diseases, osteoporosis, and gastrointestinal diseases are attributed to dietary excesses and imbalances.[41] The heightened awareness of nutrition-related health issues generated several Department of the Army Military Nutrition Initiatives,[42] which are consistent with national health objectives. Since 1985, the U.S. Army has introduced nutrition initiatives into the Armed Forces Recipe Service,[43] the Army Master Menu,[44] and the Army Food Service Program[45] in an attempt to provide soldiers with a variety of nutritious menu alternatives lower in fat, cholesterol, and sodium. Furthermore, the initiatives were designed to heighten soldiers' awareness of the importance of nutrition and to educate soldiers and their families to make appropriate food choices.

Between 1988 and 1993, there were significant improvements in the menu provided at the military dining facility at Fort Jackson, SC.[6] Energy provided by fat was reduced from 38 to 33% (energy from saturated fat in 1993 was 10%), while energy provided from carbohydrate was increased from 50 to 56%. These changes align the menu with the current MRDA, which recommends 50 to 55% from carbohydrate, 10 to 15% from protein, and 35% or less from fat,[21] and with the goals of the Military Nutrition Initiatives to provide no more than 30% of energy from fat (no more than 10% of energy from saturated fat) by 1998.[42] The 1993 menu also was lower in dietary cholesterol than the 1988 menu (928 mg vs. 1299 mg). However, 928 mg remains considerably higher than the recommended goal of 300 mg or less by 1993. The reduction in sodium content of the menu from 1731 mg/1000 kcal in 1988 to 1640 mg/1000 kcal brought the menu within the target of an average of 1700 mg/1000 kcal of food served in military food service systems.

Table 10 summarizes the 1988 and 1993 female soldiers' nutritional intake data depicting the nutrition initiatives' 5-year progress.[6] Limitations of the 1988 nutrient data base precluded analyses of vitamin B_6, folic acid, magnesium, and zinc. The increased dietary cholesterol intake was due to the increased visible egg consumption. The number of female soldiers consuming more than three eggs per week increased from 50% in 1988 to 64% in 1993. In 1988, 39% of the total dietary cholesterol was contributed by visible eggs, while in 1993, visible eggs accounted for 43% of the total dietary cholesterol (1993 data base dietary cholesterol value adjusted to the 1988 data base). This finding underscores the need for nutrition education programs.

TABLE 10
Nutrition Initiatives: 1988 vs. 1993 Female Soldiers' Nutritional Intakes

	Fort Jackson	
	1988 (n = 40)	**1993** (n = 49)
Energy/kg of body wt (kcal)	41.7	41.0
Mean energy intake (kcal/% MRDA)	2467/103	2592/108
Nutrients with mean intake <100% MRDA	Ca[a]	Vitamin B_6, folic acid, Ca, Mg, Fe, Zn
Percent of total kcal (%)		
Protein	16	12
Fat	34	32
Carbohydrate	52	56
Soldiers with energy fat intake (%)		
<25	0	6
25–29	23	22
30–34	30	47
35–39	40	18
40–44	7	6
Mean cholesterol intake (mg)	418	466
Mean sodium intake (mg)	4420	3994

[a] Limitations of the 1988 nutrient data base precluded analyses of several nutrients, such as vitamin B_6, folic acid, magnesium, zinc, and potassium.

From Rose, R. W., Baker, C. J., Salter, C., Wisnaskas, W., Edwards, J. S. A., and Rose, M. S., *Dietary Assessment of U.S. Army Basic Trainees at Fort Jackson, S.C.*, Technical Report No. T6-89, U.S. Army Research Institute of Environmental Medicine, Natick, MA, 1989; King, N., Arsenault, J. E., Mutter, S. H., Murphy, T. C., Champagne, C., Westphal, K. A., and Askew, E. W., *Nutritional Intake of Female Soldiers During the U.S. Army Basic Combat Training*, Technical Report No. T94-17, U.S. Army Research Institute of Environmental Medicine, Natick, MA, 1994.

The Military Nutrition Initiatives are being revised to include increasing the consumption of fruits and vegetables for all military personnel. Furthermore, the initiatives will emphasize achieving adequate consumption of calcium, iron, and folic acid for female members. The Committee on Military Nutrition Research has recommended that a nutrition program be established for military women emphasizing the importance of dietary calcium and how to select calcium-rich foods, and the provision of low-fat, calcium-rich food choices in the dining halls.[42]

Low-fat milk and other dairy products are already integral parts of the A-ration. In an effort to increase the calcium content of the other military rations, ultra high temperature-treated (UHT) milk has been added to the T-ration. Furthermore, dry milk products (filled milk products) are being developed at the Natick Research, Development and Engineering Center in Natick, MA. These products will be added to the B-ration and MRE once testing is completed. A dehydrated dairy shake which, when reconstituted with water, provides 416 kcal, 18.7 g of protein, 65 g of carbohydrate, 9 g of fat, and 630 mg of calcium per serving is now available and can be used with the rations. A new product that is also available for military field feeding is the MRE pouch bread. One bread (200 kcal, 5.8 g of protein, 28 g of carbohydrate, and 7.4 g of fat) is relatively high in calcium (74 mg) and iron (1.9 mg).

However, just improving the nutritional content of the military rations would not be sufficient to meet the Military Nutrition Initiatives' goals. Nutrition education remains the cornerstone in motivating soldiers and families to (1) select diets consistent with current knowledge relative to healthy eating practices and (2) adopt healthier eating habits. Nutrition education programs in military dining facilities include information on the caloric value of each menu component, nutrition posters, and table tents. During their 8-week Basic Combat Training, female soldiers at Fort Jackson, SC receive one 1-h nutrition briefing based upon the Dietary Guidelines for Americans from *The Surgeon General's Report on Nutrition and Health*.[41] The Army Nutrition Policy Council, chaired by the Chief Dietitian of the Army, is developing lesson plans that include nutrient composition and fortification information of the military rations, in an effort to disseminate field feeding nutrition information to all Armed Forces members. Furthermore, the Council is developing guidelines for a nutrition education program for military women. This program will emphasize increasing calcium and iron intakes while maintaining desirable body weight. In addition, during National Nutrition Month (March) and throughout the year, Army dietitians provide nutrition education opportunities for soldiers and their families.

VII. SUMMARY AND CONCLUSIONS

It can be seen from the limited data collected on U.S. Army women that nutrition issues relevant to servicewomen are similar to those faced by their counterparts in the civilian population. Optimal calcium and iron intakes are difficult to achieve due to the density of these nutrients in the typical military and civilian diets. The emphasis that the military places upon weight control further exacerbates this problem.

Paradoxically, within the restrictive military structure soldiers are free to choose what they want to eat from what is available. Their choices are influenced by a complex interaction of factors, including the circumstances faced at the moment of eating. Since soldiers may eat what they think is good for them, nutrition education programs may be a viable solution to the nutritional problems of military women. With increased awareness, some of the behavior patterns that govern food selection and consumption may shift to a healthier diet.

VIII. RECOMMENDATIONS

More research is needed to ascertain the short- and long-term effect of sporadic and routine suboptimal nutrient intakes on nutritional status, health, and performance of military women. Considering that approximately 54% of the women in the U.S. Army are older than 25 years of age, particular emphasis should be given to including older military women in future studies.

Implementation of nutrition education programs tailored for the military woman is crucial. These programs should feature the importance of eating nutritionally balanced, varied diets, emphasizing the relevance of dietary calcium, iron, and folic acid on female health. Practical "how to" guidelines to assist military women in the selection of low-fat, nutrient-rich foods are a pivotal part of these programs.

ACKNOWLEDGMENTS

The assistance of LTC Kathleen A. Westphal and Dr. James A. Vogel in the preparation of this manuscript is gratefully acknowledged and appreciated.

REFERENCES

1. Kretsch, M. J., Conforti, P. M., and Sauberlich, H. E., *Nutrient Intake Evaluation of Male and Female Cadets at the U.S. Military Academy, West Point, New York*, LAIR Report No. 218, Letterman Army Institute of Research, Presidio of San Francisco, 1986.
2. *Combat Field Feeding System — Force Development Test and Experimentation*, Vol. 1, Basic Report No. CDEC-TR-85-006A, U.S. Army Research Institute of Environmental Medicine, Natick, MA and U.S. Army Combat Developments Experimentation Center, Fort Ord, CA, 1986.
3. Rose, R. W., Baker, C. J., Salter, C., Wisnaskas, W., Edwards, J. S. A., and Rose, M. S., *Dietary Assessment of U.S. Army Basic Trainees at Fort Jackson, S.C.*, Technical Report No. T6-89, U.S. Army Research Institute of Environmental Medicine, Natick, MA, 1989.
4. Edwards, J. S. A., Askew, E. W., King, N., Fulco, C. S., Hoyt, R. W., and Delany, J. P., *An Assessment of the Nutritional Intake and Energy Expenditure of Unacclimatized U.S. Army Soldiers Living and Working at High Altitude*, Technical Report No. T10-91, U.S. Army Research Institute of Environmental Medicine, Natick, MA, 1991.
5. Klicka, M. V., Sherman, D. E., King, N., Friedl, K. E., and Askew, E. W., *Nutritional Assessment of Cadets at the U.S. Military Academy: Part 2. Assessment of Nutritional Intake*, Technical Report No. T94-1, U.S. Army Research Institute of Environmental Medicine, Natick, MA, 1993.

6. King, N., Arsenault, J. E., Mutter, S. H., Murphy, T. C., Champagne, C., Westphal, K. A., and Askew, E. W., *Nutritional Intake of Female Soldiers During the U.S. Army Basic Combat Training*, Technical Report No. T94–17, U.S. Army Research Institute of Environmental Medicine, Natick, MA, 1994.

7. *Department of Defense Military Manpower Statistics*, June 30, 1993, Washington Headquarters Services, Directorate for Information Operations and Reports, Washington, D.C., 1993.

8. *Army Demographic Data*, Project No. M001443, Defense Manpower Data Center, Arlington, VA, 1988.

9. *Military Women in the Department of Defense*, Vol. 6, U.S. Department of Defense, Washington, D.C., 1988.

10. Gordon, C. C., Churchill, T., Clauser, C. E., Bradtmiller, B., McConville, J. T., Tebbetts, I., and Walker, R. A., *1988 Anthropometric Survey of U.S. Army Personnel: Summary Statistics Interim Report*, Technical Report NATICK/TR-89/027, U.S. Army Natick Research, Development and Engineering Center, Natick, MA, 1989.

11. *The Army Weight Control Program*, Army Regulation 600-9 (Update Change 1), Headquarters, Department of the Army, Washington, D.C., 1994.

12. Friedl, K. E., Body composition and military performance: origins of the army standards, in *Body Composition and Physical Performance*, Marriott, B. M. and Grumstrup-Scott, J., Eds., National Academy Press, Washington, D.C., 1992, chap. 3 and appendix E.

13. Vogel, J. A., Patton, J. F., Mello, R. P., and Daniels, W. L., An analysis of aerobic capacity in a large U.S. population, *J. Appl. Physiol.*, 60, 494, 1986.

14. Chandler, D. L., HCSSA Memorandum, Health Risk Appraisal, 01 Jan–31 Dec 93, Fort Sam Houston, TX, March 18, 1994.

15. Fitzgerald, P. I., Vogel, J. A., Daniels, W. L., Dziados, J. E., Teves, M. A., Mello, R. P., and Reich, P. J., *The Body Composition Project: A Summary Report and Descriptive Data*, Technical Report No. T5-87, U.S. Army Research Institute of Environmental Medicine, Natick, MA, 1986.

16. *Standards of Medical Fitness*, Army Regulation 40-501 (Change I02), Headquarters, Department of the Army, Washington, D.C., 1993.

17. *Physical Fitness Training*, Field Manual 21-20, Headquarters, Department of the Army, Washington, D.C., 1992, chap. 14.

18. Westphal, K. A., King, N., Friedl, K. E., Sharp, M. A., and Reynolds, K. L., *Health, Performance, and Nutritional Status of U.S. Army Women During Basic Training*, U.S. Army Research Institute of Environmental Medicine, Natick, MA, in press.

19. *Present and Future Operational Rations of the Department of Defense*, Natick Pamphlet 30-2, Natick Research, Development and Engineering Center, NATICK, MA, 1992.

20. Thomas, C. D., Baker-Fulco, C. J., Jones, T. E., King, N., Jezior, D. A., Fairbrother, B. N., and Askew, E. W., *Nutrition for Health and Performance — Nutritional Guidance for Military Operations in Temperate and Extreme Environments*, Technical Note No. 93-3, U.S. Army Research Institute of Environmental Medicine, Natick, MA, 1993, 2 and 42.

21. *Nutritional Allowances, Standards and Education*, Army Regulation 40-25/Naval Command Medical Instruction 10110.1/Air Force Regulation 160-95, Headquarters, Departments of the Army, the Navy, and the Air Force, Washington, D.C., 1985.

22. Food and Nutrition Board, *Recommended Dietary Allowances*, 9th ed., National Academy of Sciences, Washington, D.C., 1980.

23. Food and Nutrition Board, *Recommended Dietary Allowances*, 10th ed., National Academy of Sciences, Washington D.C., 1989.

24. Life Sciences Research Office, Federation of American Societies for Experimental Biology, *Nutrition Monitoring in the United States — An Update Report on Nutrition Monitoring*, DHHS Publ. No. (PHS) 89-1255, U.S. Department of Health and Human Services, Washington, D.C., 1989.

25. Heaney, R. P., Nutritional factors in causation of osteoporosis, *Ann. Chirur. Gynaecol.*, 77, 176, 1988.

26. Protzman, R. R. and Griffis, C. G., Stress fractures in men and women undergoing military training, *J. Bone Joint Surg.*, 59A, 825, 1977.

27. Schmidt Brudvig, T. J., Gudger, T. D., and Obermeyer, L., Stress fractures in 295 trainees: a one-year study of incidence as related to age, sex, and race, *Milit. Med.*, 148, 666, 1983.

28. Zahger, D., Abramovitz, A., Zelikovsky, L., Israel, O., and Israel, P., Stress fractures in female soldiers: an epidemiological investigation of an outbreak, *Milit. Med.*, 153, 448, 1988.

29. Block, G., Hartman, A. M., Dresser, C. M., Carroll, M. D., Gannon, J., and Gardner, L., A data-based approach to diet questionnaire design and testing, *Am. J. Epidemiol.*, 124, 453, 1986.

30. Block, G., Woods, M., Potosky, A., and Clifford, C., Validation of a self-administered diet history questionnaire using multiple diet records, *J. Clin. Epidemiol.*, 43, 1327, 1990.

31. Mazess, R. B., Barden, H. S., Bisek, J. P., and Hanson, J., Dual-energy x-ray absorptiometry for total-body and regional bone-mineral and soft-tissue composition, *Am. J. Clin. Nutr.*, 51, 1106, 1990.

32. King, N., Westphal, K. A., Friedl, K. E., Askew, E. W., Mutter, S. H., and McGraw, S., Dietary Calcium Intake and Bone Mineral Density in Young Army Women, Paper 36, presented at the 6th Conf. for Federally Supported Human Nutrition Research Units and Centers, Bethesda, MD, February 23 to 24, 1994.

33. Gardner, G. W., Edgerton, V. R., Senewiratne, B., Barnard, R. J., and Ohira, Y., Physical work capacity and metabolic stress in subjects with iron deficiency anemia, *Am. J. Clin. Nutr.*, 30, 910, 1977.

34. Lukaski, H. C., Hall, C. B., and Siders, W. A., Altered metabolic response of iron-deficient women during graded maximal exercise, *Eur. J. Exerc. Physiol.*, 63, 140, 1991.

35. Friedl, K. E., Marchitelli, L. J., Sherman, D. E., and Tulley, R., *Nutritional Assessment of Cadets at the U.S. Military Academy: Part 1. Anthropometric & Biochemical Measures*, Technical Report No. T4-91, U.S. Army Research Institute of Environmental Medicine, Natick, MA, 1990.

36. Westphal, K. A. and Friedl, K. E., unpublished data, 1994.

37. Sauberlich, H. E., Skala, J. H., Johnson, H. L., and Nelson, R. A., *Hematological Parameters and Lipid Profiles Observed in Cadets at the U.S. Military Academy, West Point, New York*, LAIR Report No. 126, Letterman Army Institute of Research, Presidio of San Francisco, 1982.

38. Scott, J. M., Kirke, P. N., and Weir, D. G., The role of nutrition in neural tube defects, *Annu. Rev. Nutr.*, 10, 277, 1990.

39. Rush, D. and Rosenberg, I. H., Folate supplements and neural tube defects, *Nutr. Rev.*, 50, 25, 1992.

40. Hoiberg, A. and White, J. F., Health status of women in the Armed Forces, *Armed Forces Soc.*, 18, 514, 1992.

41. *The Surgeon General's Report on Nutrition and Health*, Publ. No. 88-50210, U.S. Department of Health and Human Services, Washington, D.C., 1988.

42. The Committee on Military Nutrition Research, *Military Nutrition Initiatives*, Publ. IOM-91-05, National Academy of Sciences, Washington, D.C., 1991.

43. *Armed Forces Recipe Services*, Technical Manual 10-412/NAVSUP Publ. 7/AFM 146-12, Vol. 1/MCOP 10110.42A, Headquarters, Departments of the Army, the Navy, and the Air Force, Washington, D.C., 1992.

44. *The Master Menu*, Supply Bulletin No. 10-260, Headquarters, Department of the Army, Washington, D.C., published monthly.

45. *The Army Food Service Program*, Army Regulation 30-1, Headquarters, Department of the Army, Washington, D.C., 1989.

Chapter 15

NUTRITION AND THE OLDER FEMALE

**Helen Smiciklas-Wright, Irene M. Soucy,
Janet M. Friedmann, and Gordon L. Jensen**

CONTENTS

I. DEMOGRAPHY AND EPIDEMIOLOGY

Populations in the U.S. and worldwide are aging.[1-3] The U.S. population of adults 65 years and older has increased dramatically during this century. This pattern is likely to continue until at least the middle of the next century. The proportion of persons 65 years and older is projected to increase from 12.1 to 16.9% by the year 2020 and that of persons 85 years and older from 1.2 to 2.1%.[4] Older women outnumber older men and by increasing margins in successive age groups.[4] American women who are 65, 75, and 85 years can, on the average, expect to live about another 19, 12, and 6 years, respectively.[5] These simply stated demographic facts have implications for living arrangements,[4] economic status,[6-9] health status,[10,11] and nutritional well-being of older women.

Almost one half of older women live alone, about 40% of those 65 years and older and 60% of women 85 years and older. The proportion of older women in nursing homes increases significantly with age, from less than 2% for those who are 65 to 74 years to more than 10% for those 75 and older.[4,12] Economic status has generally improved for older Americans;[7,13] however, women have higher poverty rates than do men,[9,14,15] with rates increasing for those 85 years and older and for blacks and Hispanics.[8]

Heart and cerebrovascular diseases and malignant neoplasms are the leading causes of death, overall, with higher death rates in white and black women than in Hispanic, Asian, or Native American populations.[16-18] Comorbidity increases with age.[19] Many conditions, including septicemia, diabetes mellitus, pneumonia and influenza, and atherosclerosis, add to mortality risk for older women when present with other diseases. Women are major consumers of health care services. They report more symptoms of illness and have higher prevalence of nonfatal chronic diseases than do men.[20] Leading chronic conditions involve disabilities and functional decline.[20-22] Most women who are considered to be the "young old", those less than 75 years, perform daily activities with little or no difficulty; about one third of women 75 years and older report difficulties with shopping and one quarter report problems with meal preparation.[10,23] The chronic conditions that contribute to disability include arthritis, heart disease, stroke, vision and hearing disorders, and nutritional deficiencies.[20]

Demographic and epidemiological data are underscored by recent advances in gerontological research. Several themes have emerged from the research, one of which is heterogeneity. It is clear that older persons differ to a greater extent than younger persons. There is evidence of increased diversity or variability with age across physical, cognitive, and social domains.[24] It is likely that diversity will increase in many domains including ethnicity, family patterns, and roles.[25] A second theme of gerontological research relates to limits and potential... what is possible and what is not.[26] What are the limits to physical and mental well-being that are biologically imposed and what are the potentials for performance that may be modified by culture and life-style activities? Recent studies have shown significant potential for delaying declines and restoring and maintaining physical and mental functions.[26,27] We have a new outlook on health promotion for older women, an outlook that includes a prominent role for nutrition. Indeed, a recent Institute of Medicine report[28] concluded that nutrition is as important in the promotion and maintenance of health of older people as it is in younger people.

II. NUTRITION: AN OVERVIEW

Health is an increasing concern for older women. So we now find many women who are interested in nutrition and particularly in diet as it relates to prevention and treatment of chronic diseases.[29-31] Fat, cholesterol and sodium intakes rank as top dietary concerns as do questions about the use of nutrient supplements, food safety, and special diets. Physicians and publications are primary sources of information. Concerns about diet and health are frequently reflected in dietary modifications to reduce chronic disease risk.[30,32] Almost 60% of older women answered "yes" when asked if they had made lasting dietary changes in the past 5 years. Many added that they were trying to follow dietary guidelines but were often confused about which guidelines to follow.[33] This and other studies present older women as flexible and responsive to general dietary guidelines, although some changes, such as reduction of dairy products, may compromise nutrient intake.[34]

There are different estimates of prevalence of nutritional problems in older women.[35] The differences reflect, in part, the considerable heterogeneity of the populations studied. Goodwin[35] described the great diversity within one subset of older women in nursing homes. Approximately one half of nursing home residents are diagnosed with dementia or organic brain syndrome, one third are chair or bed bound, and many are disabled by cardiovascular diseases and cerebrovascular accidents. Rehabilitation patients discharged from hospitals represent an increasing population. This extreme variability has implications for energy requirements, eating dependance, and types of foods served (e.g., pureed diets),[36,37] all of which may impact on estimates of nutritional indicators. Differences in estimates of nutritional status also relate to study samples and the difficulty of distinguishing status indicators due to inadequate intake, aging, or disease-related changes.[38]

Limited nationwide data are available on nutritional status of older women, particularly the very elderly. The nutrition surveys of community-living women in the U.S. have only provided a partial perspective.[39] Food consumption surveys conducted by the U.S. Department of Agriculture assess food and nutrient intake and nutrition knowledge and beliefs but not clinical or anthropometric indices. The national Nutrition and Health Examination Surveys (NHANES) conducted by the National Center for Health Statistics assess multiple indicators of nutrition status; however, the first two of these did not sample beyond 74 years of age. The most recent, NHANES III (1986–94), was planned without an upper age limit and was designed to account for the potential nonresponse bias in studies of older persons.[40,41] Response rates frequently decline with age[33,41] and with poorer health status,[42] limiting generalizations for elderly and more frail women particularly those who are community-living and especially women who are homebound.[43]

Much of the data on nutritional status has come from local and regional samples of free-living,[44] homebound,[45] institutionalized,[36] and hospitalized[46] women. While the studies are often based on small samples and subject to limits on generalizability, they provide insights into food patterns, nutrient adequacy, and other measures of status. Overall, nutrient intake data from national and local studies show that average intakes of protein and most micronutrients meet the recommended dietary allowances,[47] while energy intakes frequently fall below recommendations. Many older women report using supplements, although the use is often irregular[48] and is seldom included in presentations of nutrient intake. Although average intakes generally are at recommended levels, intakes within groups are variable. Many women report intakes well below the recommendations for energy and micronutrients and above the guidelines for fat and saturated fat.[49,50] Few women meet the recommendations for micronutrients as well as those for fat.[51] Research models designed to explain the variability propose that demographic (e.g., education), social support, and life event variables (e.g., bereavement) account for some of the variability.[51,52] Our work with generally healthy older rural women found that two dietary pattern variables, the number of eating occasions and the variety of foods, were positively associated with energy and nutrient intakes.[156]

Body weight and body composition are important indicators of nutritional well-being.[53] Both weight and composition changes occur with aging. Women enter their older years with a "creeping up" of weight, a gain of 15 to 25 lb. that occurs until about 70 years and is followed by some loss of weight.[54,55] Body fat accumulates until 70 to 75 years;[56] adiposity gained post-menopausally tends to accumulate in the trunk and upper body.[57]

Overweight and underweight are both risk factors for older women. Approximately 35% of American women 20 years and over are categorized as overweight using the body mass index (BMI) cutoff of 27.3.[40] The prevalence of overweight for women 60 to 69 years, 70 to 79 years, and 80 years and older is approximately 42, 37, and 26%, respectively. Non-Hispanic black women and Mexican American women have higher prevalence than do non-Hispanic white women — about 60, 50, and 40%, respectively, for women 60 to 69 years. Tayback et al.[58] have questioned the specificity of the cutoff for all older women. However, extreme adiposity is associated with functional disability including basic activities of daily living such as walking, lifting, and carrying (e.g., bag of groceries).[59] Adiposity compounds the effects of hypertension and diabetes on morbidity and mortality even when cardiovascular risk factors are accounted for;[60] it presents a challenge to health care, increasing diagnostic difficulties and problems in physical handling of patients;[61] and it can contribute to increased risk for decubitus ulcers and leg vein thrombosis for bed-ridden obese elderly.[62]

Many women are concerned about weight although the motives for weight control differ by life stage, with more emphasis on health than appearance in later years.[33,63] Rodin[64] found that concern for change in body weight was second to that of concern for memory loss for older women. Lahmann[33] reported that many older women, particularly those with higher BMIs, indicated ongoing attempts to lose weight.

Underweight and involuntary weight loss are predictive of increased morbidity and mortality.[65-67] Wallace and Schwartz[68] recently reviewed the literature on low body weight and the etiology of weight loss. Age-related changes in taste and olfaction and changes in food intake regulation contribute to nonspecific "anorexia of aging". Many diseases and socioeconomic states may lead to decreased food intake. The authors recommended careful monitoring of persons with a verified loss of ≥5% of body weight over a 6- to 12-month period.

In 1990, the Institute of Medicine published a report on health promotion and disability prevention in "the second fifty years."[28] Recommendations were made for research on nutrient requirements and for the development of reliable and valid screening services predictive of nutritional risk and maintenance of functions. These two recommendations are reviewed in the following sections of this paper.

III. NUTRIENT REQUIREMENTS

It was a long held belief that older adults had a decreased energy requirement but essentially unchanged nutrient requirements when compared to younger persons. Recommendations included in the 10th edition of the *Recommended Dietary Allowances* (RDA) are based almost entirely on extrapolations from studies performed on young, healthy adults and show only minor differences between women ≥51 years and younger women.[47] The RDA for thiamin, riboflavin, and niacin are less for older than younger women, based on the assumption of lower energy needs in the elderly. The reduced recommendation for iron is based on post-menopausal changes.

Nutrient requirements of older adults have been a common theme of recent nutrition aging research.[38] Thorough reviews of the nutrient requirements of older adults based on current knowledge of macronutrient,[69,70] vitamin,[71] mineral,[72] and trace metal[73] requirements are available elsewhere. Two surveys in the past decade have added tremendously to our knowledge of nutrient status of the elderly: the Boston Nutritional Status Survey[74] and the Survey in Europe on Nutrition and the Elderly, a Concerned Action (SENECA Survey).[75-82] We can also anticipate more information in the next few years from the third National Health and Nutrition Examination Survey (NHANES III), now in progress.[40,83] The available data suggest that requirements for energy and vitamin A may decrease with age. Requirements for thiamin, riboflavin, niacin, and folate seem to be unchanged with age. Requirements for protein, vitamin B_6, vitamin B_{12}, calcium, and vitamin D appear to be higher in older adults. For other nutrients, including zinc, vitamin E, and copper, there is insufficient evidence of requirements for older adults.

Energy requirements have been most recently considered in multiples of basal metabolic rate (BMR). The FAO/WHO/UNU has suggested that the average requirement is 1.5 times the BMR.[84] Regression equations used to predict BMR in older individuals have been extrapolated from studies done on younger adults and/or have been based on studies done with small sample sizes of elderly. The ability to accurately assess energy needs for older women by this method remains uncertain. Furthermore, these estimates are based on nutrient intake data, which tend to underestimate actual consumption. Goran and Poehlman[85] have measured as much as 30% underreporting of energy intake in older women. New predictive equations for assessing the energy needs of elderly women have been proposed by Poehlman[86] to include body weight, standing height, and menopausal status and have been able to predict resting metabolic rate (RMR) within a standard error of estimate of 66 kcal/d. This predictive equation may be helpful in the future if it can be correlated to other more direct measures of RMR.

Direct measurements of energy expenditure of free living young adults and elderly men by Roberts et al.[87] have determined daily energy expenditure in the elderly to be 1.75 times the BMR. Research done by Vaughan et al.[88] demonstrates a definitive decrease in energy needs with increasing age. Sixty percent or more of the daily energy requirement is thought to be due to basal metabolism. BMR is reduced in the elderly presumably due to the age-related loss of lean body mass.

The doubly labeled water technique is a promising method for estimating daily energy requirements in the free-living elderly population. This method is advantageous over those used in the past for several reasons. First, it measures total daily energy expenditure including not only the effect of RMR, but also those of physical activity and the thermic effect of food which must now only be approximated. Additionally, these measurements can provide information about free-living energy expenditure and are repeated over time to acquire more unbiased information. Unfortunately, current use of this method is limited due to expense and the availability of the necessary isotope.

The current RDA for vitamin A in older women is 800 retinol equivalents (RE). There is some evidence that requirements may be lower for older adults than for younger ones. Older women have been shown to have increased absorption of vitamin A compared to their younger counterparts.[89] There are greater endogenous reserves in older adults than those in the young. Finally, an age-related delay in clearing retinyl esters in chylomicron has been demonstrated, suggesting that decreased clearance plays as much of a role in elevated serum vitamin A levels as increased absorption.[90] Although increased intake of this vitamin has been associated with lower risk levels for cancer, care must be taken in supplementation. These studies suggest that aging is associated with greater storage pools and a lower margin of safety for vitamin A intake.

Recommended allowances for several nutrients, including riboflavin, are set at lower levels for older women. The RDA for riboflavin is 1.2 mg/d for women ≥51 years and 1.3 mg/d for younger women. This is based on the assumption that riboflavin needs would mirror lower energy needs. The classic riboflavin studies by Horwitt et al.[91] demonstrated the tissue saturation point of riboflavin to be 1.1 mg/d for young adults. Experiments by Boisvert et al.[92] have shown necessary levels for the elderly to be 1.1 to 1.3 mg/d, dependent on the macronutrient content of the diet, and suggest that the requirement for riboflavin is the same for older adults as it is in younger adults. The current recommendation appears to leave little margin for error in intakes of riboflavin.

Protein needs of the elderly may be higher than for younger adults.[93] Metabolic studies by Uauy et al.[94,95] found that body nitrogen balance required intakes of 0.8 g egg protein per kilogram per day or more. Gersovitz et al.[96] showed that a significant number of subjects were unable to achieve or maintain nitrogen balance at this level. A short-term nitrogen balance study and recalculation of data from three previous studies using the WHO balance formula done by Campbell et al.[97] suggest a safe recommended protein intake for elderly adults to be 1.00 to 1.25 g/kg/d. This does not answer the question of optimal protein intakes to minimize loss of lean body mass with age. The decline in energy intake along with the consequence of reduced protein utilization also tends to increase the protein need of older adults as compared to that for more physically active younger adults. Since energy needs diminish progressively with age, while protein needs remain constant, protein should be consumed as a higher proportion of total dietary energy with advancing age. Young[69] has suggested that not less than 12 to 14% of caloric intake should be consumed as high biological value protein. Infection and metabolic stress will increase this requirement for individuals, while renal or hepatic insufficiency may necessitate protein restriction.

Surveys in the U.S. and in Europe have documented the prevalence of biochemical vitamin B_6 deficiency as between 10 and 20% of free-living elderly.[74,98] Vitamin B_6 status of women is reduced with aging.[99] The recommendation for vitamin B_6 for women 51 years and older was decreased between the 1980 and 1989 RDA from 2.0 to 1.6 mg/d.[47,100] Since that time, Ribaya-Mercado et al.[101] have demonstrated the actual physiological need in healthy, elderly volunteers to be 1.9 mg/d. Related experiments have shown the amount of vitamin B_6 necessary to restore immune function in depleted individuals is 20 to 45 times the current RDA. Studies of older adults suffering from vitamin B_6 responsive carpal tunnel syndrome also suggest there is an age-related increase in need for this nutrient.[102]

The 1989 RDA for vitamin B_{12} for elderly women was lowered to 1.6 µg from the 1980 value of 3.0 µg.[47,100] A relatively high prevalence of vitamin B_{12} deficiency has been reported in free-living elderly adults.[103] Many elderly persons malabsorb only the protein-bound vitamin and may, therefore, have a normal Schilling's test for megaloblastic anemia, making them difficult to identify for treatment. A large number of elderly have atrophic gastritis, as many as 25% of persons aged 60 to 69 and 40% of persons who are 80 and older. This condition impairs release of B_{12} from food and production of intrinsic factor.[104] Many elderly also have gastrointestinal disease or surgery that will compromise vitamin B_{12} status. Given the potentially devastating neurological effects of vitamin B_{12} deficiency and the uncertainties of diagnosing deficiency, increasing the value to 3.0 mg/d has been recommended.[105] However, there is uncertainty about the extent to which raising the RDA would reduce the prevalence of deficiency in those for whom the primary cause of depletion is malabsorption.[104]

The current RDA for vitamin D is 5 µg or 200 IU cholecalciferol daily. This RDA is the same for women of all ages, yet elderly women appear to have an increased need for vitamin D. Older women have been found to have low serum levels of 1, 25-dihydroxyvitamin D.[106] This has been attributed to decreased consumption of dairy products, less outdoor activity, and a reduced ability of the kidney to synthesize the active form. Other researchers have noted a decreased capacity of the skin to produce provitamin D_3.[107] Finally, it is known that the aged intestine is less responsive to the calciotrophic effect.

Many experts agree that the elderly should receive at least 10 μg/d.[105] A recent study has shown that 400 IU supplement per day for 1 year can increase spinal bone density in older women.[108] This may be a prudent recommendation. Hungary recently increased its recommended dietary intake (RDI) from 2.5 to 6 μg/d and the Nordic countries have increased their recommendation to 10 μg/d.[109,110] There is a danger of excess supplementation of vitamin D resulting in hypercalcemia and toxicity and elderly women may be particularly prone to this effect due to their increased fat stores.[111] Supplementation of vitamin D beyond two times the RDA is not advisable.

The current RDA for calcium is 800 mg. Studies have suggested requirements may be 1500 mg/d in postmenopausal women.[112] There is considerable concern that appropriate levels of calcium intake may not be achievable by elderly women without supplementation. NHANES II data suggest that over half of the elderly surveyed were consuming less than the current RDA of 800 mg.[112] The recommendations for calcium in the elderly woman vary considerably throughout the world. Japan's current RDI is 600 mg, with consideration of increasing to 800 mg.[113] The Nordic countries have increased their recommendation to 800 mg.[110] Hungary recently increased its RDI from 500, to 800 to 1000 mg/d.[109] Excessive supplementation of calcium is to be avoided, as the risk of calcium stone formation is great with excessive doses.[114] Calcium supplementation is contraindicated in persons with a history of calcium stones, hyperparathyroidism, sarcoidosis, or renal hypercalcuria. A discussion of bone and osteoporosis in elderly women is given elsewhere in this volume.

Inadequate evidence is available about zinc requirements in elderly women to make any substantive recommendations about the current RDA. Many studies show that older women consume less than the RDA of zinc.[112] Although decreased zinc absorption has been observed in the elderly, net losses are also decreased such that zinc balance is not different in older women than in young.

There is evidence that α-linolenic acid should be considered as an essential dietary constituent. Internationally, the Nordic countries have established an RDI for α-linolenic acid and long chain ω3 fatty acids at 0.5% of total dietary calories.[110] Some researchers have suggested that the daily need may be as high as 1% of energy from ω3 fatty acids.[115] No RDA has been established in the U.S. for these nutrients, although the National Research Council has concluded that "the possibility of establishing an RDA for these fatty acids should be considered in the near future."[47] This may be particularly relevant for older adults because fatty acid deficiency has been demonstrated in persons with medical problems affecting fat absorption and those receiving long-term parenteral or enteral feedings. These persons should be receiving supplementation of ω3 fatty acids.

The American Dietetic Association has made ten recommendations to the Institute of Medicine's Food and Nutrition Board for consideration in revising the RDAs.[116] Several of these recommendations would specifically make the RDAs more appropriate for the older population. First is the establishment of RDAs to address the needs of elderly persons with recommendations that consider both biological function and chronological age; second, to consider providing a range of nutrients rather than a single value to reflect the diverse needs of the population; third, to target the RDAs more specifically with realistic applications, such as providing more than one set of recommendations for categories such as health maintenance, prevention of chronic disease, increased metabolic states, and parenteral feedings, finally, to establish research priorities and initiatives regarding application of the RDAs that specifically evaluate how the goals for which they are intended are being met.

IV. NUTRITION RISK AND SCREENING

The prevalence of malnutrition in hospitalized and long term care elderly patients is approximately one third of all admissions.[117-121] Significant numbers of older adults living at home may also be malnourished with estimates of <5%.[122] The consequences of poor nutrition are manifested by impaired immunocompetence, prolonged recovery periods, dysfunctioning organ systems, depressed metabolic response to injury, delayed wound healing, and even death.[119,121,123-126]

Malnutrition is often undetected in older women.[46,127] There has been a growing effort to identify older persons who are at risk of malnutrition. Davies and Knutson[128] define a nutritional risk factor as "a major, identifiable biological or environmental circumstance or event that increases the risk of malnutrition and therefore suggests the need for special care and attention." These authors also consider "warning signals" as conditions that if left unchecked may cause an at-risk individual to become malnourished.

Nutritional risk can be categorized in various ways. Long-standing risk represents the latent period between deficiency and the physical signs of malnutrition. Acting in response to warning signals during this period may prevent the resulting consequences of dietary deficiencies. Acute risk brought on by sudden stressors can deplete previously adequate nutritional reserves.[129]

Certain risk factors are core to all elderly persons (Table 1).[35,130-135] These risks cross over all living situations and can contribute to the complications associated with malnutrition. In addition, there are some risks that are more specific to community dwelling older adults and others to those in hospitals and institutions. Older adults in the community need to be concerned not only with food intake, but food acquisition. For this reason, issues such as food security, income, cooking facilities, and social support systems are key to ensuring nutritional adequacy in the home.[50,52,122,136-143] Institutionalized elderly persons have increased nutritional requirements due to surgery, decubitus ulcers, and medical complications.[133,144-150]

Nutritional risk assessment is increasing in frequency among acute care hospitals, as there is growing recognition of the role of nutrition in patient outcome. Nutrition screening upon admission offers baseline data for follow-up care and allows for outcome assessment. Several researchers have used nutritional screening criteria in predictive models of mortality and duration of

TABLE 1
Core Risk Factors for Malnutrition in Older Adults

Food intake and digestion	Physical	Health and Behavior
Decreased appetite	Unintentional weight	Presence of chronic disease
Difficulty chewing/swallowing	loss	Bone pain
	Recent weight change	
Mouth, teeth, or gum pain	Inappropriate weight for	Depression
Dyspersia	height	Mental impairment
Vomiting	Sensory loss	Polypharmacy
Constipation	Skin changes	Anemia
Dietary modifications		Smoking
Food alergy		Activity level
Vitamin supplement use		Triceps skinfold, muscle arm
		circumference values greater
		than 95%, or less than 5%

hospital stay.[144,151] Screening of the elderly patient is especially critical. Elderly persons at nutritional risk manifest greater health care utilization as evidenced by longer length of hospital stay and greater readmission rates.[127,146] Several investigators have shown the decline in nutritional status among elderly patients when hospitalized.[118-120,127] In older women, increasing age has been associated with more severe protein energy malnutrition than in younger women.[144] Although evidence for the necessity of aggressive nutritional screening and intervention in the hospital is growing, screening programs are not mandatory and often not implemented. Further analysis of the cost/benefit ratio and validation of nutritional status measures is needed to expand the use of nutrition screening programs in acute care hospitals.

Nutrition screening in long-term-care institutions requires specific considerations for serial measurements, eating dependency, medications, and diagnoses. Tramposch and Blue[152] reported on the development, implementation, and evaluation of a *Geriatric Nutritional Screening and Data Collection Form* for use in long term care. The authors reported this screening and assessment tool was effective in meeting the goals of a comprehensive, concise, and efficient system.

Although tools have been available to identify nutritional risk, it was not until the Nutrition Screening Initiative was established in 1991 that great efforts were made to heighten the awareness of health professionals in regard to nutritional concerns of elderly persons in the community. The Nutrition Screening Initiative is a collaborative effort by the America Dietetic Association, the American Academy of Family Physicians, and the National Council on the Aging, Inc. to promote nutritional screening, assessment, and intervention in the elderly. This program utilizes three instruments designed for use in different settings. The *Checklist* can be used by the older population and their caregivers to increase awareness of nutritional well-being; it urges those at risk to seek help to address nutritional problems and implement intervention.

The *Level I Screen* is designed for use by social service and other health care professions. BMI, socioeconomic conditions, living circumstances, and dietary habits provide the indicators of nutritional risk in this tool. If risk is identified, interventions available to community living elderly persons (e.g., home delivered meals, congregate meals, homemaker services) can be initiated. The final screening tool of this program is the *Level II Screen*. This is more specific, requiring information that may only be available in a clinical setting: skinfold measures, laboratory data, clinical assessment, and cognitive status assessment. These measures are best obtained by qualified health care professionals.[130,131,134,153] Further testing and validation of these instruments will be necessary.

Another community-based approach was created to account for the interactions of various warning signs associated with nutrition risk. The *grid system*, developed by Davies and Knutson,[128] considers applicable risk factors and warning signs. This tool has been suggested for use by care providers, social service professionals, and in clinical practice to identify potential malnutrition among the older population.

A *Nutritional Risk Index* was designed and validated in 1985 by Wolinsky et al.[135,154] This 16-item additive scale is available to identify elderly individuals at nutritional risk. Wolinsky's risk index considers the mechanics of food intake, prescribed dietary restrictions, morbid conditions affecting food intake, discomfort associated with food intake, and significant changes in dietary habits.

The benefits of nutrition screening include the opportunity for early intervention to promote improved outcomes and decreased health care utilization. However, little work has been completed on evaluating the effectiveness of the nutrition screening tools. Posner et al.[153] investigated the *Checklist* as a tool to predict poor nutrient intakes and low perceived health status. This tool was able to identify only 36% of patients who reported inadequate intakes (presumed to be at increased nutritional risk). Questions as to the appropriate use of this instrument in nutrition screening have been asked based on its low sensitivity and specificity, ability to detect and confer treatment early, and benefits to the economy and public health system.[155] Future research is needed to focus on the validity and reliability of screening tools used in all settings, as well as the benefits of early nutrition intervention initiated through nutrition screening.

V. SUMMARY

The U.S. and other societies are indeed aging. Women comprise a majority of the older U.S. population and will continue to do so; this will be especially true for the very old. Older women face special circumstances in terms of their resources, living situations, social role expectations, and health status. Limitations in any of these areas may compromise nutritional well-being.

Poor nutrition can also negatively impact on one's quality of life. Various recommendations have been proposed for enhancing the contribution of nutrition to improved life quality. These include recommendation for research, for clinical and community care, and for nutrition education. One recommendation is to determine the appropriate nutrient requirements for older women based on the diversity of their age and health status, with consideration of life quality and functional abilities. Another recommendation is to improve on the current impetus for nutrition risk screening in clinical care and community services. The result of these efforts should be improved life quality and decreased health care utilization. Further efforts must be directed to validate screening tools, to evaluate interventions on such measurable outcomes as hospital readmissions, and to educate health and social service professionals in geriatric nutrition. Finally, educational models must be developed to assist older women in nutrition and self-care for the ultimate goals of enhanced quality of life and nutritional well-being.

ACKNOWLEDGMENTS

This work was supported by the Howard Heinz Endowment and the USDA Northeast Regional Project No. 172.

REFERENCES

1. U.S. Department of Commerce, Bureau of the Census, *An Aging World,* International Population Reports, Series P-95, 1987.
2. Golini, A. and Lori, A., Aging of the population: demographic and social changes, *Aging,* 2, 319, 1990.
3. Miles, T. P. and Brody, J., International aging, in *Health Data in Older Americans: U.S. 1992,* Vol. 3, Van Nostrand, J. F., Furner, S. E., and Suzman, R., Eds., Vital Health Statistics, National Center for Health Statistics, Washington, D.C., 1993, 289.
4. Brock, D. B., Guralnik, J. M., and Brody, J. A., Demography and epidemiology of aging in the U.S., in *Handbook of the Biology of Aging,* 3rd ed., Schneider, E. L. and Rowe, J. W., Eds., Academic Press, San Diego, 1990, chap. 1.
5. Van Nostrand, J. F., Furner, S. E., and Suzman, R., Eds., *Health Data in Older Americans: U.S., 1992,* Vital Health Statistics, National Center for Health Statistics, Vital Health Stat. Washington D.C., 1993.
6. Schwenk, F. N., Income and expenditures of older widowed, divorced, and never-married women who live alone, *Fam. Econ. Rev.,* 5, 2, 1992.
7. Schwenk, F. N., Changes in the economic status of American's elderly population during the last 50 years, *Fam. Econ. Rev.,* 6, 18, 1993.
8. Radner, D. B., The economic status of the aged, *Soc. Sec. Bull.,* 55, 3, 1992.
9. McLaughlin, D. and Jensen, L., Poverty among older Americans: the plight of nonmetropolitan elders, *J. Gerontol. Soc. Sci.,* 48, S44, 1993.
10. Guralnik, J. M. and Simonsick, E. M., Physical disability in older Americans, *J. Gerontol.,* 48, 3, 1990.

11. Strawbridge, W. J., Camacho, T. C., Cohen, R. D., and Kaplan, G. A., Gender differences in factors associated with change in physical functioning in old age: a 6-year longitudinal study, *Gerontologist,* 33, 603, 1993.

12. Coward, R. T., Cutler, S. J., and Schmidt, F. E., Differences in the household composition of elders by age, gender and area of residence, *Gerontologist*, 29, 814, 1989.

13. Hurd, M. D., The economic status of the elderly, *Science,* 244, 659, 1989.

14. Holden, K. C., Poverty and living arrangements among older women: are changes in economic well-being underestimated? *J. Gerontol.*, 43, S22, 1988.

15. Ford, A. B., Haug, M. R., Roy, A. W., Jones, P. K., and Folmar, S. J., New cohorts of urban elderly: are they in trouble? *J. Gerontol. Soc. Sci.,* 47, S297, 1992.

16. Brody, J. A. and Brock, D. B., Trends in the health of the elderly population, *Annu. Rev. Public Health*, 8, 211, 1987.

17. Furner, S. E., Maurer, J., and Rosenberg, H., Mortality, in *Health Data in Older Americans: U.S. 1992*, Vol. 3, Van Nostrand, J. F., Furner, S. E., and Suzman, R., Eds., Vital Health Statistics, National Center for Health Statistics, Washington, D.C., 1993, 77.

18. Fingerhut, L. A. and Makuc, D. M., Mortality among minority populations in the U.S., *Am. J. Public Health*, 82, 1168, 1992.

19. Guralnik, J. M., LaCroix, A. Z., Everett, D. F., and Kovar, M. G., Aging in the eighties: the prevalence of comorbidity and its association with disability, *Adv. Data,* 170, 1, 1989.

20. Lonergan, E. T., Ed., *Extending Life, Enhancing Life: A National Research Agenda in Aging*, National Academy Press, Washington, D.C., 1991.

21. Boult, C., Kane, R. L., Louis, T. A., Boult, L., and McCaffrey, D., Chronic conditions that lead to functional limitations in the elderly, *J. Gerontol.*, 49, M28, 1994.

22. Penning, M. J. and Strain, L. A., Gender differences in disability assistance and subjective well-being in later life, *J. Gerontol. Soc. Sci.*, 49, S202, 1994.

23. Prohaska, T., Mermelstein, R., Miller, B., and Jack, S., Functional status and living arrangements, in: *Health Data in Older Americans: U.S. 1992*, Van Nostrand, J. F., Furner, S. E., and Suzman, R., Eds., Vital Health Statistics, National Center for Health Statistics, Washington D.C., 1993, 23.

24. Nelson, E. A. and Dannefer, D., Aged heterogeneity: fact or fiction? The fate of diversity in generontological research, *Gerontologist*, 32, 17, 1992.

25. Moeng, P., Robison, J., and Fields, W., Women's work and caregiving roles: a life course approach, *J. Gerontol. Soc. Sci.*, 49, S176, 1994

26. Baltes, P. B., The aging mind: potentials and limits, *Gerontologist,* 33, 580, 1993.

27. Fiatorone, M., O'Neill, E. F., Ryan, N. D., Clements, K. M., Solares, G. R., Nelson, M. E., Roberts, S. E., Kehayias, J. J., Lipsitz, L. A., and Evans, W. J., Exercise training and nutritional supplementation for physical frailty in very elderly people, *N.Engl. J. Med.*, 330, 1769, 1994.

28. Berg, R. L. and Cassells, J. S., Eds., *The Second Fifty Years: Promoting Health and Preventing Disability*, National Academy Press, Washington D.C., 1990.

29. Worsley, A., Lay persons' evaluation of health: an exploratory study of an Australian population, *J. Epidemiol. Comm. Health*, 44, 7, 1990.

30. Goldberg, J. P., Gershoff, S. N., and McGandy, R. B., Appropriate topics for nutrition education for the elderly, *J. Nutr. Elder.*, 22, 303, 1990.

31. Krinke, U. B., Nutrition information topic and format preferences of older adults, *J. Nutr. Educ.*, 22, 292, 1990.

32. Fanelli, M. T., Kannon, G. A., and McDuffie, J. R., An assessment of the nutrition education needs of congregate meal program participants, *J. Nutr. Elder.*, 19, 131, 1987.

33. Lahmann, P., The Association of Attitudes about Weight and Health with Dietary Quality of Older Women, Doctoral dissertation, Pennsylvania State University, University Park, 1993.

34. Horwath, C. C., Dietary changes reported by a random sample of elderly people, *J. Nutr. Elder.*, 12, 13, 1992.

35. Goodwin, J. S., Social, psychological, and physical factors affecting the nutritional status of elderly subjects: separating cause and effect, *Am. J. Clin. Nutr.*, 50, 120, 1989.

36. Johnson, R. M., Nutritional Status of Female Nursing Home Residents; Independent and Dependent Eating, Doctoral Dissertation, Pennsylvania State University, University Park, 1993.

37. Johnson, R. M., Smiciklas-Wright, H., Soucy, I. M., and Rizzo, J., Nutrient intake of nursing-home residents receiving pureed foods on a regular diet, *J. Am. Geriatr. Soc.*, 43, 1, 1995.

38. Feldman, E., Aspects of the interrelations of nutrition and aging — 1993, *Am. J. Clin. Nutr.*, 58, 1, 1993.

39. Interagency Board of Nutrition Monitoring and Related Research, *Nutrition Monitoring in the U.S.: The Directory of Federal and State Nutrition Monitoring Activities,* Wright, J., Ed., Public Health Service, Hyattsville, MD, 1992.

40. Kuczmarski, R. J., Flegal, K. M., Campbell, S. M., and Johnson, C.L., Increasing prevalence of overweight among U.S. adults: the National Health and Nutrition Examination Surveys, 1960 to 1991, *J.A.M.A.*, 272, 205, 1994.

41. Harris, T., Cook, E. F., Garrison, R., Higgins, M., Cannell, W., and Goldman, L., Body mass index and mortality among nonsmoking older persons, *J.A.M.A.*, 259, 1520, 1988.

42. Norris, F. H., Characteristics of older nonrespondents over five waves of a panel study, *J. Gerontol.*, 40, 627, 1985.

43. Smiciklas-Wright, H., Aging, in *Present Knowledge in Nutrition,* 6th ed., Brown, M. L., Ed., International Life Sciences Institute, Washington D.C., 1990, chap. 39.

44. Koehler, K. M., Hunt, W. C., and Garry, P. J., Meat, poultry, and fish consumption and nutrient intake in the healthy elderly, *J. Am. Diet. Assoc.*, 92, 325, 1992.

45. Bernardo, V. D., The Nutritional Status of Homebound Elderly Persons, Master of Science thesis, Pennsylvania State University, University Park, 1988.

46. Mowe, M. and Bohmer, T., The prevalence of undiagnosed protein-calorie undernutrition of hospitalized elderly patients, *J. Am. Geriatr. Soc.*, 39, 1089, 1991.

47. National Research Council, *Recommended Dietary Allowances*, 10th ed., National Academy Press, Washington, DC, 1989.

48. Ervin, R.B., Smiciklas-Wright, H., and Fosmire, G. J., Intra-individual variation in zinc intake among elderly women: the effect of diet and supplements, *Nutr. Res.*, 9, 613, 1989.

49. Smiciklas-Wright, H., Lago, D. J., Bernardo, V., and Beard, J. L., Nutritional assessment of homebound elderly, *J. Nutr.*, 120, 1535, 1990.

50. Fanelli, M. T. and Woteki, C. F., Nutrient intakes and health status of older Americans, *Ann. N.Y. Acad. Sci.*, 561, 94, 1989.

51. Murphy, S. P., Davis, M. A., Neuhaus, J. M., and Lein, D., Factors influencing the dietary adequacy and energy intake of older Americans, *J. Nutr. Educ.*, 22, 284, 1990.

52. McIntosh, A. W. and Shifflett, P. A., Social support, stressful events, strain, dietary intake, and the elderly, *Med. Care*, 27, 140, 1989.

53. Kuczmarski, R. J., Need for body composition information in elderly subjects, *Am. J. Clin. Nutr.*, 50, 1150, 1989.

54. Steen, B., Lundgren, B. K., and Isaksson, B., Body composition at age 70, 75, 79, and 81; a longitudinal population study, in *Nutrition Immunity and Illness in the Elderly*, Chandra, R. K., Ed., Pergaman Press, New York, 1985, 49.

55. Frankle, R. T., A rational approach to long-term management of obesity for the elderly, in *Health Promotion and Disease Prevention in the Elderly*, Chernoff, R. and Lipschitz, D. A., Eds., Raven Press, New York, 1988, 131.

56. Young, C. M., Blondin, J., Tensuan, R., and Fryer, J. H., Body composition of older women, *J. Am. Diet. Assoc.*, 43, 344, 1963.

57. Roche, A. F., Abdel-Malek, A. K., and Mukherjee, D., New approaches to clinical assessment of adipose tissue, in *Body Composition Assessment in Youth and Adults*, Ross Laboratories, Columbus, OH, 1985.

58. Tayback, M., Kumanyika, S., and Chee, E., Body weight as a risk factor in the elderly, *Arch. Intern. Med.,* 150, 1065, 1990.

59. Galanos, A., Piper, C. F., Coroni-Huntley, J. C., Bales, C. W., and Fillenberg, G. G., Nutrition and function: is there a relationship between body mass index and the functional capabilities of community dwelling elderly?, *J. Am. Geriatr. Soc.,* 42, 368, 1994.

60. DiPietro, L., Ostfeld, A. M., and Rosner, G. L., Adiposity and stroke among older adults of low socioeconomic status: the Chicago Stroke Study, *Am. J. Public Health*, 84, 14, 1994.

61. Steen, B., Obesity in the aged, in *Handbook of Nutrition in the Aged*, 2nd ed., Watson, R. R., Ed., CRC Press, Boca Raton, FL, 1994, chap. 1.

62. Haleem, M. A., The problem of obesity in the elderly, *Br. J. Clin. Pract.*, 32, 45, 1978.

63. Devine, C., Women's Perceptions about Diet and Chronic Disease Risk: The Influence of Life Stage and Social Roles, Doctoral dissertation, Cornell University, Ithaca, NY, 1990.

64. Rodin, J., Yale Health and Patterns of Living Study: A Longitudinal Study on Health, Stress, and Coping in the Elderly, unpublished paper, Yale University, New Haven, 1984.

65. Dwyer, J. T., Coleman, K. A., Krall, E., Yang, G. A., Scanlan, M., Galper, L., Winthrop, E., and Sullivan, P., Changes in relative weight among institutionalized elderly adults, *J. Gerontol.*, 42, 246, 1987.

66. Fischer, J. and Johnson, M. A., Low body weight and weight loss in the aged, *J. Am. Diet. Assoc.*, 90, 1697, 1990.

67. Mowe, M., Bomer, T., and Kindt, E., Reduced nutritional status in an elderly population (>70y) is probable before disease and possibly contributes to the development of disease, *Am. J. Clin. Nutr.*, 59, 317, 1994.

68. Wallace, J. I. and Schwartz, R. S., Involuntary weight loss in the elderly, in *Handbook of Nutrition in the Aged*, 2nd ed., Watson, R. R., Ed., CRC Press, Boca Raton, FL, 1994, chap. 6.

69. Young, V. R., Macronutrient needs in the elderly, *Nutr. Rev.*, 50, 454, 1992.

70. Carter, W. J., Macronutrient requirements for elderly persons, in *Geriatric Nutrition*, Chernoff, R., Ed., ASPEN Publishers, Little Rock, AR, 1991, 11.

71. Suter, P. M., Vitamin requirements, in *Geriatric Nutrition*, Chernoff, R., Ed., ASPEN Publishers, Little Rock, AR, 1991, 25.

72. Lindeman, R. D. and Beck, A. A., Mineral requirements, in *Geriatric Nutrition,* Chernoff, R., Ed., ASPEN Publishers, Little Rock, AR, 1991, 53.

73. Fosmire, G. J., Trace metal requirements, in *Geriatric Nutrition*, Chernoff, R., Ed., ASPEN Publishers, Little Rock, AR, 1991, 77.

74. Hartz, S. C., Rosenberg, I. H., and Russel, I. M., Nutrition in the elderly, *Boston Nutritional Survey*, Smith-Gordon, Ltd, London, 1992.

75. **Anon.,** Summary and recommendations for further analysis. Euronut SENECA investigators, *Eur. J. Clin. Nutr.,* 45S, 183, 1991.

76. Cruz, J. A., Moreiras-Varela, O., van Stavern, M. A., Trichopoulous, A., and Roszkowski, W., Intake of vitamins and minerals. Euronut SENECA investigators, *Eur. J. Clin. Nutr.,* 45S, 121, 1991.

77. de Groot, L. C., Sette, S., Zajkas, G., Carbajal, A., and Anorim, J. A., Nutritional status: anthropometry. Euronut SENECA investigators, *Eur. J. Clin. Nutr.*, 45S, 31, 1991.

78. Dirren, H., Decarli, B., Lesourd, B., Schlienger, J. L., Deslypere, J. P., and Kiepurski, A., Nutritional status: haematology and albumin. Euronut SENECA investigators, *Eur. J. Clin. Nutr.*, 45 S, 43, 1991.

79. Haller, J., Lowik, M. R., Ferry, M., and Ferro-Luzzi, A., Nutritional status: blood vitamins A, E, B-6, B-12, folic acid, and carotene. Euronut SENECA investigators, *Eur. J. Clin. Nutr.,* 45S, 63, 1991.

80. Kafatos, A., Schlienger, J. L., Deslypere, J. P., Ferro-Luzzi, A., and Cruz, J. A., Nutritional status: serum lipids. Euronut SENECA investigators, *Eur. J. Clin. Nutr.*, 45S, 53, 1991.

81. Moreiras, O., van Stavern, W. A., Cruz, J. A., Nes, M., and Lund-Larsen, K., Intake of energy and nutrients. Euronut SENECA investigators, *Eur. J. Clin. Nutr.*, 45S, 105, 1991.

82. Schlettwein-Gsell, D., Barclay, D., Osler, M., and Trichopoulous, A., Dietary habits and attitudes. Euronut SENECA investigators, *Eur. J. Clin. Nutr.*, 45S, 83, 1991.

83. Harris, T., Woteki, C., Briefel, R. R., and Kleinman, J. C., NHANES III for older persons: nutrition content and methodological considerations, *Am. J. Clin. Nutr.*, 50, 1145, 1993.

84. FAO/WHO/UNU, Energy and protein requirements. Report of a joint FAO/WHO Ad Hoc Expert Committee, Technical Report Serial No. 522, World Health Organization, Geneva, 1985.

85. Goran, M. I. and Poehlman, E. T., Total energy expenditure and energy requirements in healthy elderly persons, *Metabolism*, 41, 744, 1992.

86. Poehlman, E. T., Energy expenditure and requirements in aging humans, *J. Nutr.*, 122, 2057, 1992.

87. Roberts, S. B., Young, V. R., Fuss, P., Heyman, M. B., Fiatorone, M., Dalla, G. E., Cortiella, J., and Evans, W. J., What are the dietary energy needs of elderly adults?, *Int. J. Obesity*, 16, 969, 1992.

88. Vaughan, L., Zurlo, F., and Ravussin, E., Aging and energy expenditure, *Am. J. Clin. Nutr.*, 53, 821, 1991.

89. Hollander, D. and Morgan, D., Aging: its influence on vitamin A intestinal absorption in vivo by the rat, *Exp. Gerontol.*, 14, 301, 1979.

90. Krasinski, S. D., Russell, R. M., and Otradovec, C. L., Relationship of vitamin A and vitamin E intake to fasting plasma retinol, retinol-binding protein, retinyl esters, carotene, α-tocopherol, and cholesterol among elderly people and young adults: increased plasma retinyl esters among vitamin A supplement users, *Am. J. Clin. Nutr.*, 49, 112, 1989.

91. Horwitt, M. K., Harvey, C. G., Hills, O. W., and Liebert, E., Correlation of urinary excretion of riboflavin with dietary intake and symptoms of ariboflavinosis, *J. Nutr.*, 41, 247, 1950.

92. Boisvert, W. A., Mendoza, I., Castaneda, C., De Portocarrero, L., Solomons, N. W., Gershoff, S. N., and Russell, R. M., Riboflavin requirement of healthy elderly humans and its relationship to the macronutrient composition of the diet, *J. Nutr.*, 123, 915, 1993.

93. Young, V. R., Amino acids and proteins in relation to the nutrition of elderly people, *Age Ageing*, 19, S10, 1990.

94. Uauy, R., Scrimshaw, N. S., and Young, V. R., Human protein requirments: nitrogen balance response to graded levels of egg protein in elderly men and women, *Am. J. Clin. Nutr.*, 31, 779, 1978.

95. Uauy, R., Scrimshaw, N. S., Rand, W. M., and Young, V. R., Human protein requirements: obligatory urinary and fecal nitrogen losses and the factorial estimation of protein needs in elderly males, *J. Nutr.*, 108, 97, 1978.

96. Gersovitz, M., Motil, K., Munro, H. N., Schrimshaw, N. S., and Young, V. R., Human protein requirements: assessment of the adequacy of the current recommended dietary allowance for dietary protein in elderly men and women, *Am. J. Clin. Nutr.*, 35, 6, 1982.

97. Campbell, W. W., Crim, M. C., Dallal, G. E., Young, V. R., and Evans, W. J., Increased protein requirements in the elderly: new data and retrospective reassessments., *Am. J. Clin. Nutr.*, 60, 501, 1994.

98. Kant, A. K. and Block, G., Dietary vitamin B-6 intake and food sources in the U.S. population: NHANES II, 1976–1980, *Am. J. Clin. Nutr.*, 52, 707, 1990.

99. Lee, C. M. and Leklem, J. E., Differences in vitamin B-6 status indicator responses between young and middle aged women fed constant diets with two levels of vitamin B-12, *Am. J. Clin. Nutr.*, 42, 226, 1985.

100. National Research Council, *Recommended Dietary Allowances*, 9th ed., National Academy Press, Washington, D.C., 1980.

101. Ribaya-Mercado, J. D., Russell, R. M., Sahyoun, N., Morrow, F. D., and Gershoff, S. N., Vitamin B-6 requirements of elderly men and women, *J. Nutr.*, 121, 1062, 1991.

102. Blumberg, J. B., Changing nutrient requirements in older adults, *Nutr. Today*, September, October, 15, 1992.

103. Lindenbaum, J., Rosenberg, I. H., Wilson, P. W. F., Stabler, S. P., and Allen, R. H., Prevalence of cobalamin deficiency in the Framingham elderly population, *Am. J. Clin. Nutr.,* 60, 2, 1994.

104. Allen, L. H. and Casterline, J., Vitamin B-12 deficiency in elderly individuals: diagnosis and requirements, *Am. J. Clin. Nutr.,* 60, 12, 1994.

105. Russell, R. M. and Suter, P. M., Vitamin requirements of elderly people: an update, *Am. J. Clin. Nutr.,* 58, 4, 1993.

106. Francis, R. H., Peacock, M., Storer, J. H., Davies, A. E. J., Brown, W. B., and Nordin, B. E. C., Calcium malabsorption in the elderly: the effect of treatment with oral 25-hydroxyvitamin D3, *Eur. J. Clin. Nutr.,* 13, 391, 1983.

107. Webb, A. K., Kline, L., and Hollick, M. F., Influence of season and latitude on the cutaneous synthesis of vitamin D_3. Exposure to winter sunlight in Boston and Edmonton will not promote vitamin D_3 synthesis in human skin, *J. Clin. Endocrinol. Metab.,* 67, 373, 1988.

108. Dawson-Hughes, B., Dalla, G. E., Krall, E. A., Harris, S., Sokoll, L. J., and Falconer, G., Effect of vitamin D supplementation on wintertime and overall bone loss in healthy postmenopausal women, *Ann. Intern. Med.,* 115, 505, 1991

109. Biro, G., Recommended dietary intakes in Hungary, *Eur. J. Clin. Nutr.,* 46, 151, 1992.

110. Bruce, A., Recommended dietary allowances: the Nordic experience, *Eur. J. Clin. Nutr.,* 44(Suppl.), 27, 1990.

111. Gupta, K. L., Dworkin, B., and Gambert, S. R., Common nutritional disorders in the elderly: atypical manifestations, *Geriatrics,* 43, 87, 1988.

112. Barrett-Connor, E., The RDA for calcium in the elderly: too little, too late, *Calcif. Tissue Int.,* 44, 303, 1989.

113. deSouza, A. C., Nakamura, T., Stergiopoulos, K., Ouchi, M., and Orimo, H., Calcium requirement in elderly Japanese women, *Gerontology,* 37(suppl), 43, 1991.

114. Heaney, R. P., Gallagher, J. C., and Johnston, C. C., Calcium nutrition and bone health in the elderly, *Am. J. Clin. Nutr.,* 36, 986, 1982.

115. Bjerve, K. S., Requirements of adults and elderly, *World Rev. Nutr. Diet.,* 66, 26, 1991.

116. St Jeor, S. T., Chernoff, R., Geiger, C. J., Miller, J. L., Schwartz, N. E., Simko, M., Sims, L., Stauss, J. A., and Thomson, C., ADA testifies on need for revised RDAs, *J. Am. Diet. Assoc.,* 93, 864, 1993.

117. Bistrian, B. R., Blackburn, G. L., Hallowell, E., and Heddle, R., Protein status of general surgical patients, *J.A.M.A.,* 230, 858, 1974.

118. Coats, K. G., Morgan, S. L., Bartolucci, A. A., and Weinsier, R. L., Hospital-associated malnutrition: a reevaluation 12 years later, *J. Am. Diet. Assoc.,* 93, 27, 1993.

119. Reilly, J. J., Hull, S. F., Albert, N., Waller, A., and Bringardener, S., Economic impact of malnutrition: a model system for hospitalized patients, *J. Paren. Enter. Nutr.,* 12, 371, 1988.

120. Sullivan, D. H., Moriarty, M. S., Chernoff, R., and Lipschitz, D. A., Patterns of care: an analysis of the quality of nutritional care routinely provided to elderly hospitalized veterans, *J. Paren. Enter. Nutr.,* 13, 249, 1989.

121. Weinsier, R. L., Hunker, E. M., Krumdieck, C. L., and Butterworth, C. E., Hospital malnutrition. A prospective evaluation of general medical patients during the course of hospitalization, *Am. J. Clin. Nutr.,* 32, 418, 1979.

122. Thorslund, S., Toss, G., Nilsson, I., Schenck, H. V., Symreng, T., and Zetterqvist, H., Prevalence of protein-energy malnutrition in a large population of elderly people at home, *Scand. J. Prim. Health Care,* 8, 243, 1990.

123. Chandra, R. J., 1990 McCollum award lecture. Nutrition and immunity: lessons from the past and new insights Into the future, *Am. J. Clin. Nutr.,* 53, 1087, 1991.

124. Sullivan, D. H., Patch, G. A., Walls, R. C., and Lipschitz, D. A., Impact of nutrition status on morbidity and mortality in a select population of geriatric rehabilitation patients, *Am. J. Clin. Nutr.,* 51, 749, 1990.

125. Sullivan, D. H., Walls, R., and Lipschitz, D. A., Protein-energy undernutrition and the risk of mortality within 1 year of hospital discharge in a select population of geriatric rehabilitation patients, *Am. J. Clin. Nutr.,* 53, 599, 1991.

126. Woo, J., Chan, S. M., Mak, Y. T., and Swaminathan, R., Biochemical predictors of short term mortality in elderly residents of chronic care institutions, *J. Clin. Pathol.*, 42, 1241, 1989.

127. Burns, J. T. and Jensen, G. L., Malnutrition among geriatric patients admitted to medical and surgical services in a tertiary care hospital: frequency, recognition, and associated disposition and reimbursement outcomes, *Nutrition*, 11, 245, 1995.

128. Davies, L. and Knutson, K.C., Warning signals for malnutrition in the elderly, *J. Am. Diet. Assoc.*, 91, 1413, 1991.

129. Davies, L., Nutrition and the elderly: identifying those at risk, *Proc. Nutr. Soc.*, 43, 295, 1984.

130. Ham, R. J., Indicators of poor nutritional status in older Americans, *Am. Fam. Physician*, 45, 219, 1992.

131. Lipschitz, D. A., Ham, R. J., and White, J. V., An approach to nutrition screening for older Americans, *Am. Fam. Physician*, 45, 601, 1992.

132. Ryan, V. C. and Bower, M. E., Relationship of socioeconomic status and living arrangements to nutritional intake of the older person, *J. Am. Diet. Assoc.*, 89, 1805, 1989.

133. Vellas, B. J., Albarede, J. L., and Garry, P. J., Diseases and aging: patterns of morbidity with age; relationship between aging and age-associated diseases, *Am. J. Clin. Nutr.*, 55, 1225S, 1992.

134. White, J. V., Risk factors for poor nutritional status in older Americans, *Am. Fam. Physician*, 44, 2087, 1991.

135. Wolinsky, F. D., Coe, R. M., McIntosh, W. A., Kubena, K. S., Prendergast, J. M., Chavez, M. N., Miller, D. K., Romeis, J. C., and Landmann, W. A., Progress in the development of a nutritional risk index, *J. Nutr.*, 120, 1549, 1990.

136. Betts, N. M. and Vivian, V. M., Factors related to the dietary adequacy of noninstitutionalized elderly, *J. Nutr. Elderly*, 4, 3, 1985.

137. Davis, M. A., Randall, E., Forthofer, R. N., Lee, E. S., and Margen, S., Living arrangements and dietary patterns of older adults in the U.S., *J. Gerontol.*, 40, 434, 1985.

138. deCastro, J. M. and deCastro, E. S., Spontaneous meal patterns of humans: influence of the presence of other people, *Am. J. Clin. Nutr.*, 50, 237, 1989.

139. Horwath, C. C., Dietary intake studies in elderly people, *World Rev. Nutr. Diet.*, 59, 1, 1989.

140. Lowik, M. R. H., Schrijver, J., Odink, J., van den Berg, H., Wedel, M., and Hermus, R. J. J., Nutrition and aging: nutritional status of "apparently healthy" elderly (Dutch nutrition surveillance system), *J. Am. Coll. Nutr.*, 9, 18, 1990.

141. McIntosh, W. A. and Shifflett, P. A., Influence of social support systems on dietary intake of the elderly, *J. Nutr. Elderly*, 4, 5, 1984.

142. Ryan, A. S., Craig, L. D., and Finn, S. C., Nutrient intakes and dietary patterns of older Americans: a national study, *J. Gerontol.*, 47, M145, 1992.

143. Stevens, D. A., Grivetti, L. E., and McDonald, R. B., Nutrient intake of urban and rural elderly receiving home-delivered meals, *J. Am. Diet. Assoc.*, 92, 714, 1992.

144. Constans, T., Bacq, Y., Brechot, J. F., Guilmot, J. L., Choutet, M. D., and Lamisse, F., Protein-energy malnutrition in elderly medical patients, *J. Am. Geriatr. Soc.*, 40, 263, 1992.

145. Franklin, C. A. and Karkeck, J., Weight loss and senile dementia in an institutionalized elderly population, *J. Am. Diet. Assoc.*, 89, 790, 1989.

146. Hanson, L. C., Weber, D. J., and Rutala, W. A., Risk factors for nosocomial pneumonia in the elderly, *Am. J. Med.*, 92, 161, 1992.

147. Henderson, C. T., Nutrition and malnutrition in the elderly nursing home patient, *Clin. Geriatr. Med.*, 4, 527, 1988.

148. Kerstetter, J. E., Holthausen, B. A., and Fitz, P. A., Malnutrition in the institutionalized older adult, *J. Am. Diet. Assoc.*, 92, 1109, 1992.

149. Lowik, M. R. H., Schneijder, P., Hulshof, K. F. A. M., Kistemaker, C., Sleutel, L., and van Houten, P., Institutionalized elderly women have lower food intake than do those living more independently (Dutch nutrition surveillance system), *J. Am. Coll. Nutr.*, 11, 432, 1992.

150. Silver, A. J., Morley, J. E., Strome, L. S., Jones, D., and Vickers, L., Nutritional status in an academic nursing home, *J. Am. Geriatr. Soc.*, 36, 487, 1988.

151. Sullivan, D. H., Risk factors for early hospital readmission in a select population of geriatric rehabilitation patients: the significance of nutritional status, *J. Am. Geriatr. Soc.*, 40, 792, 1992.

152. Tramposch, T. S. and Blue, L. S., A nutrition screening and assessment system for use with the elderly in extended care, *J. Am. Diet. Assoc.*, 87, 1207, 1987.

153. Posner, B. M., Jette, A. M., Smith, K. W., and Miller, D. R., Nutrition and health risks in the elderly: the nutrition screening initiative, *Am. J. Public Health*, 83, 972, 1993.

154. Wolinsky, F. D., Prendergast, J. M., Miller, D. K., Coe, R. M., and Chavez, M. N., A preliminary validation of a nutritional risk measure for the elderly, *Am. J. Prev. Med.*, 1, 53, 1985.

155. Rush, D., Evaluating the nutrition screening initiative, *Am. J. Public Health*, 83, 944, 1993.

156. Smiciklas-Wright, H., personal communication.

Chapter 16

WOMEN AS A COMMUNITY WITH NUTRITIONAL NEEDS

Paula Zemel and Betsy Haughton

CONTENTS

0-8493-8502-4/96/$0.00+$.50
© 1996 by CRC Press, Inc.

I. WOMEN AS A COMMUNITY
WITH PUBLIC HEALTH NEEDS

A community is any group of people that has some common bond or shared characteristic. This broad definition engenders a variety of different perceptions depending on the frame of reference.[1-4] In public health, community often refers to those persons who live within certain geographic or political boundaries, such as a city (Atlanta), region (southern Appalachia), or service area (the eight southeastern states that comprise U.S. Department of Health and Human Services' Region IV). A community can refer also to persons who share a common language (Hispanic Americans), culture (African Americans), or characteristic or trait. In this latter case and for the purposes of this chapter, women constitute a community whose common characteristic is their gender and who are either of reproductive age or postmenopausal and live within the U.S.

In 1988 the Institute of Medicine (IOM) published a report, *The Future of Public Health*,[5] that reviewed the current state of public health and made recommendations for strengthening it. The definition of public health, its mission, and identification of responsibilities also form the basis for this chapter's organization. The IOM report stated that the mission of public health is to fulfill society's interest in assuring conditions in which people can be healthy. Communities, therefore, must be proactive in identifying health problems and goals, and developing plans, programs, and services to attain these goals. Women must play an active role in determining their own health values and what is important to them about their health status.

Organizationally, three community sectors are responsible for the public's health:

- Federal, state, and local governments
- Public sector
- Private sector

Therefore, the traditional frame of reference for public health and public health responsibilities, as those programs and services that are planned, implemented, and evaluated by official health agencies or departments, is antiquated. All community sectors are responsible for the public's health, but how those responsibilities are delegated and implemented varies.

This chapter, then, focuses on women as a community, who have some health problems, conditions, or needs similar to those of men due to physiologic effects of aging, but who also have unique health concerns and interests (Table 1). Descriptions of programs, services, and activities that address women's health concerns are organized categorically by community sectors responsible for public health, or the government, public, and private sectors.

TABLE 1
Criteria Used to Identify a Health Problem
or Condition as a Women's Health Issue

Diseases or conditions *unique* to women or some subgroups of women
Diseases or conditions *more prevalent* in women or some subgroup of women
Diseases or conditions *more serious* among women or some subgroup of women
Diseases or conditions for which *risk factors* are different for women or some subgroup of women
Diseases or conditions for which the *interventions* are different for women or some subgroup of women

From U.S. Department of Health and Human Services, Public Health Service, Office of Women's Health, Action Plan for Women's Health, DHHS Publ. No. (PHS) 91-50214, U.S. Government Printing Office, Washington, D.C., 1991, 149.

II. GOVERNMENT'S RESPONSIBILITY FOR WOMEN'S HEALTH

A. THE PUBLIC HEALTH INFRASTRUCTURE

Government's unique public health responsibility is to assure conditions in which women can be healthy and its focus is on the entire population of women. This is accomplished by maintaining a public health infrastructure that includes the core public health functions of assessment, policy development, and assurance (Figure 1).[6-8]

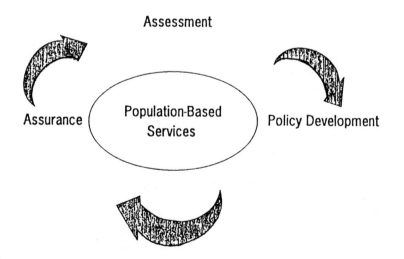

FIGURE 1. Core Public Health Functions: Assessment, Assurance, and Policy Development. (Adapted from Washington State Core Government Public Health Functions Task Force, *Core Public Health Functions*, National Association of County Health Officials, Washington, DC, 1993, 5.)

1. Core Public Health Function: Assessment

Assessment requires systematic data collection and analysis, monitoring, and surveillance to describe not only women's health status, but also factors affecting their health and the resources available to address needs. This information is used then as part of the policy development and planning process.[7,9]

The federal government has a variety of nutrition monitoring activities, which are described in *Nutrition Monitoring in the U.S. The Directory of Federal and State Nutrition Monitoring Activities*.[10] This complex array of surveys and surveillance systems provides much information about the whole U.S. population, but also certain target populations, including women.[11] A variety of survey questions, designs, and data collection tools and strategies are employed by a number of federal agencies. To strengthen this system of monitoring, Congress passed the National Nutrition Monitoring and Related Research Act of 1990. This act required development of a 10-Year Comprehensive Plan for Nutrition Monitoring and Related Research and formation of an Interagency Board for Nutrition Monitoring and Related Research to oversee the plan's implementation. These national nutrition monitoring activities are categorized as:

- Nutrition and related health measurements
- Food and nutrient consumption
- Knowledge, attitudes, and behavior assessment
- Food composition and nutrient data bases
- Food supply determination

Few of the surveys or surveillance systems are unique to women (Table 2), although women are part of the target population of many (Table 3). Furthermore, those studies unique to women focus on childbearing alone, with no attention to the nutritional needs and concerns of older women, such as breast cancer and osteoporosis.

Although federal agencies are responsible for designing these surveys and surveillance systems, analyzing data, and reporting results, state and local governmental agencies have important responsibilities for collecting local data and preparing it for submission to the respective federal agencies for analysis. Information from these surveys and surveillance systems are used in developing policies and programs based on the most current and relevant data about existing health problems and concerns.

2. Core Public Health Function: Policy Development

Assessment data are only as valuable as the extent to which they are employed in the planning process and used with communities to help understand each community's unique health needs and determine its health-related values. These community values are key to policy development and are expressed as public statements, principles, or guidelines about what communities believe is important about health, including health promotion, disease

TABLE 2

Nutrition Monitoring and Related Research Focused on Women

Survey or Surveillance System	Target Problem	Sponsoring Agency
Nutrition and related health measurements		
National Survey of Family Growth (NSFG)	Women of reproductive age (15–44 years)	NCHS, CDC
National Maternal and Infant Health Survey (NMIHS)	Study of women, hospitals and prenatal care providers associated with live births, still births, infant deaths — 1988	NCHS, CDC
Longitudinal follow-up to the National Maternal and Infant Health Survey	Participants of the 1988 NMIHS	NCHS, CDC
Pregnancy Nutrition Surveillance System (PNSS)	Low-income, high-risk pregnant women	NCCDPHP, CDC
Food and nutrient composition		
Continuing Survey of Food Intakes of Individuals (CFSII), 1985–1986	Persons of selected sex and age residing in 48 conterminous states or households with incomes at any level (basic survey) and with incomes <130% poverty (low income survey); in 1985, women 19-50 years and their children 1-5 years, and men 19-50 years; and in 1986, women 19-50 years and their children 1-5 years	
National Seafood Consumption Survey	1973-1974 panel representative of families, young children and pregnant women. 1980-1981 panel representative of households and individuals in U.S.	NMFS, NOAA, USDC
An evaluation of the special supplemental Food Program for Women, Infants, and Children (an evaluation of WIC)	Pregnant women in first two trimesters of pregnancy and their children who were participating in WIC, and WIC-eligible but non-participating women from the same geographic region	FNS, USDA
Knowledge, attitudes and behavior assessment		
Infant Feeding Practices Survey	New mothers and healthy, full-term infants from birth to 1 year	FDA

Note: CDC = Centers for Disease Control and Prevention; FDA = Food and Drug Administration; FNS = Food and Nutrition Service; NCCDPHP = National Center for Chronic Disease Prevention and Health Promotion; NCHS = National Center for Health Statistics; NMFS = National Marine Fisheries Service; NOAA = National Oceanic and Atmospheric Administration; USDA = U.S. Department of Agriculture; USDC = U.S. Department of Commerce

TABLE 3
Nutrition Monitoring and Related Research:
Target Populations that Include Women and Others

Nutrition and related health measurements

National Health Examination Surveys (NHES I, II, III)
National Health and Nutrition Examination Surveys (NHANES I, II, III)
Hispanic Health and Nutrition Examination Survey (HHANES)
National Health and Nutrition Examination Survey I Epidemiologic Followup Study (NHEFS)
HANES Mortality Follow-up Studies
National Health Interview Survey (NHIS)
National Health Interview Survey on Aging
National Health Interview Survey on Health Promotion and Disease Prevention (NHISHPDP)
1991 National Health Interview Survey on Health Promotion and Disease Prevention
National Health Interview Survey on Vitamin and Mineral Supplements
National Health Interview Survey on Cancer Epidemiology and Cancer Control
National Health Interview Survey on Youth Behavior Supplement (NHIS-YBS)
National Hospital Discharge Survey (NHDS)
National Ambulatory Medical Care Survey (NAMCS)
National Hospital Ambulatory Medical Care Survey (NHAMCS)
National Nursing Home Survey (NNHS)
National Home and Hospice Care Survey (NHHCS)
Vital Statistics Program
National Mortality Follow Back Survey (NMFS)
Navajo Health and Nutrition Survey

Food and nutrient composition

National Food Consumption Survey (NFCS)
Continuing Survey of Food Intakes by Individuals (CSFII), 1989–1991
Vitamin and Mineral Supplement Intake Survey
Nutritional Evaluation of Military Feeding Systems and Military Populations
Feeding the Homeless: Does the Prepared Meal Provision Help?
Evaluation of the Food Distribution Program on Indian Reservations (FDPIR)
Food Stamp Supplemental Security Income/Elderly Cash-Out Demographic
  Evaluation
Adult Day Care Program Study
Consumer Expenditure Survey
Survey of Income and Program Participation (SIPP)

Knowledge, attitudes, and behavior assessments

Behavioral Risk Factor Surveillance System (BRFSS)
National Adolescent Student Health Survey (NASHS)
Consumer Food Handling Practices and Awareness of Microbiological Hazards
Point of Purchase Labeling Studies
Survey of Weight-Loss Practices
Diet and Health Knowledge Survey (DHKS)
Health and Diet Survey
Cancer Prevention Awareness Survey
National Knowledge, Attitudes, and Behavior Survey
National Label Format Studies

prevention, and treatment. State and local health agencies are responsible to help communities formulate these principles, which then are incorporated in the development of comprehensive health policies.[7] This process requires both leadership and management roles and includes:

- Statement of mission
- Definition of the women's health problem
- Community assessment and value clarification on priority issues
- Identification of goals and objectives to address priority issues
- Development of an action plan and management system
- Budget development
- Implementation of the plan
- Monitoring and evaluation[12,13]

A comprehensive delineation of national health goals and objectives and related implementation plan were published in several documents beginning in 1979 with *Healthy People: The Surgeon General's Report on Health Promotion and Disease Prevention*,[14] and followed by *Promoting Health/Preventing Disease: Objectives for the Nation*[15] and *Promoting Health/Preventing Disease: Implementation Plans for Attaining the Objectives for the Nation*.[16] These documents focused on health status objectives to be achieved by 1990 and provided a model for state and local health agencies to use in their own planning.

The current federal document delineating health goals and objectives for the U.S. to be attained by the year 2000 is titled *Healthy People 2000*.[17] Three broad goals provide the framework for the supporting objectives:

- Increase Americans' healthy life span
- Reduce health disparities among Americans
- Achieve access to preventive services for all Americans

Within each of the 22 health priority areas, 332 primary health objectives are categorized as health promotion, health protection, preventive services, and surveillance and data systems. Of these objectives 18 are nutritionally related and targeted to women (Table 4) and most concern the health status of or risk reduction strategies for pregnant or breastfeeding women and not those of older women. As with national surveys and surveillance systems, women are included in other health objectives, but are not necessarily targeted.

In 1985 the U.S. Department of Health and Human Services' Public Health Services began to develop a women's health agenda. Its Coordinating Committee on Women's Health Issues published *Women's Health: Report of the PHS Task Force on Women's Health Issues* with 16 recommendations for developing a women's health policy. This served as the basis for the subsequent 1991 publication of the Office of Women's Health, *PHS Action Plan for Women's Health*.[18] This 2-year plan and its 1-year progress review[19] clearly

TABLE 4
Healthy People 2000. Nutrition-Related Health
Objectives Targeted to Women

Healthy People 2000 objective no.

Health Status Objectives

2.3a	Reduce overweight to a prevalence of no more than 25% among low-income women aged 20 and older
2.3b	Reduce overweight to a prevalence of no more than 30% among black women aged 20 and older
2.3c	Reduce overweight to a prevalence of no more than 25% among Hispanic women aged 20 and older
2.3f	Reduce overweight to a prevalence of no more than 41% among women with high blood pressure
14.1	Reduce the infant mortality rate to no more than 7/1000 live births
14.2	Reduce the fetal death rate (20 or more weeks of gestation) to no more than 5/1000 live births plus fetal deaths
14.3	Reduce the maternal mortality rate to no more than 3.3/100,000 live births
16.3	Reduce breast cancer deaths to no more than 20.6/100,000 women
17.1 0	Reduce the most severe complications of diabetes as follows

Perinatal mortality — 2%
Major congenital malformation — 4%

Risk Reduction Objectives

2.8	Increase calcium intake so at least 50% of youth aged 12 through 24 and 50% of pregnant and lactating women consume three or more servings daily of foods rich in calcium, and at least 50% of people aged 25 and older consume two or more servings daily
2.10	Reduce iron deficiency to less than 3% among children aged 1 through 4 and among women of childbearing age
2.11	Increase to at least 75% the proportion of mothers who breastfeed their babies in the early postpartum period and to at least 50% the proportion who continue breastfeeding until their babies are 5 to 6 months old
14.5	Reduce low birth weight to an incidence of no more than 5% of live births and very low birth weight to no more than 1% of live births
14.6	Increase to at least 85% the proportion of mothers who achieve the minimum recommended weight gain during their pregnancies
14.7	Reduce severe complications of pregnancy to no more than 15/100 deliveries

Services and Protection Objectives

14.1 1	Increase to at least 90% the proportion of all pregnant women who receive prenatal care in the first trimester of pregnancy
14.1 2	Increase to at least 60% the proportion of primary care providers who provide age-appropriate preconception care and counseling
14.1 4	Increase to at least 90% the proportion of pregnant women and infants who receive risk-appropriate care

From U.S. Department of Health and Human Services, Public Health Service, Healthy People 2000, U.S. Government Printing Office. Washington, D.C., 1991.

support women's health as a national public health priority by incorporating objectives from each of the Public Health Services' agencies and offices into a unified plan.

Although *Healthy People 2000* identifies national goals and objectives, these are obtained only through the efforts of states and local communities. *Healthy Communities 2000: Model Standards*[20] is a tool developed by the American Public Health Association to help local communities tailor objectives to their unique community needs and values. It recommends an 11-step process[20] that includes the basic public health core functions as a framework for local community planning.

Several other models for assessment and planning are available, including *Assessment Protocol for Excellence in Public Health (APEXPH)*[21] and *Planned Approach to Community Health* (PATCH).[22-24] The *APEXPH* document and PATCH process can be used by local health agencies to:

- Assess their own and the community's organizational needs and capacity to address women's health problems and promote health
- Improve the agency's and community's capacity to promote public health
- Establish strong community relations and support
- Develop community coalitions in the government, public, and private sectors for community-based systems of health care[25]

Policy development also relates to population-based dietary recommendations for women. Scientific evidence supports the notion that nutritional practices significantly affect women's overall health and is documented in a number of consensus reports: *The Surgeon General's Report on Nutrition and Health*,[26] the National Academy of Sciences' *Diet and Health*,[27] the U.S. Department of Agriculture and U.S. Department of Health and Human Services' *Dietary Guidelines for Americans*,[28] and, with specific reference to women, the IOM's three publications, *Nutrition During Pregnancy*,[29] *Nutrition During Lactation*,[30] and *Nutrition During Pregnancy and Lactation: An Implementation Guide*.[31] Although the latter documents provide recommendations for preconceptional, perinatal, and postpartum women, Abrams and Berman[32] argue that these same recommendations should be made for all women to reduce chronic disease risk. These recommendations include four consensus-based nutrition recommendations:

- Consume five or more servings of vegetables (including legumes) and fruits a day and six or more servings of grains, emphasizing whole grain foods
- Avoid obesity and maintain a healthy weight by balancing food intake and physical activity
- Gain appropriate weight during pregnancy based on pre-pregnancy weight-for-height

- Reduce total dietary fat intake to less than 30% of calories
- Consume adequate calcium based on age, menopausal status, and use of exogenous calcium

3. Core Public Health Function: Assurance

The third core function of public health agencies is to assure that high quality and effective services are available and accessible.[7] This mandates quality improvement systems and regulatory responsibilities. Although the federal government is responsible for assuring that actions and services are in the whole nation's public health interest, state and local official health agencies have specific responsibilities related to assuring not only that there are adequate statutory bases for health activities, but also that essential public health services are available and accessible, and a minimum set of essential health services are guaranteed. This has led to a primary focus on direct service provision rather than other assurance functions. In its vision for public health the American Public Health Association's Subcommittee on Community Prevention Programs and Public Health Vision[33] reported in 1993 that state and local health agencies should:

- Provide public health and environmental health services
- Encourage, purchase, or provide additional population-based services
- Maintain the capacity to respond to emergencies
- Administer quality assurance programs
- Recruit and retain health care practitioners
- Maintain administrative capacity

Currently, to help assure the provision of necessary health services, local official health agencies provide personal health services, including nutrition services, to women. This is especially true in areas where the public and private sectors have not provided or have been unable to provide primary and secondary prevention services.[34,35] The components of nutrition services[36] include:

- Screening and assessment to identify nutrition problems
- Prevention, treatment, and follow-up services, including

    Nutrition counseling
    Nutrition education
    Referrals to community food assistance resources
    Assessment of individual care plans
    Assessment of nutrition program services, or quality improvement

With the advent of a revised health care system, it is anticipated that these personal health and nutrition services will be financed through some insurance funding mechanism yet to be determined, allowing health departments to focus on the public health core functions of assessment, policy development, and assurance. The challenge of health care reform is that state and local health agencies will need to shift away from the role of providing direct care services and reassert public health leadership with a population focus using the core functions.

Title V of the Social Security Act, or the Maternal and Child Health (MCH) Program, is an example of targeted assurance for *all* mothers, infants, and children, but especially those of low income and with limited access to health care services. It was authorized in 1935 with a particular focus on reducing infant mortality.[37] It is the only federal program developed exclusively for the maternal and child population. Two key provisions relate to the assurance responsibilities of all levels of government. First, Title V provides the federal statutory basis for MCH services in each state and territory and, second, it provides resources necessary to support state and local public health infrastructure for these services.[38]

Title V requires each state to (1) provide direct MCH support for available and accessible community health services and (2) assure statewide systems of community-based quality health care. The new Title V block grants also require a statewide needs assessment to support funding requests and provide a baseline for program evaluation. Direct support for MCH services is achieved through grants, contracts, and reimbursement to providers and, where not feasible, direct care service provision. Community-based health care systems can be developed by applying the core functions of community assessment and policy development, and providing technical assistance, information and education, and training. While other federal programs may help improve women's health by, for example, the provision of food assistance, Title V is unique as the only comprehensive health program for mothers and children.[38-41]

4. Federal, State, and Local Public Health Responsibilities for the Public Health Infrastructure

Although all levels of government are responsible for the public health core functions, each has unique responsibilities. States, however, are the central focus of public health functions with responsibility for:

- Assessment of state needs
- Assurance of a statutory base for public health activities
- Establishment of statewide health objectives
- Assurance of state efforts to develop and maintain health services, provide access to services, and solve problems that threaten the public's health
- Guarantee of essential health services
- Support of local public health service capacity[42]

Local official health agencies help support state public health efforts by focusing on their own community's needs and fostering community support. They, too, have responsibility for core public health functions, but focused at the local level. At the other end of the spectrum, the federal government is responsible for knowledge development and dissemination, establishment of national objectives and priorities, provision of technical assistance, funding to strengthen state capacity for services and achieve national objectives, and assurance of actions and services of national public health interest.

An excellent example of how these responsibilities are delegated and applied to women using the public health core functions is the MCH Title V Block Grant. As indicated previously, Title V of the Social Security Act provides funding to states to improve the health of all mothers and children and reduce infant mortality. Each state's health agency must have a unit responsible for MCH program administration. In 1981 Title V was amended to consolidate seven categorical programs into a single MCH Services Block Grant and give states discretion for how they allocate funding within their respective states.[43] Although Title V provides federal assurance for MCH programs and services, states have central responsibility for how this assurance is manifested in comprehensive systems of care to meet identified MCH population needs. These systems of care are assured through assessment, planning, and policy development; community-based systems development; interagency coordination; setting and monitoring of standards of care; and provision of information, education, training, and technical assistance. Further amendments in 1989 as part of the Omnibus Reconciliation Act of 1989 (OBRA '89) strengthened the states' roles and responsibilities by requiring, specifically:

- Assurance of access to quality and community-based prevention and primary care for pregnant women, infants, children, and youth and specialized health and family support services for children with special health care needs
- Comprehensive needs assessment and plan consistent with applicable health status goals and national health objectives
- Development of family-centered, coordinated, community-based systems of care
- Enhanced interagency coordination, especially with Medicaid, and
- Annual reporting[38]

Each state must have programs in five areas: (1) maternity and infant care, (2) intensive infant care, (3) family planning, (4) health care for children and youth, and (5) dental care for children.[44] Nutrition-related activities include nutrition assessment, counseling, and education; referral to food assistance programs; care coordination; home visits, especially in association with nursing; and integration of multiple services, or one-stop shopping.[38,41]

Local health agencies, in turn, are responsible for providing local leadership and assuring that these high quality services are available and accessible to all women and consistent with not only statewide health objectives and plans, but also local community needs. Therefore, local MCH initiatives can vary widely. Ideas and new initiatives from the nearly 100 urban health departments are shared at annual CityMatCH Urban Maternal and Child Health Leadership Conferences. Examples of profiles of urban health department initiatives are categorized in the areas of outreach, access to care, and comprehensive systems of care (Table 5).[45]

How the federal appropriations are allocated also reflects respective governmental responsibilities. For federal appropriations of $600 million or less, 85% is allocated to the states to enable assurance of access, implementation, and services, while 15% is a set-aside for Special Projects of Regional and National Significance (SPRANS), research, and training. For appropriations totaling more than $600 million, an additional 12.75% set-aside is for six types of demonstration projects. States allocate their MCH block grant funds based on state needs, which are in turn based on local needs.[38,43]

B. GOVERNMENT PROGRAMS FOR WOMEN

Although Title V MCH programs are the only comprehensive systems of health care for women, there are a number of other government nutrition programs that directly affect women's health. These are primarily administered through the U.S. Department of Health and Human Services and U.S. Department of Agriculture.

1. Health and Nutrition Programs of U.S. Department of Health and Human Services (DHHS)

DHHS' mission is to promote, protect, and advance the nation's physical and mental health. The Public Health Service is the primary agency within DHHS responsible for national public health concerns. Within its Health Resources and Services Administration, two key programs are administered: Title V MCH within the Maternal and Child Health Bureau and the Community Health Centers Program within the Community Health Services Bureau.

It is estimated that over one half million women receive Title V prenatal care, including 14% of all babies born and more than one third of births to low income women.[38] The primary source of medical care for those receiving Medicaid, the uninsured, and underinsured is MCH programs. Title V programs have contributed significantly not only to reducing low birth weight, maternal and infant mortality, and disability for those who are mentally retarded or developmentally disabled, but also to improving children's overall health status.[46-50]

The Community Health Services program is a categorical program initiated by the Office of Economic Opportunity and authorized by the Public Health Service Act in 1966. Community health centers provide health services and related training in medically underserved areas and are free-standing health clinics not connected with a hospital or medical center. Service sites include migrant health centers, Appalachian health demonstration projects, rural health initiative projects, and urban health initiative projects. Both preventive health

TABLE 5
Selected Profiles of Urban Health Department Initiatives, 1993

Reaching Out to Urban MCH Populations

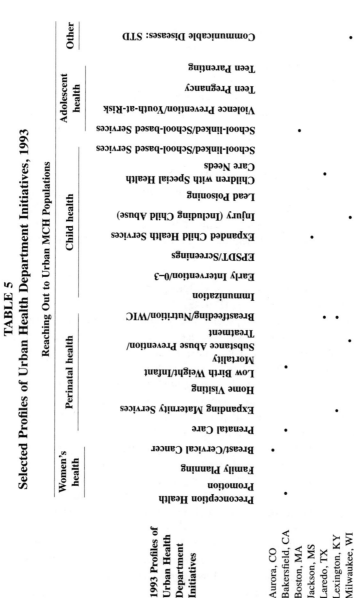

1993 profiles of Urban Health Department initiatives

Improving access to care for urban children and families:

- Overcoming Racial/Ethnical/language/Cultural Barriers
- Reducing Transportation Barriers
- Expanding Private Sector Linkages
- Clergy and Health Connections
- Housing and Health Connections
- Schools and Health Connections
- One-Stop Shopping, Co-location of Services
- Using Mobile Vans, Clinics for Outreach
- Other Outreach Activities
- Increasing Social Support Systems
- Case Management/Care Coordination
- Increasing Access to Medicaid

Strengthening urban public health system for MCH:

- Staff Training
- Strategic Planning for Urban MCH
- Reshaping Financing for Urban MCH
- Securing Urban MCH Technical Assistance
- Managed Care Initiatives
- Building Coalitions and Partnerships
- Building MCH Data Capacity
- Immunization Tracking, Recall Systems
- Infant/Child Death Review Activities

Cities:

- Aurora, CO
- Bakersfield, CA
- Boston, MA
- Jackson, MS
- Laredo, TX
- Lexington, KY
- Milwaukee, WI
- Nashville, TN
- Phoenix, AZ
- St. Petersburg, FL
- Washington, D.C.
- Wilmington, DE

From Peck, M. G., *Improving Urban MCH Linkages: Highlights of the 1993 Urban Maternal and Child Health Leadership Conference*, City MalCH of the University of Nebraska Medical Center, Omaha, 1994, 40.

and comprehensive primary health care services are provided, including nutrition.[51,52]

Another DHHS program that can provide nutrition services for women under 21 years of age is the early periodic screening, diagnosis, and Treatment Program (EPSDT) of Medicaid. Medicaid was created in 1965 as Title XIX of the Social Security Act. It is administered at the federal level by the Health Care Financing Administration (HCFA), but each state administers its own program and determines which provider services are reimbursed. Amendments in 1969 stipulated that states must provide EPSDT to improve low income children's health status. EPSDT requires primary and secondary preventive services, including nutrition status assessment of eligible children. If a physical or mental defect is detected in screening, then Medicaid funds services, including nutrition services, to correct and ameliorate that condition, even if the services required are not covered traditionally by Medicaid.[41,53-55] For example, if a nutrition problem such as obesity or iron deficiency anemia is identified, then nutrition intervention is required.

Elderly women exclusively are not targeted for nutrition programs by DHHS programs. Two food assistance programs administered by DHHS' Administration on Aging, however, do reach women over 60 years of age, regardless of income: congregate meals and home-delivered meals. The Nutrition Program for Older Americans, or Title III of the Older Americans Act, is designed to help maintain independent living and improve quality of life for the elderly. Program components include meals, established and planned with the advice of dietitians, opportunities for social interaction, nutrition education at least semiannually, counseling and referral to social services, and transportation services. Meals are available at a minimum once a day, 5 d/week, and must be consistent with the Dietary Guidelines for Americans and provide at least one third of the RDA.[56-58] Congregate meals provide the opportunity for social interaction, while home-delivered meals provide the opportunity for nutritious foods for those who are home-bound. Although there is no required cost, program participants are encouraged to contribute to each meal's cost. USDA, through its Nutrition Program for the Elderly, contributes to these programs by providing cash and commodity foods to participating senior citizen centers. Title VI of the Older Americans Act provides nutrition and social service programs comparable to Title III, but for Native Americans, including American Indians, Alaskan, and Hawaiian native elders.

2. Food and Nutrition Programs of U.S. Department of Agriculture (USDA)

USDA is responsible for national food and agricultural programs. A number of its agencies provide support for community nutrition programs, including the Human Nutrition Information Service (HNIS), Food and Nutrition Service (FNS), Food Safety Inspection Service, Cooperative Extension Service, and National Agricultural Library. The HNIS administers USDA's nutrition-monitoring activities (Tables 2 and 3) and develops a variety of educational materials for use with the *Dietary Guidelines for Americans*.

The Cooperative Extension Service's Expanded Food and Nutrition Education Program (EFNEP) is designed to provide nutrition education for low income families in rural and urban communities. Although not specifically targeted to women, in 1968 it was authorized to provide food and nutrition education to homemakers and their young children. Paraprofessionals provide food and nutrition education under the supervision of cooperative extension home economists.[59,60]

In response to the growing number of health care concerns, the Cooperative Extension System adopted a national Extension Health Agenda, Decisions for Health, for FY 1994. Its purpose is to promote healthy lifestyles, improve access to affordable health care, and expand communities' capacity to strengthen their health and health-related infrastructure. Three goals articulated by the National Extension Health Agenda Task Force[61] are operational:

- People will adopt healthy lifestyles by reducing high-risk behaviors and taking responsibility for health decisions
- Individuals and community organizations, making informed decisions, will improve access to and affordability of health care
- Communities will improve their capacity to analyze and take action related to health and health-related infrastructure needs

Although targeted to all people and communities with limited resources, special emphasis is given to children, youth, and the aging; culturally diverse populations; limited resource populations; and agricultural populations with physical disabilities. Since many of the poor are women and more poor families are headed by single mothers, it can be assumed that women will be the recipients of activities and services that result from this initiative.[62,63]

In 1969 FNS was created to administer USDA's food assistance programs. Its goals are to provide low income people access to a nutritious diet, improve children's eating habits, and stabilize farm prices through distribution of surplus foods. The focus, therefore, is on addressing issues related to access to food, hunger, and food security. The federal government provides states funding to cover administrative costs, while states determine how food benefits will be distributed and to whom. For FY 1993 FNS was appropriated $35.9 billion to operate its 14 food assistance programs (Table 6) and participate in national advisory councils associated with its program areas.[64]

The FNS program that has received widespread national attention in relation to program benefits is the Supplemental Food Program for Women, Infants, and Children (WIC). WIC was authorized in 1972 by P.L. 92-433 as an amendment to the Child Nutrition Act of 1966. It is an adjunct to health care and provides food assistance, nutrition education, and referrals to health care services to pregnant, postpartum, and breastfeeding women, infants, and children up to the age of 5 years who are low income (100 to 185% federal

Table 6
Food Assistance Programs Available to Women

Program	Service provided	Target population	Service provider
Food Stamp Program	Monthly coupon allotments redeemable at retail food stores for foods, or food products for human consumption, and seeds and plants for home gardens to produce foods, amount based on Thrifty Food Plan	Low income households that meet income and work eligibility requirements and provide proof of household circumstance	Local public assistance or social services offices
Nutrition Assistance Program	Cash and coupons for food purchases	Low income persons in Puerto Rico and northern Marianas, replaced Food Stamp Program	Commonwealth of Puerto Rico; commonwealth of northern Mariana Islands
Child and Adult Care Food Program	Cash and commodity food assistance to centers, free and reduced-price meals at centers based on household size and income of participants	Children $\leq$12 years; children of migrant workers $\leq$15; chronically impaired adults, disabled adults $\geq$18; persons $\geq$60 years in group setting outside home on <24-h basis	Nonresidential child and adult day care centers and, through sponsor organizations, family and group day care homes for children
Special Supplemental Food Program for Women, Infants, and Children (WIC)	Supplemental food, nutrition education, and referrals for health services, participants receive vouchers redeemable at retail food stores for specified foods high in protein, caldium, iron, and vitamins A and C	Pregnant, breastfeeding, and postpartum women, infants, and children up to 5 years old who are income eligible (100–185% poverty) or participate in AFDC, Food Stamp, or Medicaid programs and are at nutritional risk	Health agencies, social services, community action agencies
WIC Farmers Market Nutrition Program	Fresh produce redeemed by vouchers at authorized farmers markets	WIC participants (infants must be 4 months old)	Local WIC agencies in association with authorized farmers or farmers markets

Commodity Supplemental Food Program	Commodity food packages tailored to participants' nutritional needs	Low income (≤185% poverty) infants; children up to age 6; pregnant, post-partum, and breast-feeding women; persons ≥60 years	Public and private nonprofit agencies, including health departments, social services, education, or agriculture agencies
Food Distribution Program on Indian Reservations and Trust Territories	Commodity food packages	Native American families who live on or near Indian reservations, and to Pacific Islanders	Local agency
Nutrition Program for the Elderly	Cash reimbursements for meals and commodity foods to senior citizen centers of meals-on-wheels program for meals and snacks consistent with Dietary Guidelines for Americans; nutrition education; access to social and rehabilitative services; transportation	Persons ≥60 years and their spouses regardless of age	DHHS programs for elderly, e.g., area agency on aging or other aging services provider
Food Distribution Program for Charitable Institutions	Commodity and USDA-donated foods	Needy persons receiving food at eligible charitable institutions	Nonprofit charitable institutions that serve meals regularly to needy persons, e.g., food banks, meals-on-wheels programs, summer camps, orphanages
Emergency Food Assistance Program	USDA — donated foods	Low income and unemployed persons who meet state-specific eligibility criteria	Public and private nonprofit agencies (community action agencies, councils on aging, local health or local school districts) designated by state

poverty level) and at nutritional risk. The categories of nutritional risk are medically related risks (e.g., anemia, underweight, history of high-risk pregnancies, and maternal age), diet-related risks (e.g., inadequate dietary pattern), or conditions that predispose the individual to medically related or diet-related risks (e.g., substance abuse).[65] The program has grown from $20 million in FY 1974 to $2.1 billion, and reaching 4.5 million eligible women, infants, and children in FY 1990.[66] WIC is not an entitlement program and, therefore, only approximately 55% of the estimated 8.4 million eligible participants were being served in 1990 due to limited funding.[67]

Congressional and community support for WIC has been maintained, especially through documentation of the program's benefits and cost effectiveness.[68] For example, a 1984 General Accounting Office study[69] reported that WIC reduced the incidence of low birth weight by 16 to 20%; the 1986 National WIC Evaluation Study found that WIC contributed a reduced incidence of premature births among high risk women and 20 to 33% reduction in fetal mortality;[70] and a 1990 USDA study of more than 100,000 mothers and babies found that birth weights increased significantly while on WIC.[71] A frequently cited cost/benefit statistic from the General Accounting Office[72] is that for every dollar spent on WIC for pregnant women, $4.21 can be saved in Medicaid costs. Although an important food assistance program, it is important to remember that WIC is not a comprehensive health care program for women. Rather it is a food assistance and nutrition education program targeted to address select nutritional needs of high risk women.

III. PUBLIC AND PRIVATE SECTOR PROGRAMS FOR WOMEN

Nongovernmental providers of community nutrition programs have been organized by Kaufman[4] into three areas: voluntary health and education organizations, professional organizations, and food industry/trade organizations. Organizations in each of these three groups can be either involved in program delivery or educational material development that addresses the nutritional needs of women.

Thus, community nutritionists need to assess the needs of women, evaluate the programs and educational materials developed by voluntary health and education organizations, professional organizations, and food industry/trade organizations, and incorporate them into their overall program if the programs or materials can meet needs. Nutrition education programs and educational materials can be used to provide the components of nutrition services,[36] including screening and assessment to identify nutrition problems and prevention, treatment, and follow-up services. Nutrition programs and educational materials can contribute to primary and secondary prevention services as well as tertiary treatment.[4,35]

Primary prevention or health promotion efforts work to change the environment and the community as well as family and individual life-styles and behaviors, to enhance and maintain a state of wellness.[4] Programs designed to prevent osteoporosis or obesity among women are examples of primary prevention efforts. Secondary prevention means risk appraisal and reduction. Interventions are designed to reduce risk among those who may be more susceptible to a health problem because of their family history, life-style, environment, or age.[4] Interventions which focus on secondary prevention include screening, detection, early diagnosis, treatment, and follow-up before the woman experiences symptoms of the disease. Low fat diet interventions for women at risk of breast cancer are an example of secondary prevention.

Tertiary prevention is directed at treating and rehabilitating persons with diagnosed health conditions in order to prevent or delay their disability, pain, suffering, and premature death.[4] Dietary treatment of hypercholesterolemia following carotid endarterectomy is an example of tertiary prevention.

Primary and secondary prevention can be offered through federal, state and local health agencies and other agencies/institutions involved in community nutrition. Some secondary prevention and almost all tertiary prevention are generally provided to individuals by medical nutrition therapists in hospitals, ambulatory care clinics, or through home health care.[4]

Representative programs and materials produced by organizations in each of these three groups that address the nutrition-related needs of women will be presented. These nutrition programs can involve various levels of community action, including the individual or family, agency, neighborhood, city/county, district, state, or nation. A primary prevention program can focus on a state or national level. For example, Project LEAN (Low fat Eating for America Now), a national media campaign to promote low fat eating habits, is currently being sponsored by The American Dietetic Association.[73] A secondary prevention program was also recently developed to detect new cases of hypertension in at-risk neighborhoods in Knoxville, TN.[74] Community leaders, such as housing project managers, were trained to measure blood pressure and distribute educational and referral materials in the community.

Existing nutrition programs and educational materials can be evaluated and their use can be assessed as to the degree to which they meet the needs of women. For example, a pamphlet on prevention of osteoporosis may be written for an adult audience and may be appropriate for use in primary or secondary prevention activities. The pamphlet may be used in counseling individual women who receive feedback following a health and nutrition screening activity in a primary care clinic. This is an example of secondary prevention. The pamphlet may also be distributed at a cafeteria display as part of a work site wellness program. This is an example of primary prevention. Profiling programs and materials in this manner enables determination of the fit between materials developed by voluntary health and education organizations, professional organizations, and food industry/trade organizations, and the nutrition-related needs of women.

In addition to evaluating materials to determine whether they meet a nutritional need of women, materials and programs must be assessed to determine if they are appropriate for the educational levels and cultural backgrounds within the community. The American Diabetes Association and The American Dietetic Association have developed a series of booklets on ethnic and regional food practices.[75-78] The Stanford Health Promotion Resource Center[79] has addressed health promotion in diverse cultural communities and The Center for Research on Women at the University of Memphis has developed a training program for enhancing cultural awareness and communication skills for health care providers.[80] Further, The National Center for Education in Maternal and Child Health recently published a booklet entitled *Celebrating Diversity: Approaching Families Through Their Food*,[81] which specifically addresses culture within a food and nutrition context.

A. NUTRITION PROGRAMS AND MATERIALS FROM PROFESSIONAL ORGANIZATIONS ADDRESSING NEEDS OF WOMEN

A variety of programs and materials have been developed by voluntary health and education organizations for women across the life cycle. Voluntary health and education organizations include organizations such as The American Heart Association, The American Cancer Society, The American Diabetes Association, The March of Dimes, and La Leche League. Some religious organizations also are involved in presenting nutrition programs to their members, usually with involvement of health care professionals.

La Leche League chapters offer programs and educational materials that can help breastfeeding mothers learn about the benefits of breastfeeding and specific information about feeding their infants and breast care. Peer counseling has been used by La Leche League International to successfully increase breastfeeding among women in low income urban populations.[82] The March of Dimes provides educational materials about perinatal nutrition and healthy pregnancy.[83] Some work site wellness programs include components designed for pregnant and lactating women in their overall health promotion programs.[84] Strategies used at The Harvard Community Health Plan to support working women who choose to breastfeed their infants were shared[85] in *Connections*, a newsletter designed to share government and private sector community efforts which promote and support breastfeeding.

The Baltimore Church High Blood Pressure Program offers a behaviorally oriented weight control program for black women.[86] An evaluation of the program indicated that 8 months following intervention, moderate weight loss and reduced blood pressure persisted.

Some community-university partnerships also result in nutrition programs for women. The Cancer and Diet Intervention Project was popular among women over 44 years of age in the Minnesota city where the intervention took place.[87] In addition, an audiovisual program for English and Spanish-speaking women positively affected knowledge of women concerning AIDS in California.[88]

B. NUTRITION PROGRAMS AND MATERIALS FROM PROFESSIONAL ORGANIZATIONS ADDRESSING NEEDS OF WOMEN

Professional organizations which develop programs and materials that address the nutrition-related needs of women include The American Diabetes Association, The American College of Obstetrics and Gynecology, and The Society for Nutrition Education. The March of Dimes has produced programs and materials to promote optimal nutrient intake during pregnancy.[83] The American College of Obstetrics and Gynecology provides patient education materials, including pamphlets that address nutritional issues such as breast-feeding and preventing osteoporosis.[89,90]

A nutrition screening program for the elderly has been developed as a collaborative effort by The American Dietetic Association, The American Academy of Family Physicians, and the National Council on Aging in order to promote early intervention as part of routine health care.[91] The Nutrition Screening Initiative has developed a ten-question self-assessment "checklist", a level I screen, that can be distributed to groups or individuals. The level II screen can then be conducted by a health care professional with older adults who have a potentially serious medical or nutritional problem.

The American Dietetic Association, through its National Center for Nutrition and Dietetics (NCND), provides services, programs, and materials for the public. A nutrition hotline provides consumers with up-to-date information about nutrition and is staffed by registered dietitians. The center also publishes fact sheets on topics related to women's health, including tips for pregnant teens, fitness and bone health and osteoporosis.[92,94] NCND also is involved with Project LEAN (Low fat eating for America now), a national public awareness campaign to promote low fat eating.[73]

C. NUTRITION PROGRAMS AND MATERIALS FROM THE PRIVATE SECTOR, THE FOOD INDUSTRY, AND TRADE ORGANIZATIONS ADDRESSING NEEDS OF WOMEN

Materials to address community needs of young adults may be available through the private sector. Nasco Nutrition Teaching Aids,[94] a distributor of educational programs and materials, and National Health Video[95] offer educational materials to provide young women with information about eating disorders as well as topics related to health promotion for women.

In some areas, private sector programs parallel public sector programs when they are not able to meet the needs in a community. The Meals-On-Wheels America program, for example, is a similar but separate program to the federal home-delivered meals program. Its purpose is to help fill gaps in services provided by the federal programs by either reaching older adults in communities not fully serviced by the federal program or by adding weekend and holiday meals in addition to the standard five luncheon meals. Funding may come from corporations, religious or other organizations, or individual donations.[96] Food banks also solicit donations or "irregular" food items that are safe for consumption but cannot be sold to the consumer and provide these to the needy through emergency feeding systems. Many food bank users are women, since poverty disproportionately affects single mothers and elderly women.[97] Home health agencies that supply nursing and homemaking services are increasing. It has been reported that 50 to 75% of the clients referred for home health services may need nutrition services.[98] Some agencies employ nutritionists and assessment of these groups may identify the need for nutrition programs.

Many food industry corporations and other trade organizations develop programs and materials that address the nutrition-related needs of women, including The National Dairy Promotion and Research Board, The Produce Marketing Association, Nabisco Foods Group, and Kraft Foods. Nutrition Update receives financial support from Nabisco Foods Group and produces a publication that provides patient education tearsheets on topics of interest to women, such as dietary supplements.[99] Kraft General Foods' *A Matter of Balance: Using the New Food Labels* is a consumer brochure which uses the themes of balance and moderation to explain how to use the new food label to plan a healthful diet.[100]

Many registered dietitians are self-employed and develop nutrition programs and educational materials that are useful in meeting the needs of women. Supermarket tours, videos, brochures, and other materials have been developed as either self-contained programs or individual components that can be used to address womens' needs in the community.[101-103]

The National Dairy Promotion and Research Board has developed programs and educational materials that address nutrition-related needs of women. Pamphlets have also been developed and address general health issues relevant to women (obesity, osteoporosis, premenstrual syndrome, and iron deficiency) and brochures specific to osteoporosis, dietary sources of calcium, and hypertension.[104,105] Lifesteps is a comprehensive weight management program that is conducted by trained professionals in a variety of community and work site locations.[106] Other weight control programs in the private sector include Weight Watchers International, which may provide access to group programming at community and work site locations.[107] Weight Watchers International formed a partnership with the American Dietetic Association to achieve a healthy weight and help prevent heart disease, breast cancer, and osteoporosis.[108]

IV. POTENTIAL IMPACT OF HEALTH CARE REFORM ON PUBLIC AND PRIVATE SECTOR RESPONSIBILITY FOR WOMEN'S HEALTH AND NUTRITION

As the health care financing system undergoes a transition from a fee-for-service system to a more managed-care system, there are implications for nutrition programs for women as a community. Direct care service provision in some community nutrition programs and services in official health agencies or departments may become part of services and programs delivered in the private and voluntary sectors rather than through the federal, state, or local government sector. Therefore, all community sectors will be responsible for women's health, but how those responsibilities are delegated and implemented will vary. The government's responsibility will be to assure the conditions in which all women can be healthy through the core public health functions of assessment, policy development, and assurance.[6-8] Government will need systematic data collection and analysis, monitoring, and surveillance to describe women's health status, assess needs, and develop policy that assure that women's nutrition-related needs are met. For example, a local health department may develop a policy to promote breastfeeding in their community and form a partnership with local health maintenance organizations and employers to provide mothers with programs, services, and workplace environments that make successful breastfeeding possible.

Public health nutritionists will have primarily a population-based focus with the responsibility for monitoring programs and services delivered by all community sectors, including assuring the quality of care provided by registered dietitians, nutritionists, and other health care professionals. Embracing a broad definition of women as a community and using the core functions of public health (assessment, policy development, and assurance) provide a framework for understanding and evaluating community nutrition programs for women. A review of existing programs indicates that the federal, state, and local government sector provides programs that include food, education/social service, or financial assistance to women who have financial and/or nutritional need. Elderly women also have access to various government-based community nutrition programs. The public and private sectors offer some programs and services for women, but they are not comprehensive in nature. The changes anticipated in the health care system provide an opportunity for all three sectors to contribute to identifying the needs of women as a community, setting policies related to these needs, developing programs and services to reduce the needs, and working with the government sector to monitor the system and assure that women's needs are addressed.

REFERENCES

1. Boyle, M. A. and Morris, D. H., *Community Nutrition in Action*, West Publishing Company, Minneapolis/St. Paul, MN, 1994, chap. 1.
2. Hillery, G. A., Jr., Definitions of community: areas of agreement, *Rural Sociol.*, 20, 111, 1955.
3. Frankle, R. T. and Owen, A. L., *Nutrition in the Community. The Art of Delivering Services*, C.V. Mosby, St. Louis, MO, 1993, 362.
4. Kaufman, M., Assessing the community's needs for nutrition services, in *Nutrition in Public Health. A Handbook for Developing Programs and Services*, Kaufman, M., Ed., Aspen Publishers, Rockville, MD, 1990, 46.

5. Institute of Medicine, Committee for the Study of the Future of Public Health, *The Future of Public Health*, National Academy Press, Washington, D.C., 1988.

6. Assistant Secretary for Health's Public Health Service Task Force to Strengthen Public Health in the U.S., A plan to strengthen public health in the U.S., *Public Health Rep.*, 106 (Suppl. 1,) 1, 1991.

7. Institute of Medicine, Committee for the Study of the Future of Public Health, *The Future of Public Health*, National Academy Press, Washington, D.C., 1988, chap. 5 and 6.

8. Washington State Core Government Public Health Functions Task Force, *Core Public Health Functions*, National Association of County Health Officials, 1993.

9. Kaplan, J. P., Public health in the new American health system, *Digest*, Summer, 1, 1993.

10. Interagency Board for Nutrition Monitoring and Related Research, *Nutrition Monitoring in the U.S. The Directory of Federal and State Nutrition Monitoring Activities*, DHHS Publ. No. (PHS) 92-1255-1, U.S. Department of Health and Human Services, Hyattsville, MD, 1992.

11. Interagency Board for Nutrition Monitoring and Related Research, *Nutrition Monitoring in the United States Chartbook I: Selected Findings from the National Nutrition Monitoring and Related Research Program*, Ervin, B. and Reed, D., Eds., U.S. Public Health Service, Hyattsville, MD, 1993.

12. Kaufman, M., Planning and evaluating nutrition services for the community, *Nutrition in Public Health. A Handbook for Developing Programs and Services*, Kaufman, M., Ed., Aspen Publishers, Rockville, MD, 1990, chap. 14.

13. Kettner, P. M., Moroney, R. M., and Martin, L. L., *Designing and Managing Programs. An Effectiveness-Based Approach*, Sage Publications, Newbury Park, CA, 1990, 13.

14. U.S. Department of Health and Human Services, Public Health Service, Healthy People: The Surgeon General's Report on Health promotion and Disease Prevention, PHS Publ. No. 79-55071, U.S. Government Printing Office, Washington, D.C., 1979.

15. U.S. Department of Health and Human Services, Public Health Service, Promoting Health/Preventing Disease: Objectives for the Nation, U.S. Government Printing Office, Washington, D.C., 1980.

16. U.S. Department of Health and Human Services, Public Health Service, Office of Disease Prevention and Health Promotion, Promoting Health/Preventing Disease, PHS implementation plans for attaining the objectives for the nation, *Public Health Rep.*, 98 (Suppl. 1), 1, 1983.

17. U.S. Department of Health and Human Services, Public Health Service, Healthy People 2000, U.S. Government Printing Office, Washington, D.C., 1990.

18. U.S. Department of Health and Human Services, Public Health Service, Office of Women's Health, PHS Action Plan for Women's Health, DHHS Publication No. (PHS) 91-50214, U.S. Government Printing Office, Washington, D.C., 1991.

19. U.S. Department of Health and Human Services, Public Health Service, PHS Action Plan for Women's Health: 1991 Progress Review, DHHS Publ. No. (PHS) 93-50215, U.S. Government Printing Office, Washington, D.C., 1992.

20. American Public Health Association, *Healthy Communities 2000: Model Standards. Guidelines for Community Attainment of the Year 2000 National Health Objectives*, American Public Health Association, Washington, D.C., 1991.

21. National Association of County Health Officials, *APEXPH, Assessment Protocol for Excellence in Public Health*, National Association of County Health Officials, Washington, D.C., 1991.

22. Cook, T. J., Schmid, T. L., Braddy, B. A., and Orenstein, D., Evaluating community-based program impacts, *J. Health Educ.*, 23, 183, 1992.

23. Green, L. W. and Kreuter, M. W., CDC's planned approach to community health as an application of PRECEED and an inspiration for PROCEED, *J. Health Educ.*, 23, 140, 1992.

24. Kreuter, M. S., PATCH: its origin, basic concepts, and links to contemporary public health policy, *J. Health Educ.*, 23, 135, 1992.

25. Model Standards Project, American Public Health Association, *Community Strategies for Health*, American Public Health Association, Washington, D.C., undated.
26. U.S. Department of Health and Human Services, Public Health Services, The Surgeon General's Report on Nutrition and Health, DHHS Publ. No. 88-50210, U.S. Government Printing Office, Washington, D.C., 1988.
27. National Research Council, *Diet and Health: Implications for Reducing Chronic Disease Risk*, National Academy Press, Washington, D.C., 1989.
28. USDA, *Nutrition and Your Health: Dietary Guidelines for Americans*, Home and Garden Bulletin No. 232, U.S. Department of Agriculture, U.S. Department of Health and Human Services, Washington, D.C., 1990.
29. Institute of Medicine, *Nutrition During Pregnancy, Weight Gain and Nutrient Supplements*, Food and Nutrition Board, National Academy Press, Washington, D.C., 1990.
30. Institute of Medicine, *Nutrition During Lactation*, Food and Nutrition Board, National Academy Press, Washington, D.C., 1991.
31. Institute of Medicine, *Nutrition During Pregnancy and Lactation: An Implementation Guide*, Food and Nutrition Board, National Academy Press, Washington, D.C., 1992.
32. Abrams, B. and Berman, C., Women, nutrition, and health, *Obstet. Gynecol. Fertil.*, 163, 1993.
33. American Public Health Association, Subcommittee on Community Prevention Programs and Public Health Vision, APHA's vision: publication health and a reformed health care system. Strengthening community prevention programs when individual health services are available to all, *Nation's Health*, July, 9, 1993.
34. Kaufman, M., Understanding public health, in *Nutrition in Public Health. A Handbook for Developing Programs and Services*, Kaufman, M., Ed., Aspen Publishers, Rockville, MD, 1990, 3.
35. U.S. Preventive Services Task Force, *Guide to Clinical Preventive Services: An Assessment of the Effectiveness of 169 Interventions*, Williams & Wilkins, Baltimore, MD, 1990.
36. Brennan, R. E. and Traylor, M. N., *Call to Action. Better Nutrition for Mothers, Children, and Families*, Sharbaugh, C. S., Ed., National Center for Education in Maternal and Child Health, Washington, D.C., 1991, 243.
37. Magee, E. M. and Pratt, M. W., *1935–1985: 50 Years of U. S. Federal Support to Promote the Health of Mothers, Children and Handicapped Children in America*, Information Sciences Research Institute, Vienna, VA, 1985, 2.
38. Aliza, B. and Fine, A., *Making a Difference: A Report on Title V Maternal and Child Health Services Programs' Role in Reducing Infant Mortality*, The Association of Maternal and Child Health Programs, Washington, D.C., 1991.
39. Garza, C. and Cowell, C., *Call to Action. Better Nutrition for Mothers, Children, and Families*, Sharbaugh, C. S., Ed., National Center for Education in Maternal and Child Health, Washington, D.C., 1991, 135.
40. Select Panel for the Promotion of Child Health, *Better Health for Our Children: A National Strategy*, Vol. 2, U.S. Department of Health and Human Services, Washington, D.C., 1981, 18.
41. U.S. Department of Health and Human Services, Public Health Services, *The Surgeon General's Report on Nutrition and Health*, DHHS Publ. No. 88-50210, U.S. Government Printing Office, Washington, D.C., 1988, 544.
42. Institute of Medicine, Committee for the Study of the Future of Public Health, *The Future of Public Health*, National Academy Press, Washington, D.C., 1988, chap. 6.
43. Magee, E. M. and Pratt, M. W., *1935–1985: 50 Years of U. S. Federal Support to Promote the Health of Mothers, Children and Handicapped Children in America*, Information Sciences Research Institute, Vienna, VA, 1985, 11.
44. Select Panel for the Promotion of Child Health, *Better Health for Our Children: A National Strategy*, Vol. 2, U.S. Department of Health and Human Services, Washington, D.C., 1981, 17.

45. Peck, M. G., Ed., *Improving Urban MCH Linkages. Highlights of the 1993 Urban Maternal and Child Health Leadership Conference*, CityMatCH at the University of Nebraska Medical Center, Omaha, NE, 1994, 40.

46. Buescher, P. A., Smith, C., Holliday, J. L., and Levine, R. H., Source of prenatal care and infant birth weight: the case of a North Carolina county, *Am. J. Obstet. Gynecol.*, 156, 204, 1987.

47. Buescher, P. A. and Ward, N. I., A comparison of low birth weight among Medicaid patients of public health department and other prenatal care in North Carolina and Kentucky, *Public Health Rep.*, 107, 54, 1992.

48. O'Hare, D., Testimony at Hearing, *Children, Youth, and Families in the Northeast*, Select Committee on Children, Youth, and Families, U.S. House of Representatives, Washington, D.C., July 25, 1983.

49. Select Panel for the Promotion of Child Health, *Better Health for Our Children: A National Strategy*, vol 2, U.S. Department of Health and Human Services, Washington, D.C., 1981, 21.

50. Sokol, R. J., Woolf, R. B., Rosen, M. G., and Weingarden, K., Risk antepartum care, and outcome: Impact of a maternity and infant care project, *Obstet. Gynecol.*, 56, 150, 1980.

51. Boyle, M. A. and Morris, D. H., *Community Nutrition in Action. An Entrepreneurial Approach*, West Publishing Company, St. Paul, MN, 1994, 401.

52. Kaufman, M., Providing nutrition services in primary care, in *Nutrition in Public Health. A Handbook for Developing Programs and Services*, Kaufman, M., Ed., Aspen Publishers, Rockville, MD, 1990, chap. 11.

53. American Academy of Pediatrics, Committee on Child Health Financing, *Medicaid's EPSDT Program: A Pediatrician's Handbook for Action*, American Academy of Pediatrics, Elk Grove Village, IL, 1987, 1.

54. Association of Maternal and Child Health Program, *Medicaid. MCH Related Federal Programs: Legal Handbooks for Program Planners*, Association of Maternal and Child Health Programs, Washington, D.C., 1990.

55. Kelley, M. B. H., Clements, D. F., Horsley, J. W., and Young, M. R., *Nutrition Survey Report. Virginia Department of Health, September 1990*, Virginia Department of Health, Richmond, 1990.

56. Boyle, M. A. and Morris, D. H., *Community Nutrition in Action. An Entrepreneurial Approach*, West Publishing Company, St. Paul, 1994, 481.

57. Institute of Medicine, *The Second Fifty Years: Promoting Health and Preventing Disability*, National Academy Press, Washington, D.C., 1992, 182.

58. Legislative highlights: Older Americans Act passes, *J. Am. Diet. Assoc.*, 92, 1458, 1992.

59. Randall, M. J., Brink, M. S., and Joy, A. B., EFNEP: an investment in America's future, *J. Nutr. Educ.*, 21, 276, 1989.

60. Select Panel for the Promotion of Child Health, *Better Health for Our Children: A National Strategy*, Vol. 1, U.S. Department of Health and Human Services, Washington, D.C., 1981, 156.

61. Report of the National Extension Health Agenda Task Force, in *Decisions for Health. An Extension System Agenda,* U.S. Department of Agriculture and the University of Wisconsin-Extension, Madison, WI, 1992.

62. Frankle, R. T. and Owen, A. L., *Nutrition in the Community. The Art of Delivering Services*, C. V. Mosby, St. Louis, MO, 1993, 27.

63. U.S. Bureau of the Census, Poverty in the U.S., 1987, Current Population Reports (Series P-60, No. 163), U.S. Government Printing Office, Washington, D.C., 1989.

64. U.S. Department of Agriculture, Food and Nutrition Service, Food Assistance Programs. Food Program Facts, U.S. Government Printing Office, Washington, D.C., 1992.

65. Batten, S., Hirschman, J., and Thomas, D., Impact of the Special Supplemental Food Program on infants, *J. Pediatr.*, 117, S101, 1990.

66. U.S. Department of Agriculture, Food and Nutrition Service, Study of WIC Participation and Program Characteristics, 1990, U.S. Government Printing Office, Washington, D.C., 1992.

67. Congressional Budget Office, *Estimated Costs to Provide Full Funding to the Special Supplemental Food Program for Women, Infants, and Children (WIC)*, Congressional Budget Office, Washington, D.C., March 13, 1991.

68. Brown, J. L., Gershoff, S. N., and Cook, J. T., The politics of hunger: when science and ideology clash, *Int. J. Health Serv.*, 22, 221, 1992.

69. General Accounting Office, *WIC Evaluations Provide Some Favorable But No Conclusive Evidence on the Effects Expected for the Special Supplemental Food Program for Women, Infants, and Children*, GAO/PEMD-84-4, U.S. General Accounting Office, Washington, D.C., January 30, 1984.

70. Rush, D., The National WIC Evaluation: evaluation of the Special Supplemental Food Program for Women, Infants, and Children, *Am. J. Clin. Nutr.*, 48, 389, 1988.

71. Mathematica Policy Research, *The Savings in Medicaid Costs for Newborns and Their Mothers from Prenatal Participation in the WIC Program*, report prepared for the U.S. Department of Agriculture, Food and Nutrition Service, Office of Analysis and Evaluation, Washington, D.C., 1990.

72. General Accounting Office, *Early Interventions: Federal Investments Like WIC Can Produce Savings*, GAO/HRD-92-18, U.S. General Accounting Office, Washington, D.C., 1992.

73. *LEAN Toward Health*, National Center for Nutrition and Dietetics, Chicago, IL, 1993.

74. Horton, K., personal communication, 1994.

75. *Ethnic and Regional Food Practices: A Series (Mexican American Food Practices, Customs and Holidays)*, American Dietetic Association, Chicago, IL, 1989.

76. *Ethnic and Regional Food Practices: A Series (Jewish Food Practices, Customs and Holidays and Chinese American Food Practices, Customs and Holidays)*, American Dietetic Association, Chicago, IL, 1990.

77. *Ethnic and Regional Food Practices: A Series (Navajo Food Practices, Customs and Holidays and Hmong American Food Practices, Customs and Holidays)*, American Dietetic Association, Chicago, IL, 1992.

78. *Ethnic and Regional Food Practices: A Series (Alakda Native Food Practices, Customs and Holidays)*, American Dietetic Association, Chicago, IL, 1994.

79. Gonzalez, V. M., Gonzalez, J. T., Freeman, V. and Howard-Pitney, B., *Health Promotion in Diverse Cultural Communities*, Stanford Health Promotion Resource Center, Palo Alto, CA, 1991.

80. Holmes, L., Bernstein, P., Rodrigues-Trias, H., and Rusek, S. B., Enhancing Cultural Awareness and Communication Skills: A Training Program for Health Care Providers and Educators, Memphis State University, Center for Research on Women, Memphis, TN, 1989.

81. Eliades, D. C. and Suitor, C. W., *Celebrating Diversity: Approaching Families Through Their Food*, National Center for Education in Maternal and Child Health, Arlington, VA, 1994.

82. Boyle, M. A. and Morris, D. H., *Community Nutrition in Action*, West Publishing Company, St. Paul, MN, 1994, chap. 1.

83. *Eating for Two*, March of Dimes Foundation, White Plains, NY, 1994.

84. Barber-Madden, B., Cowell, C., Petschek, M.A., and Glanz, K., Nutrition for pregnant and lactating women: implications for worksite health promotion, *J. Nutr. Educ.*, 18(2), S72, 1986.

85. Walker, M., Supporting working women: an HMO example, *Connections*, 1(2), 5, 1993.

86. Kumanyika, S. K. and Charleston, J. B., Lose weight and win: a church-based weight loss program for blood pressure control among black women, *Patient Educ. Counsel.*, 19(1), 19, 1992.

87. Finnegan, J. R., Rooney, B., Viswanath, K., Elmer, P., Graves, K., Baxter, J., Hertog, J., and Mullis, R., Process evaluation of a home-based program to reduce diet-related cancer risk: the "WIN at Home Series", *Health Educ. Q.*, 19, 233, 1992.
88. Flaskerud, J. H. and Nyamathi, A. M., Effects of an AIDS education program on the knowledge, attitudes and practices of low income black and Latina women, *J. Community Health,* 15, 343, 1990.
89. *Breastfeeding Your Baby*, American College of Obstetricians and Gynecologists, Washington, D.C., 1993.
90 *Preventing Osteoporosis*, 2nd Ed., The American College of Obstetricians and Gynecologists, Washington, D.C., 1993.
91. White, J. V., Dwyer, J. T., Wellman, N. S., Blackburn, G. L., Barrocus, A., Chernoff, R., Cohen, D. L., Lysen, L., Moore, S., Moyer, B., Pla, G., and Roe, D., Beyond nutrition screening: a systems approach to nutrition intervention, *J. Am. Diet. Assoc.*, 93, 405, 1993.
92. *Nutrition Fact Sheet: Osteoporosis*, National Center for Nutrition and Dietetics, Chicago, IL, 1993.
93. *Nutrition Fact Sheet: Fitness and Bone Health*, National Center for Nutrition and Dietetics, Chicago, IL, 1994.
94. *Home Economics and Life Skills Catalogue*, NASCO, Fort Atkinson, WI, 1994.
95. *National Health Video Catalogue*, National Health Video, Los Angeles, CA, 1994.
96. *Meals-on-Wheels America: More Meals for the Homebound Through Public/Private Partnerships — A Technical Assistance Guide*, New York City Department for the Aging, New York, NY, 1989.
97. Boyle, M. A. and Morris, D. H., *Community Nutrition in Action*, West Publishing Company, Minneapolis/St. Paul, 1994, 389.
98. Gaffney, J. T. and Singer, G. R., Diet needs of patients referred to home health, *J. Am. Diet. Assoc.,* 85, 198, 1985.
99. Morgan, K. J., Ed., *Nutrition Update*, 4, 1994.
100. *A Matter of Balance: Using the New Food Labels*, Kraft General Foods, Chicago, IL, 1993.
101. Reed, L., *Supermarket SAVVY*, Herndon, VA, 1994.
102. Strehl, M., *Worksite Health Competitions*, Rochester Hills, MI, 1994.
103. Lyford, J., *Educators Advantage, Inc.*, Portland, OR, 1994.
104. *Every Woman's Guide to Health and Nutrition*, National Dairy Council, Rosemont, IL, 1993.
105. *Osteoporosis: Are You at Risk?, 2nd Ed.*, National Dairy Council, Rosemont, IL, 1993.
106. *Lifesteps. Personal Plans For Healthy Living, Weight Management*, 2nd Ed., National Dairy Council, Rosemont, IL, 1992.
107. *This is Weight Watchers*, Weight Watchers International, New York, 1994.
108. *Nutrition and Health Campaign for Women*, the American Dietetic Association and Weight Watchers International, Chicago, IL, 1994.

INDEX

A

F

G

W

X

Z